Infectious Disease in the Aging

Infectious Disease

SERIES EDITOR: *Vassil St. Georgiev*

National Institute of Allergy and Infectious Diseases
National Institutes of Health

Drug Interactions in Infectious Diseases, edited by
  Stephen C. Piscitelli, PharmD and *Keith A. Rodvold,* PharmD, 2001
Management of Antimicrobials in Infectious Diseases: *Impact of Antibiotic*
  Resistance, edited by *Arch G. Mainous III,* PhD and *Claire Pomeroy,* MD, 2001
Infectious Disease in the Aging: *A Clinical Handbook,* edited by
  Thomas T. Yoshikawa, MD and *Dean C. Norman,* MD, 2001
Infectious Causes of Cancer: *Targets for Intervention,* edited by
  James J. Goedert, MD, 2000

Infectious Disease in the Aging

A Clinical Handbook

Edited by

Thomas T. Yoshikawa, MD

*Charles R. Drew University of Medicine and Science
and Martin Luther King, Jr.–Charles R. Drew Medical Center
Los Angeles, CA*

Dean C. Norman, MD

*Greater West Los Angeles Healthcare System
and UCLA School of Medicine
Los Angeles, CA*

Humana Press ✳ Totowa, New Jersey

© 2001 Humana Press Inc.
999 Riverview Drive, Suite 208
Totowa, New Jersey 07512

Due diligence has been taken by the publishers, editors, and authors of this book to assure the accuracy of the information published and to describe generally accepted practices. The contributors herein have carefully checked to ensure that the drug selections and dosages set forth in this text are accurate and in accord with the standards accepted at the time of publication. Notwithstanding, as new research, changes in government regulations, and knowledge from clinical experience relating to drug therapy and drug reactions constantly occurs, the reader is advised to check the product information provided by the manufacturer of each drug for any change in dosages or for additional warnings and contraindications. This is of utmost importance when the recommended drug herein is a new or infrequently used drug. It is the responsibility of the treating physician to determine dosages and treatment strategies for individual patients. Further it is the responsibility of the health care provider to ascertain the Food and Drug Administration status of each drug or device used in their clinical practice. The publisher, editors, and authors are not responsible for errors or omissions or for any consequences from the application of the information presented in this book and make no warranty, express or implied, with respect to the contents in this publication.

This publication is printed on acid-free paper. ∞
ANSI Z39.48-1984 (American Standards Institute) Permanence of Paper for Printed Library Materials.

Cover design by Patricia F. Cleary.

For additional copies, pricing for bulk purchases, and/or information about other Humana titles, contact Humana at the above address or at any of the following numbers: Tel: 973-256-1699; Fax: 973-256-8341; E-mail: humana@humanapr.com, or visit our Website: http://humanapress.com

Printed in the United States of America. 10 9 8 7 6 5 4 3 2 1

Library of Congress Cataloging in Publication Data

Infectious disease in the aging: a clinical handbook / edited by Thomas T. Yoshikawa, Dean C. Norman
         p.;cm.--(Infectious disease)
     Includes bibliographical references and index.
     ISBN 0-89603-744-4 (alk. paper)
     1. Communicable disease in old age. I. Yoshikawa, Thomas T. II. Norman, Dean C. III. Infectious disease (Totowa, N.J.)
     [DNLM: 1. Infection--Aged. 2. Communicable Diseases--Aged. 3. Infection Control--Aged. WC 195 I439 2000]
     RC112.I4585 2001
     618.97'69--dc21

                                                                                                    00-024929

To our wives,

Catherine Yoshikawa and Jane Norman,

for their love and support

Preface

With the beginning of the third millennium, the rapid growth of the aging population will accelerate. The expansion of the number of older people mandates that clinicians and other health care providers become familiar with and knowledgeable about the biology and health-related problems of aging.

One major health problem of the elderly is infection. The incidence and prevalence of infections increase with aging. In addition, the clinical manifestations, morbidity, mortality, and functional recovery are quite different in the elderly, compared with younger patients. In many instances, the microbial causes of infection in older adults may differ from what is usually expected in younger adults with the same infection. With the physiological changes associated with aging, the pharmacokinetics and pharmacodynamics of drugs will invariably be affected; thus, drug selection and dosages have to be carefully assessed in older patients. With increasing age, frailty and functional incapacity become more common, often resulting in the need for long-term care. Long-term care, especially long-term institutionalization, poses special problems and challenges in the diagnosis, management, and prevention of infections in the very old. Finally, preventive strategies will be the primary focus in the future to reduce the incidence, morbidity, and mortality of infectious diseases in the elderly.

In this new work, *Infectious Disease in the Aging: A Clinical Handbook,* the editors have invited clinicians and researchers who are acknowledged experts in the field of aging and infectious diseases. Each contributor has provided the most up-to-date scientific information and clinical data on the approach to the diagnosis, treatment, and prevention of a specific infectious disease problem. The book is divided into three major parts: Part I discusses the important concepts and principles of aging and infections, including the epidemiology, predisposing factors, clinical features, and antimicrobial therapy as they relate to infectious diseases in the elderly. Part II describes the most important and common infectious diseases encountered in elderly patients. These range from common organ system infections (e.g., pneumonia, urinary tract infection, ocular infections) to more specific microbial types of infections (tuberculosis, fungal infections, viral infections). Each chapter is formatted similarly so that the reader can quickly and easily find the desired information. Part III highlights some of the special and unique aspects of infections in the elderly population, such as infections in long-term care facilities, infections in diabetics, and sexually transmitted diseases, as well as concepts of prevention with regard to vaccination and nutrition.

The editors attempted to present to the readers a book in which the information is informative, current, and easily accessible. Substantial number of figures, photos, tables, and charts have been included for quick retrievability of information. The most pertinent and current references have been included. Clinicians, nurses, pharmacists, and health care trainees involved with care of the elderly will find *Infectious Disease in the Aging: A Clinical Handbook* a useful and quick guide to the understanding, diagnosis, treatment, and prevention of infections and infectious diseases-related problems in the elderly. We welcome your comments and suggestions.

Thomas T. Yoshikawa, MD
Dean C. Norman, MD

Acknowledgments

The editors wish to thank all of the contributing authors, who made this book a reality. We also want to extend our gratitude to Ms. Patricia Thompson for typing and retyping the manuscripts.

Contents

Contributors

RICHARD S. BAKER, MD • *Department of Ophthalmology, Charles R. Drew University of Medicine and Science and the Jules Stein Eye Institute, and Department of Ophthalmology, UCLA School of Medicine, Los Angeles, CA*

BRADLEY S. BENDER, MD • *GRECC, VA Medical Center and the University of Florida College of Medicine, Gainesville, FL*

DAVID W. BENTLEY, MD • *Division of Geriatric Medicine, St. Louis University School of Medicine, and VA Medical Center, GRECC, St. Louis, MO*

STEVEN BERK, MD • *Regional Dean, University of Texas Tech Health Sciences Center, Amarillo, TX*

ROBERT A. BONOMO, MD • *Geriatric Care Center, Fairhill Institute of the Elderly, Cleveland, OH*

SUZANNE F. BRADLEY, MD • *GRECC, VA Medical Center, Ann Arbor, MI*

HELENE CALVET, MD • *Division of Infectious Diseases, Department of Internal Medicine, Charles R. Drew University of Medicine and Science, and King-Drew Medical Center, Los Angeles, CA*

BRIAN SCOTT CAMPBELL, MD • *Orange, CA*

JIRAYOS CHINTANADILOK, MD • *Geriatric Research, Education, and Clinical Center, VA Medical Center, University of Florida College of Medicine, Gainesville, FL*

CHESTER CHOI, MD • *Department of Medical Education, St. Mary Medical Center, Long Beach, CA*

ANTHONY W. CHOW, MD • *Division of Infectious Diseases, Department of Medicine, University of British Columbia, and Vancouver Hospital Health Sciences Centre, Vancouver, British Columbia*

BURKE A. CUNHA, MD • *Chief, Division of Infectious Diseases, Winthrop-University Hospital, Mineola, NY*

VINOD K. DHAWAN, MD • *Division of Infectious Diseases, Department of Internal Medicine, Charles R. Drew University of Medicine and Science, and King-Drew Medical Center, Los Angeles, CA*

BRYAN DOO, MD • *Department of Internal Medicine, Charles R. Drew University of Medicine and Science, and King-Drew Medical Center, Los Angeles, CA*

ANN R. FALSEY, MD • *Department of Medicine, Rochester General Hospital, and University of Rochester School of Medicine, Rochester, NY*

CHARLES W. FLOWERS, MD • *Department of Ophthalmology, Charles R. Drew University of Medicine and Science, and King-Drew Medical Center, Los Angeles, CA*

KEVIN P. HIGH, MD, MSC • *Sections on Infectious Diseases and Hematology/Oncology, Wake Forest University School of Medicine, Winston-Salem, NC*

CAROL A. KAUFFMAN, MD • *Division of Infectious Diseases, VA Medical Center, and the University of Michigan Medical School, Ann Arbor, MI*

NATALIE C. KLEIN, MD, PHD • *Infectious Disease Division, Winthrop-University Hospital, Mineola, NY*

THOMAS J. MARRIE, MD • *Department of Medicine, Walter C. MacKenzie Health Sciences Centre, Edmonton, Alberta Canada*

JACK D. McCUE, MD • *Department of Medical Education, St. Mary's Medical Center, San Francisco, CA*

JAMES W. MYERS, MD • *Department of Internal Medicine, James H. Quillen College of Medicine, East Tennessee State University, Johnson City, TN*

LINDSAY E. NICOLLE, MD • *Department of Medicine, Health Sciences Centre, Winnipeg, Manitoba, Canada*

DEAN C. NORMAN, MD • *Office of the Chief Medical Officer, West Los Angeles VA Medical Center, and UCLA School of Medicine, Los Angeles, CA*

SHOBITA RAJAGOPALAN, MD • *Division of Infectious Diseases, Department of Internal Medicine, King-Drew Medical Center, and Charles R. Drew University of Medicine and Science, Los Angeles, CA*

LOUIS B. RICE, MD • *Louis B. Stokes Veterans Affairs Medical Center, Cleveland, OH*

FRANCISCO L. SAPICO, MD • *Division of Infectious Diseases, Rancho Los Amigos Medical Center, Downey, CA*

MARGARET S. TERPENNING, MD • *GRECC, VA Medical Centre, Ann Arbor, MI*

SAMUEL E. WILSON, MD • *Chairman, Department of Surgery, University of California at Irvine, Orange, CA*

THOMAS T. YOSHIKAWA, MD • *Department of Internal Medicine, Charles R. Drew University of Medicine and Science, and King-Drew Medical Center, Los Angeles, CA*

I
Concepts and Principles
of Infections and Aging

Epidemiology of Aging and Infectious Diseases

Thomas T. Yoshikawa

1. INFECTIOUS DISEASES AND HISTORY OF MANKIND

Throughout recorded history, mankind has always faced the scourges of infectious diseases. Infections were the major causes of mortality prior to the modern era of antimicrobial chemotherapy, and even today, infectious diseases worldwide account for over one-third of the deaths. Until the mid-20th century, such diseases as typhus, plague, typhoid fever, cholera, diphtheria, smallpox, and tuberculosis caused major outbreaks of illnesses and accounted for deaths of millions of people throughout the world. Moreover, rheumatic fever, scarlet fever, measles, mumps, pertussis, poliomyelitis, and syphilis not only resulted in mortality but also caused disability, deformities, limitation in functional capacity, and social rejection (1). During the Civil War, infections caused more deaths than battle injuries—for both the Confederate and Union armies; similar statistics have been described for combatants in World War II (2). Poor sanitation, close contact, lacking in acquired immunity to diseases, and high stress levels left military combatants vulnerable to typhoid, malaria, dysentery, tuberculosis, smallpox, and measles.

With the establishment of the germ theory of diseases, medical advances followed, i.e., sanitation, public health measures, antisepsis, antibiotics, and immunization, that reduced the mortality and morbidity of infectious diseases after the middle of the 20th century. The modern era of antimicrobial therapy beginning in the last half of 20th century and vaccination successes of smallpox and poliomyelitis appear to herald the "conquering" of the lethal effects of infections (2). However, in 1981, the first cases of acquired immunodeficiency syndrome (AIDS) were reported by the Centers for Disease Control and Prevention, which in 1984 would be identified to be caused by the human immunodeficiency virus (HIV) (2). This infection has become a global health care problem, striking the young, old, rich, poor, men, women, and people of all ethnic and racial backgrounds. HIV infection and its complications have clearly become the single most publicized and (perhaps) important disease of recent modern times. Finally, newer pathogens have emerged during this past one or two decades, e.g., Hanta virus, Ebola virus, and herpes simplex type 6, as well as mutant strains of antibiotic-resistant organ-

From: *Infectious Disease in the Aging*
Edited by: Thomas T. Yoshikawa and Dean C. Norman
© Humana Press Inc., Totowa, NJ

isms such as methicillin-resistant *Staphylococcus aureus*, penicillin-resistant *Streptococcus pneumoniae*, vancomycin-resistant enterococci, and multiple drug-resistant *gram-negative* bacilli *(3)*. The impact of these and other new and changing infectious disease agents on both young and old will be in the future the interest and focus of many infectious diseases specialists and clinicians caring for children, adults and the elderly.

2. DEMOGRAPHICS OF AGING

In 1900 the average life expectancy at birth in the United States (U.S.) was approximately 47 years (46 years for males and 48 years for females) *(4)*. Only 4% of the total U.S. population was aged 65 years and older *(5)*. With the reduction in childhood mortality, due primarily to infectious diseases, the average life expectancy dramatically increased during the latter half of the 20th century. Presently, the average life expectancy at birth in the U.S. is approximately 75 years (73 years for males and 80 years for females) *(4)*. Furthermore, the elderly (aged 65 years and older) now account for approximately 13% of the entire U.S. population *(5)*. It is anticipated that over the next 30 years, those persons 65 years and older will account for 21% of all Americans, with the older elderly (80 years and older) experiencing the most rapid growth based on percentage of elderly persons.

3. EPIDEMIOLOGY OF MORTALITY, INFECTIONS AND AGING

3.1. Causes of Death

Up until the beginning of the 20th century, half of the top 10 causes of death in the U.S. was attributed to infections. Children, unfortunately, were disproportionately affected. As stated earlier, with the advent of immunization, sanitation, public health practices, antisepsis, and antibiotics, many of the lethal infectious diseases were prevented or mitigated. With the reduction of childhood mortality, life expectancy drastically increased (see earlier discussion). Similarly, there were decreases in infectious disease deaths and complications in adults as well. With adults living longer, other diseases have now become common and prevalent. For the entire U.S. population, heart disease, cancer, and stroke are the most common causes of death. In the elderly population, these same three diseases hold the same level of prominence. However, in the elderly, pneumonia and influenza are the fourth leading cause of death; diabetes mellitus and its complications including infections is the sixth leading cause of death; and bacteremia is responsible for the ninth most common cause of death *(6)*.

3.2. Common Infections in the Elderly

Although older persons are at greater risk for acquiring infections (*see also* Chapter 2,), there are little data to indicate that aging is associated with greater susceptibility to all infections. Whether aging alone versus age-related diseases (that adversely impact host resistance to infections) is responsible for vulnerability to infections remains controversial and unproven *(7)*.

There are considerable data indicating that certain infections appear to occur more often in older persons and/or are associated with higher mortality and morbidity *(8–11)*. These infections include lower respiratory infections, primarily bacterial pneumonia; urinary tract infections; skin and soft tissue infections including infected pressure ulcers; tuberculosis; infective endocarditis; sepsis with known and unknown causes; intraabdominal infections, primarily cholecystitis, diverticulitis, appendicitis, and ab-

**Table 1. Common Infections
in the Elderly and Comparative Mortality with Younger Adults**

Infections	Mortality rate in elderly vs. young adult
Pneumonia	3*
Tuberculosis[a]	10
Urinary tract infection[b]	5–10
Infective endocarditis	2–3
Intraabdominal infection	
Cholecystitis	2–8
Appendicitis	15–20
Bacterial meningitis	3
Bacteremia/sepsis	3
Septic arthritis	2–3

*Indicates that mortality rate is three times greater in elderly compared with young adult.
[a]Compared to nonhuman immunodeficiency virus-infected persons.
[b]Kidney infection.
Source: Refs. *8, 12,* and *13.*

scesses; bacterial meningitis; and herpes zoster *(8)*. (Specific and in-depth details of these infections can be found in the appropriate chapters.)

The majority of these infections are associated with higher death rates in the elderly when compared with younger adults with the same diseases. **Table 1** provides a summary of these findings *(8,12,13)*.

3.3. Infections in Long-Term Care Setting

As mentioned earlier, it is anticipated that with the rapid increase in the aging population, there will be disproportionate growth in the very old segment of this group. With extreme old age comes frailty, cognitive impairment, and physical dependence. It has been stated that persons aged 65 years and older have approximately 45% risk during their lifetime to becoming institutionalized in a long-term care facility such as a nursing facility (nursing home) *(14)*. Furthermore, frail elderly residents in nursing facilities are substantially vulnerable to infections because of age-related immune changes and diseases and physical disabilities. A closed, institutional environment also favors constant exposure to microorganisms from frequent contacts with personnel and other residents; limited ventilation, filtration, and removal of recirculated air, which could contain microorganisms; and unrestricted movement of infected residents *(15)*.

It is estimated that approximately 1.5 million infections occur annually in nursing facilities in the U.S. *(16)*. The incidence of infections has been reported to range from approximately 10 to 20 infections per 100 residents per month *(17)*. The most frequently encountered infections in residents of long-term care facilities are lower respiratory infections (pneumonia most often), urinary tract infections, and skin and soft tissue infections (including infected pressure ulcers). These three infections constitute nearly 70–80% of nursing facility-associated infections *(17)*. Moreover, fever is one of the most common reason residents of a nursing facility are transferred to an acute care facility. Furthermore, infections are often the cause of acute confusion or delirium in older persons *(18)*. Thus, the presence of fever and/or an acute change in clinical/functional status of a resident in a long-term care facility should prompt a careful search for an infectious etiology. Finally, the increasing use of antimicrobial agents in residents of long-term care facilities has been associated with an alarming rise in mutant strains of bacteria resistant to a variety of antibiotic agents *(3)*. Stringent adherence to infection control policies and measures and appropriate prescribing of antimicrobial agents will be necessary to prevent major outbreaks of life-threatening and untreatable infections. (*See* also Chapters 20 and 21).

REFERENCES

1. Lyons, A.S. and Petrucelli, R.J., II (1978). *Medicine: An Illustrated History*. Harry N. Abrams, New York.
2. Kupersmith, C. (1998) *Three Centuries of Infectious Disease. An Illustrated History of Research and Treatment*, Greenwich Press, Greenwich, CT.
3. Yoshikawa, T.T. (1998) VRE, MRSA, PRP, and DRGNB in LTCF: lessons to be learned from this alphabet. *J. Am. Geriatr. Soc.* **46,** 241–243.
4. U.S. Dept. of Health and Human Services, Public Health Service, National Center for Health Statistics (1986) *Health United States 1985*. D.H.H.S. Publication No. (P.H.S.) 86–1232, Hyattsville, MD.
5. U.S. Bureau of the Census (October 1982) Decennial censuses of population, 1900–1980 and projections of the population of the United States: 1982 to 2050 (advance report). *Current Populations Reports* Series P-25, No. 922, Washington, DC.
6. National Center for Health Statistics (1996) Leading causes of death and number of deaths according to age: United States, 1980 and 1993. *Health United States, 1995*. DHHS Pub. No. (PHS) 96–1232, Hyattsville, MD, p. 108.
7. Beeson, P.B. (1985) Alleged susceptibility of the elderly to infection. *Yale J. Biol. Med.* **58,** 71–77.
8. Yoshikawa, T.T. (1981) Important infections in elderly persons. *West. J. Med.* **135,** 441–445.
9. Yoshikawa, T.T. (1983) Geriatric infectious diseases: an emerging problem. *J. Am. Geriatr. Soc.* **31,** 34–39.
10. Yoshikawa, T.T. (1997) Perspective: aging and infectious diseases: past, present and future. *J. Infect. Dis.* **176,** 1053–1057.
11. Yoshikawa, T.T. (1999) State of infectious diseases health care in older persons. *Clin. Geriatr.* **7(5),** 55–61.
12. Yoshikawa, T.T. (1994) Infectious diseases, immunity and aging. Perspectives and prospects, in *Aging, Immunity, and Infection* (Powers, D.C., Morley, J.E., Coe, R.M., eds.), Springer Publishing, New York, pp. 1–11.
13. Norman, D.C. and Yoshikawa, T.T. (1994) Infections of the bone, joint, and bursa. *Clin. Geriatr. Med.* **10(4),** 703–718.
14. Kemper, P. and Murtaugh, D.M. (1991) Lifetime use of nursing home care. *N. Engl. J. Med.* **324,** 595–600.
15. Yoshikawa, T.T. and Norman, D.C. (1995) Infection control in long-term care. *Clin. Geriatr. Med.* **11(3),** 467–480.
16. Alvarez, S. (1990) Incidence and prevalence of nosocomial infections in nursing homes, in *Infections in Nursing Homes and Long Term Care Facilities* (Verghese, A. and Berk, S.L., eds.), Karger, Basel, Switzerland, pp. 41–54.
17. Yoshikawa, T.T. and Norman, D.C. (1996) Approach to fever and infection in the nursing home. *J. Am. Geriatr. Soc.* **44,** 74–82.
18. Rockwood, K. (1989) Acute confusion in elderly medical patients. *J. Am. Geriatr. Soc.* **37,** 150–154.

2

Factors Predisposing to Infection

Dean C. Norman

It is well established that the elderly are at both increased risk for acquiring many types of infections and for increased severity of illness when an infection occurs *(1)*. Predisposing factors, which in part account for this phenomenon, include decrements in host defenses with age that are made worse by chronic disease, undernutrition, and certain medications that are commonly prescribed to older persons. Some of these factors are organ specific. For example, the increased prevalence of urinary tract infection in the elderly is due in part to age-related changes in the urinary tract, which include anatomic changes (e.g., prostatic hypertrophy) and altered physiology (e.g., increased bladder residual volume). Furthermore, the elderly are more likely to be hospitalized, undergo invasive procedures, and suffer procedure-associated complications that compromise mucocutaneous and other barriers to infection. Moreover, hospitalization and chronic illness increase the risk of colonization and subsequent infection with virulent nosocomial flora *(2)*. This chapter further identifies and summarizes factors that increase infection risk in elderly persons. Fever, as a host defense, is not covered here because it is discussed in detail in Chapter 3.

1. INFECTION RISK

The risk for developing an infection and to some extent its severity is directly proportional to the inoculum and virulence of the pathogen(s) and inversely proportional to the integrity of the host defenses. Aging and comorbidities associated with aging affect all three of these factors. It is the interplay of these three variables that account for the increased susceptibility to and severity of infections in the geriatric population.

1.1 Virulence

The virulence of a pathogen is dependent on its ability to attach to and penetrate the host and its ability to successful replicate in the host environment. Virulence factors are properties that enable a pathogen to establish itself in the host and cause disease *(3)*. For example, for certain uropathogenic strains of *Escherichia coli,* virulence is determined by the presence of P-fimbriae, which are surface structures known as

From: *Infectious Disease in the Aging*
Edited by: Thomas T. Yoshikawa and Dean C. Norman
© Humana Press Inc., Totowa, NJ

adhesins. Adhesins attach to receptors on uroepithelial cells and facilitate attachment to and colonization of uroepithelial cells *(4)*. Virulence is also dependent on the pathogen's ability to avoid being overwhelmed by the host's defenses and its ability to damage the host. In the case of *Streptococcus pneumoniae*, a common pneumonia pathogen in elderly persons, virulence is determined by pneumococcal capsular polysaccharide, which allows the bacterium to resist phagocytosis by host cells. This virulence factor is overcome if capsular-specific antibodies are present to facilitate opsonization.

The elderly are more likely to be colonized with virulent bacteria, especially those elderly who are exposed to nosocomial flora and have major breaches in barriers to infection (e.g., presence of an indwelling bladder catheter). Furthermore, for reasons that are unclear, the risk for colonization of the oropharynx by potentially virulent Gram-negative bacilli or *Staphylococcus aureus* is increased in elderly patients, and this risk increases with increasing dependence and acuity of illness *(2)*. Therefore, hospitalized elderly are at greatest risk for oropharyngeal colonization with these pathogens. Drying of upper airway secretions with age, exposure to antibiotics, and changes in local immunity may all be contributing factors.

Resistance of bacteria to antibiotics, although technically not a virulence factor, potentially increases morbidity and mortality related to infections. Frail, institutionalized elderly may suffer repeated hospitalizations and undernutrition as well as undergo repeated courses of antimicrobial therapy. Normal bacterial flora may be altered in these cases and will increase the risk for colonization by resistant bacteria.

1.2. Inoculum

The inoculum is an important determinant of risk of infection and plays a significant role in the increased risk of infection in the elderly. For example, even young, healthy individuals aspirate small amounts of oropharyngeal secretions *(5)*. However, the elderly are more likely to have neurovascular disease with resultant swallowing disorders and also at more risk to undergo tube feedings, both of which dramatically increase the risk of aspiration of copious amounts of oral secretions. Furthermore, in the elderly, the adverse effects of alcohol, long-acting benzodiazepines, and other sedating agents increase the risk for aspiration. Given the loss or alteration with age of important pulmonary host defenses including cough reflex, mucociliary clearance and changes in immune function it is not surprising that elderly patients have a markedly higher incidence of pneumonia. Endotracheal intubation and prolonged mechanical ventilation further compromise host defenses; these interventions increase the risk of aspiration of large inocula of bacteria. Such macroaspiration dramatically raises the probability for development of severe respiratory infection. Finally, the elderly are more likely to undergo intravascular catheterization and the placement of chronic dwelling bladder catheters. These catheters, even when meticulously maintained, can serve as a conduit for inocula of bacteria, thus bypassing basic host barriers to infection.

1.3. Host Defenses

Host defenses can be separated into two major divisions: nonspecific (natural) and specific (adaptive) defenses. Specific immune defenses are discussed in the following paragraphs. Nonspecific defenses include mucocutaneous barriers, comple-ment and certain effector cells such as macrophages neutrophils and natural killer (NK) cells.

1.3.1. Mucosal Defenses

Mucocutaneous tissues are more than simple mechanical barriers. The skin has antibacterial properties including a relatively low pH and glandular secretions, which have an antibacterial effect. Aging results in significant changes such as loss of dermal thickness and subcutaneous tissue as well as reduced glandular secretion, which makes the skin less capable of withstanding shearing forces. Furthermore, with age, the skin become relatively avascular, which also increases the susceptibility to injury. Also, there is a loss of Langerhans cells, and cytokine dysregulation occurs, both of which decrease the specific immune response *(6)*. Loss of mobility resulting from coexisting diseases may lead to increased pressure and shearing forces. Edema and vascular dis-eases may further compromise the integrity of this important barrier. This will facili-tate colonization and invasion with virulent bacteria.

The mucosal host defense system, like the skin, is a first-line defense against invad-ing pathogens. Mucus secretions and ciliary action continuously trap and remove bac-teria, thus preventing microbes from gaining access to deeper, normally sterile tissues. Furthermore, Peyer's patches contain T and B cells, which are capable of processing bacterial antigen necessary for the specific immune response *(7)*. Immunoglobin A antibody is the predominant immunoglobin of the mucosal immune system and does not appear to be reduced with age. However, it is not clear whether or not aging reduces the ability of the mucosa to perform as a host defense. Nevertheless, xerostomia from all causes, periodontal disease, and certain gastrointestinal disorders, such as diverticu-litis and ischemic bowel disease, occur commonly in geriatric patients and potentially damage mucosal defenses.

1.3.2. Immune Responses

The immune response is made up of two interdependent entities. These are the vari-ous components of nonspecific or natural immunity (e.g., neutrophils, macrophages, NK cells, and complement cells mentioned earlier) and specific immune responses (cellular and humoral immunity). Natural immunity is immediate and does not require prior sensitization to particular foreign antigen, does not discriminate between differ-ent antigens, and is not enhanced by repeated exposure to a particular antigen. In con-trast, the specific immune response is usually initiated by a specific foreign antigen and involves cells of lymphoid lineage including T cells (cellular immunity) and B cells (humoral immunity). Stimulus from a foreign antigen results in the generation of spe-cific molecules, which, in effect, modulate responses among the effector cells of the immune response. Repeated exposure to the specific antigen enhances the response, and this is the basis of what is an essential host defense against a wide variety of micro-bial pathogens. It should be mentioned that NK cells are presumably of lymphoid lin-eage and are an important host defense against tumor cells and possibly virus-infected cells. However, NK cells do not require prior sensitization to become cytotoxic and are considered to be an effector of natural immunity.

A summary of the specific immune response is as follows: Each mature T cell has a unique receptor that is specific for a certain antigen (epitope), and the total T-cell population provides an extensive capacity to bind with a multitude of different antigens. The T-cell receptor (TCR) does not bind directly to antigen but requires processing of the antigen by antigen-presenting cells (APC). After phagocytosis, APCs break the antigen into polypeptide components, which are complexed on the cell's surface with molecules that are coded within the major histocompatibility complex. The TCR in concert with another T-cell marker, CD3, can then initiate the cascade of signal transduction resulting in cytokine secretion, clonal expansion, and differentiation of T cells necessary for the specific T-cell response *(8–10)*.

T cells have been extensively studied in animal models and humans including aging populations. T cells are composed of two distinct cell types: T helper cells that express the CD4 marker and cytotoxic T cells that express the CD8 marker. T helper cells are further subdivided into Th1 and Th2 cells; Th1 cells secrete interleukin 2 (IL-2) and gamma interferon. Th1 cells are the major effector cells for cytotoxic activity (including killing of cells infected with intracellular pathogens such as viruses) and the inflammatory response. Th2 cells secrete IL 4, 5, 6, and 10 and have a major role modulating B-cell proliferation, differentiation, and antibody production. T cells that have not yet responded to a specific antigen are referred to as naive T cells that express the marker CD45RA and are relatively short lived. T cells, which, after clonal expansion and differentiation, have a TCR with high avidity for antigen may become long-lived memory cells. Memory T cells express the marker CD45RO.

1.4. Changes with Age

The components of natural immunity (e.g., phagocytosis by macrophages, neutrophils, complement activity, and NK activity) do not appear to be greatly affected by aging in healthy elderly patients. Although NK cellular function does not appear to be changed with age, the response of NK cells to cytokine signals may be altered *(11)*. However, there are consistent changes observed with age in the cellular and humoral components of specific immunity. First, it is firmly established that there is a shift from naive T cells to memory T cells with age and that both T-cell proliferation and IL-2 production are reduced *(8,9)*. Although IL-6 has been found to be increased with age in some studies, this is not a consistent finding. One study did find that elderly caregivers had increased levels of IL-6 during periods of stress *(12)*. Some studies have demonstrated alterations in cytokine production and increased cytokine dysregulation with age, but thus far studies in humans are inconclusive *(13,14)*. A recent study comparing infected elderly with younger patients confirmed that blood levels of certain cytokines remain elevated for prolonged periods of time in old compared with young patients. This finding may indicate prolonged inflammation response to infections in old compared with the younger patients *(15)*.

T-cell proliferation in response to mitogens and specific antigens is decreased with aging and is not explained entirely by reductions in IL-2 production *(8,9)*. Although studies consistently demonstrate reduced T-cell proliferation with age, there is wide interindividual and population variability. State of health, exercise, and nutritional status will influence measures of specific immunity *(16–18)*. Finally, B-cell production of specific, high-affinity antibodies is reduced with age. This is not simply an in vitro observation because even relatively healthy elderly persons as a population do not mount as great an antibody response to T-cell-dependent antigens such as influenza

Table 1
Effect of Aging on Immune Function

	Decrease	Increase	No change or inconclusive
T cells:			
T cell number			X
Thymus gland	X (Involutes)		
Memory T cells		X	
Naive T cells	X		
DTH[a]	X		
Cytotoxicity	X		
Proliferation	X		
Interleukin 2	X		
Interleukin 4			X
Interleukin 6			X[b]
Interleukin 10			X
Interferon-gamma			X
B cells:			
B-cell number			X
High-affinity antibodies	X		
Nonspecific antibodies		X	
Autoantibodies		X	
NK[c] cells:			
Cytotoxicity			X

[a]Delayed type hypersensitivity reaction.
[b] See Subheading 1.3.
[c]Natural killer.

vaccine compared with a younger population. It also appears that cytotoxic T-cell functions are reduced somewhat with aging. Finally, alterations of apoptosis (programmed cell death) with age have been postulated to explain some of the age-related changes in immune function; however, this theory is under active investigation *(19)*. Table 1 summarizes the foregoing discussion.

REFERENCES

1. Yoshikawa, T.T. (1997) Aging and infectious diseases: past, present and future. *J. Infect. Dis.* **176**, 1053–1057.
2. Valenti, W.M., Trudell, R.G., and Bentley, D.W. (1978) Factors predisposing to oropharyngeal colonization with gram-negative bacilli in the aged. *N. Engl. J. Med.* **298,** 1108–1111.
3. Relman, D.A. and Falkow, S. (1995) A molecular perspective of microbial pathogenicity, in *Principles and Practices of Infectious Diseases* (Mandell, G.L., Bennett, J.E., and Dolin, R. eds.), Churchill Livingstone, New York, pp. 19–29.
4. Petri, W.A. and Mann, B.J. (1995) Microbial adherence, in *Principles and Practices of Infectious Diseases* (Mandell, G.L, Bennett, J.E., and Dolin·R., eds.). Churchill Livingstone, New York, pp. 111–118.
5. Huxley, E.J., Voroslave, J., Gray, W.R., et al. (1978) Pharyngeal aspiration in normal adults and patients with depressed consciousness. *Am. J. Med.* **64**, 564–566.
6. Sunderkotter, C., Kalden, H., and Luger, T.A. (1997) Aging and the skin immune system. *Arch. Dermatol.* **133(10),** 1256–1262.

7. Iglewski, B.H., Lamm, M.E., Doherty, P.C., et al (1996) Infection, host defense and mu-cosal immunity, in *Task Force on Immunology and Aging*. National Institutes on Aging, Allergy and Infectious Diseases. U.S. Department of Health and Human Services, National Institutes of Health, Bethesda, MD, pp. 51–57.

8. Murasko, D.M. and Bersteub, E.D. (1999) Immunology of aging, in *Principles of Geron-tology* (Hazzard, W.R., Blass, J.P., Ettinger, W.H., et al., eds.), McGraw-Hill, NewYork, pp. 97–116.

9. Abraham, G.N., Davis, M.M., Bennett, M.B., et al (1996) Immune system: functions and changes associated with aging, In *Task Force on Immunology and Aging*. National Insti-tutes on Aging, Allergy and Infectious Diseases. U.S. Department of Health and Human Services, National Institutes of Health, Bethesda, MD, pp. 9–15.

10. Hodes, R.J., (1995) Molecular alterations in the aging immune system. *J. Exp. Med.* **182,** 1–3.

11. Solana, R., Alonso, M.C., and Pena, J. (1999) Natural killer cells in healthy aging. *Exp. Gerontol.* **34(3),** 435–443.

12. Lutgendorf, S.K., Garand, L., Buckwalter, K.C., et al. (1999) Life stress, mood distur-bance and elevated interleukin-6 in healthy older women. *J. Gerontol. (Med. Sci.)* **54(A),** M434–M439

13. Abbas, A.K., Weigle, W.O., and Kensil, C. (1996) Cytokines and other immunomodulators, in *Task Force on Immunology and Aging*. National Institutes on Aging, Allergy and Infec-tious Diseases. U.S. Department of Health and Human Services. National Institutes of Health, Bethesda, MD, pp. 17–22

14. Mu, X.Y. and Thoman, M.L. (1999) The age-dependent cytokine production by murine CD8+ T cells as determined by four-color flow cytometry analysis. *J. Gerontol. (Biol. Sci.)* **54A,** B116–B123

15. Bruunsgaard, H, Skinnoj, P., Qvist, J., et al. (1999) Elderly humans show prolonged in vivo inflammatory activity during pneumococcal infections. *J. Infect. Dis.* **180(2),** 551–554.

16. Woods, J.A., Ceddia, M.A., Wolters, B.W., et al. (1999) Effects of 6 months of moderate aerobic exercise training on immune function in the elderly *Mech. Ageing Dev.* **109(1),** 1–19.

17. Chandra, R.K. (1995) Nutrition and immunity in the elderly: clinical significance. *Nutr. Rev.* **53(4),** S80–S85.

18. Chandra, R.K. (1992) Effect of vitamin and trace element supplementation on immune responses and infection in the elderly. *Lancet* **340,** 1124–1127.

19. Lenardo, M.J., Mountz, J.D. and Horton, W.E. (1996) Programmed cell death and the im-munology of aging, in *Task Force on Immunology and Aging*. National Institutes on Ag-ing, Allergy and Infectious Diseases. U.S. Department of Health and Human Services. National Institutes of Health, Bethesda, MD, pp. 47–50.

3

Clinical Features of Infections

Dean C. Norman

1. OVERVIEW

Infections in the elderly often present in an atypical, nonclassical fashion. Furthermore, the differential diagnosis of infectious diseases in the elderly differs from the young because it is dependent on both the clinical setting and the patient's underlying functional status. For example, "free living," independent, healthy elderly are prone to respiratory infections, such as bacterial pneumonia, genitourinary infections and intraabdominal infections including cholecystitis, diverticulitis, appendicitis, and intraabdominal abscesses. Institution-bound elderly are more likely to develop aspiration pneumonia, urinary tract infection, (especially if a chronic indwelling bladder catheter is present), and skin and soft-tissue infections. Infections in the elderly differ from the young also because infections in this age group are often caused by a more diverse group of pathogens compared with the young. This is best exemplified by urinary tract infection, which in the young occurs almost exclusively in females and is usually caused by *Escherichia coli*. In the aged, a variety of Gram-positive cocci and Gram-negative bacilli, sometimes in combination, are potential pathogens for this infection, and at least a third of urinary tract infections occur in males. This is the reason that obtaining a urine culture prior to empirical therapy for symptomatic urinary tract infection in the elderly is recommended.

Morbidity and mortality rates for infections are usually higher in the elderly compared with the young. These observed higher mortality and morbidity rates are due in part to factors such as (1) lower physiologic reserve capacity due to biologic changes with age and comorbidities, (2) age and disease-related decrements in host defenses, (3) chronic illness, and (4) higher risk for adverse drug reactions due to multiple medications and age-related physiologic changes that alter the pharmacokinetics and pharmacodynamics of many medications. Additional contributing factors include a greater risk for hospitalization, and therefore exposure to nosocomial pathogens, a greater risk of undergoing invasive procedures, and increased likelihood of suffering a procedure-associated complication. Finally, delay in diagnosis and the initiation of appropriate empirical antimicrobial therapy is an important contributing factor. Diagnostic delays may commonly occur in this population, who can least tolerate this. However, infec-

From: *Infectious Disease in the Aging*
Edited by: Thomas T. Yoshikawa and Dean C. Norman
© Humana Press Inc., Totowa, NJ

Table 1.
Altered presentations of infection in the elderly

Potential findings with any infection	Potential findings with specific infections
Delirium	Bacteremia
Confusion	May be afebrile
Lethargy	Dyspnea, confusion, falls,
Anorexia	hypotension
"Failure to thrive"	Pneumonia
	May be afebrile
	Cough and sputum production
	may be absent
	Intraabdominal infection
	Peritoneal signs may be absent
	Anorexia
	Meningitis
	Stiff neck may be absent
	Confusion, altered consciousness
	Tuberculosis
	Weight loss, lethargy
	Failure to thrive

tions in the elderly may present in an atypical or nonclassical manner, which in turn may make early diagnosis difficult. Thus, infections in this age group provide a unique challenge to clinicians.

2. ALTERED PRESENTATION OF ILLNESS

Atypical or nonspecific responses to infection are commonly observed in older adults and has been recently reviewed extensively *(1)*. Table 1 lists some of these signs and nonclassical presenting features. Delirium, agitation, confusion, lethargy, anorexia, falls, abnormal movements, focal neurologic signs, and urinary incontinence may all be the sole symptom observed at initial presentation. Furthermore, bacteremia may be afebrile and present with dyspnea, confusion, and/or hypotension. The classical finding of a stiff neck may be absent in geriatric patients with bacterial meningitis, and the older patient with pneumonia may not have cough, sputum production, or fever. Similarly, peritoneal findings may be absent in elderly patients with intraabdominal infection *(2)*. In summary, virtually any change in functional status in the elderly may be an indication of the presence of an acute illness, which often is an infection. Furthermore, there may be a dissociation of clinical findings with severity of illness.

3. FEVER IN THE ELDERLY

Classical studies of bacteremia *(3,4)* and pneumonia *(5,6)*, as well as a recent review of tuberculosis *(7)*, demonstrate both that a higher percentage of the elderly compared with young demonstrated a blunted fever response and that up to one third of elderly patients with serious bacterial or viral infections do not mount a robust febrile response

(8,9). This is confirmed by a more recent study of acute intraabdominal infection in octogenarians in whom a large percentage with acute cholecystitis, perforation and appendicitis presented with temperatures less than 37.5°C *(10).* Additionally, a recent study of nosocomial febrile illness in a geriatric medicine unit showed that the mean "febrile" rectal temperature of elderly subjects was merely 38.1°C (100.6°F). In this last study only 8% of febrile patients had rectal temperatures greater than 38.5°C (101.3°F) *(11).* The significance of these findings is that although fever is the cardinal sign of infection its absence in elderly patients is not uncommon and may delay diagnosis and the initiation of appropriate antimicrobial therapy.

Not only is the presence of fever the single most important diagnostic feature of infection, but a febrile response or its lack thereof has other important implications. Weinstein and colleagues *(12)* demonstrated in their review of several hundred cases of bacteremia and fungemia that the more robust the fever response to these serious infections, the more likely was the survival. This and other studies have firmly established for many infectious diseases that the absence of fever in response to a serious acute infection is a poor prognostic sign for all age groups. Although the diagnostic and prognostic implications of fever are clear, it is less well established that in humans fever is an important host defense mechanism.

The best evidence that fever is an important host defense mechanism comes from animal models. Experiments that showed poikilothermic animals move to warmer environments in order to raise body temperatures in response to infection confirmed that this behavior has an impact on survival. For example, in one classic experiment, a species of lizards was placed in terrariums, which were kept at different temperatures. The body temperatures of these poikilothermic animals equilibrated with the environmental temperature of the terrarium in which they were housed. Subsequently, the animals were infected: it turned out that those kept in the higher temperature terrariums (thus higher body temperatures) had a much better chance of survival than those animals kept at lower temperatures *(13).* Similar findings were demonstrated in goldfish *(14).* Based on these and other animal data, including additional data generated from mammalian experiments, it can be inferred that fever may be an important host defense mechanism in humans. The mechanism(s) by which fever may enhance host defenses is not due to a direct effect of physiologically achievable temperature elevations for most pathogens. The exceptions are *Treponema pallidum,* the gonococcus, and certain strains of *Streptococcus pneumoniae.* In these cases normal physiologically achievable body temperatures in humans can inhibit bacterial growth directly. These exceptions aside, experimental data suggest that normal physiologically achievable elevations in body temperature enhance the production of monokines, cytokines, and other factors. These factors facilitate the adherence of granulocytes and other effector cells of the immune response to endothelial cells. Also, they promote immune effector cell migration into interstitial tissue spaces, which contain pockets of infection.

The reason(s) for the blunted fever response to infection observed in a substantial number of elderly patients have not been completely elucidated. One explanation is that the baseline body temperature is lower for this population (see discussion following) and another is the inherent inaccuracies in oral temperature measurement in a subset of elderly patients with dementia, mouth breathing, and variations in respiratory patterns. Further inaccuracies in temperature measurement may be caused by the ingestion of hot and cold foods during the time of measurement. Moreover, routine rectal temperatures are often impractical in subpopulations of debilitated, poorly cooperative patients. The availability of tympanic membrane thermometers may reduce such error in temperature measurement. Reasons for the blunted fever response other than lower baseline temperatures and difficulties in accurately measuring temperatures have not been completely established.

An understanding of potential mechanisms for the blunted fever response in the elderly may be gained by reviewing the current knowledge of the pathogenesis of fever, which has been recently reviewed *(15)*. First, pathogens activate macrophages, which produce endogenous pyrogens including tumor necrosis factor, interleukin-1 (IL-1), IL-6 and interferon-α. These pyrogens then act on the endothelium of the circumventricular organs of the anterior hypothalamus or hypothalamic cells directly and initiate a complex biochemical cascade including the production of prostaglandin E2. The resulting effect is an elevation of the "hypothalamic thermostat," which in turn results in shivering, vasoconstriction, and certain behavioral responses, all of which elevate core body temperature. When the infection subsides, the "thermostat" is reset back to normal and sweating and temperature lowering behavior ensues, restoring body temperature to baseline. Any of these pathways may be affected by aging. Animal data suggest an impaired response to endogenous pyrogens with normal aging *(16–18)* as well as diminished production of these pyrogens with age *(19)*. Evidence from one model suggests that the aging brain may respond normally to directly injected endogenous pyrogens, implying that there may be a defect in endogenous pyrogens crossing the blood–brain barrier *(20)*.

4. BASELINE TEMPERATURE, SIGNIFICANCE OF FEVER, AND FUO

It has been known for some time that baseline temperature declines significantly in the old. The clinician can remember this fact by remembering the statement "the older, the colder." Lower baseline temperatures, at least for debilitated elderly, has been reaffirmed by Castle and co-workers *(21,22)*, who demonstrated that baseline temperature was decreased among nursing facility residents. Castle and colleagues' studies further demonstrated that infections often led to "robust" or normal increases in body temperature from baseline. However, because the baseline temperature was lower, the rise in temperature, which accompanied infection, often did not reach an oral temperature of 101°F (38.3°C). Generally, 101°F (38.3°C) is the temperature level that many clinicians consider to be the definition of fever. These studies suggest that new definitions for a fever need to be established for the geriatric patient. Based on these studies, an oral temperature of 99°F (37.2°C) or greater on repeated measurements in an elderly nursing facility resident should be considered to be indicative of a fever. Similarly, a persistent rectal temperature of 99.5°F (37.5° C) would constitute a fever as would an elevation of baseline body temperature of 2°F (1.1°C). Finally, the clinician should always remember that any unexplained acute or subacute change in functional status, regardless of whether or not a fever or change in body temperature is present, may indicate the presence of an infection.

The presence of a "robust" or normal fever response to infection in an elderly person has special significance. An extensive study of over 1200 ambulatory patients showed that in contrast to younger patients in whom"benign" viral infections were common, the older febrile patient is more likely to harbor a serious bacterial infection *(19)*. This finding was confirmed by another study, which also confirmed that leukocyte elevations in response to an infection were less in the aged compared with the young *(24)*. Based on these studies, it is recommended that any elderly patient with an oral temperature of 101°F (38.3°C) or greater be evaluated for a serious bacterial infection.

Fever of unknown origin (FUO) in the elderly differs from the young because a diagnosis can be made in a higher percentage of cases. Furthermore, infections are more likely to cause FUO in the elderly. It is well worthwhile investigating FUO in the elderly because treatable conditions are often found *(25,26)*.

REFERENCES

1. Leinicke, T., Navitsky, R., Cameron, S., et. al. (1999). Fever in the elderly: how to surmount the unique diagnostic and therapeutic challenges. *Emerg. Med. Pract.* **1(5)**, 1–24.
2. Norman, D. C. and Yoshikawa, T. T. (1984) Intraabdominal infection: diagnosis and treatment in the elderly patient. *Gerontology* **30**, 327-338.
3. Gleckman, R. and Hibert, D. (1982) Afebrile bacteremia. a phenomenon in geriatric patients. *JAMA* **248**, 1478–1481.
4. Finkelstein, M., Petkun ,W. M., Freedman, M. L., et al. (1983) Pneumococcal bacteremia in adults: age-dependent differences in presentation and outcome. *J. Am. Geriatr. Soc.* **31**, 19–27.
5. Bentley, D. W. (1984) Bacterial pneumonia in the elderly: clinical features, diagnosis, etiology and treatment. *Gerontology* **30**, 297–307.
6. Marrie, T. S., Haldane, E. V., Faulkner, R. S., et al. (1985) Community-acquired pneumonia requiring hospitalization: is it different in the elderly? *J. Am. Geriatr. Soc.* **33**, 671–680.
7. Perez-Guzman, C., Vargas, M.H., Torres-Cruz, A., et. al. (1999) Does aging modify pulmonary tuberculosis? A meta-analytical review. *Chest* **116(4)**, 961–967.
8. Yoshikawa, T. T. and Norman, D. C. (1998) Fever in the elderly. *Infect. Med.* **15(10)**, 704–706.
9. Norman, D. C. (1998) Fever and aging. *Infect. Dis. Clin. Pract.* **7(8)**, 387–390.
10. Potts, F. E., IV and Vukov, L. F. (1999) Utility of fever and leukocytosis in acute surgical abdomens in octogenarians and beyond. *J. Gerontol. (Med. Sci.)* **54A(2)**, M55–M58.
11. Trivalle, C., Chassagne, P., Bouaniche, M., et al. (1998) Nosocomial febrile illness in the elderly: frequency, causes, and risk factors. *Arch. Intern. Med.* **158(14)**, 1560–1565.
12. Weinstein, M. P., Murphy, J. R., Reller, R. B., et al. (1983) The clinical significance of positive blood cultures: a comprehensive analysis of 500 episodes of bacteremia and fungemia II: clinical observations with special reference to factors influencing prognosis. *Rev. Infect. Dis.* **5**, 54–70.
13. Kluger, M. J., Ringler, D. M., and Anver, M. R. (1975) Fever and survival. *Science* **188**, 166–168.
14. Covert, J. B. and Reynolds, W. M. (1977) Survival value of fever in fish. *Nature* **267**, 43–45.
15. Dinarello, C. A. (1999) Cytokines as endogenous pyrogens. *J. Infect. Dis.* **179(Suppl 2)**, S294–S304.
16. Norman, D. C., Yamamura, R. H. and Yoshikawa, T. T. (1988) Fever response in old and young mice after injection of interleukin. *J. Gerontol.* **43**, M80–M85.
17. Miller, D., Yoshikawa, T. T., Castle, S. C., et al. (1991) Effect of age in fever response to recombinant tumor necrosis factor alpha in a murine model. *J. Gerontol.* **46**, M176– M179.
18. Miller, D. J., Yoshikawa, T. T., and Norman, D. C. (1995) Effect of age on fever response to recombinant interleukin-6 in a murine model. *J. Gerontol.* **50A**, M276–M279.
19. Bradley, S. F., Vibhagool, A., Kunkel S. L., et al. (1989) Monokine secretion in aging and protein malnutrition. *J. Leukocyte Biol.* **45**, 510–514.
20. Satinoff, E., Peloso, E., and Plata-Salamn, C. R. (1999) Prostaglandin E2-induced fever in young and old Long-Evans rats. *Physiol. Behav.* **67(1)**, 149–152.

21. Castle, S. C., Norman, D. C., Yeh, M., et al. (1981) Fever response in elderly nursing home residents: are the older truly colder? *J. Am. Geriatr. Soc.* **39,** 853–857.
22. Castle, S. C., Yeh, M., Toledo, S., et al. (1993) Lowering the temperature criterion improves detection of infections in nursing home residents. *Aging Immunol. Infect. Dis.* **4,** 67–76.
23. Keating, J. H., III, Klimek, J. J., Levine, D. S., et. al. (1984) Effect of aging on the clinical significance of fever in ambulatory adult patients. *J. Am. Geriatr. Soc. 32,* 282–287.
24. Wasserman, M., Levenstein, M., Keller, E., et. al. (1989) Utility of fever, white blood cells, and differential count in predicting bacterial infections in the elderly. *J. Am. Geriatr. Soc.* **37,** 537–543.
25. Espositio, A. L. and Gleckman, R. A. (1978) Fever of unknown origin in the elderly. *J. Am. Geriatr. Soc.* **26,** 498–505.
26. Knockaert, D. C., Vanneste, L. J., and Bobbaers, J. H. (1993) Fever of unknown origin in elderly patients. *J. Am. Geriatr. Soc.* **41,** 1187–1192.

4

Principles of Antimicrobial Therapy

Bryan Doo and Thomas T. Yoshikawa

From the first three chapters of this book, it is quite apparent that with aging comes a substantial susceptibility to and incidence of serious infections, as well as an increased risk of complications from these infections, including death. Moreover, subsequent chapters of this book describe in detail the most important and serious infectious disease problems of elderly people, and how these infections should be diagnosed and treated. In this chapter, the discussion focuses on general principles and some unique aspects of antimicrobial therapy in older infected patients. Comments will also be made on some of the more useful classes of antimicrobial agents for treating infections in the elderly. For a more in–depth review of various classes of antibiotics and their usage in the elderly, several current references are recommended *(1–3)*.

1. SPECIAL CONSIDERATIONS

Throughout this book, a common theme is that older patients with infection, compared with younger adults, suffer greater complications including a higher mortality. Factors contributing to these greater complications include presence of chronic underlying diseases, diminished host defense responses, delays in diagnosis and treatment, complications from diagnostic and therapeutic interventions, and adverse reactions to antibiotics *(1)*. Early and rapid diagnosis of infection and prompt initiation of appropriate antimicrobial therapy are fundamental to reducing the mortality and morbidity from infections. However, the problem of atypical and nonspecific clinical manifestations of infections in the elderly poses a major challenge to clinicians (Chapter 3).

Other sections of this book describe microbial causes of select infections that can vary from those usually anticipated in younger adults. Under these clinical circumstances, it becomes essential that the initial empiric therapy include coverage for such pathogens. For example, the most common pathogen isolated in bacterial meningitis in the general adult population is *Streptococcus pneumoniae* and *Neisseria meningitidis*; viral meningitis also occurs. In elderly patients with this infection, not only is *S. pneumoniae* recovered but Gram–negative bacilli and *Listeria monocytogenes* are relatively common meningopathogens; viral meningitis is distinctly uncommon (Chapter 11). Consequently, in elderly meningitis patients, initial empiric treatment must include antibiotics active against these three types of bacteria.

From: *Infectious Disease in the Aging*
Edited by: Thomas T. Yoshikawa and Dean C. Norman
© Humana Press Inc., Totowa, NJ

Select age–related physiological changes impact on the pharmacokinetics and pharmacodynamics of drugs in general. It is beyond the scope of this chapter to describe all of these changes, but reviews have been published elsewhere *(4,5)*. The primary concern regarding prescribing of antibiotics in elderly patients is the decline in renal function associated with aging. Those antibiotics that are renally excreted—especially if they are associated with serious dose–related toxicities—must have dosages adjusted according to the patient's kidney function. The classical examples are the aminoglycoside antibiotics (streptomycin, gentamicin, tobramycin, amikacin, and netilmicin). These agents have toxicities that affect primarily the kidney and eighth nerve. Coincidentally, with aging, there is a general decline in renal function and loss of hearing. Thus, the elderly are especially at risk for serious and debilitating adverse effects from aminoglycosides. The other major concern in prescribing antibiotics to older patients is the potential harmful effects of drug interactions *(6)*. Examples of adverse interactions include erythromycin with terfenadine or astemizole (life–threatening cardiac dysrhythmias); aminoglycosides and furosemide (increase in ototoxicity); quinolones and multivalent–ion–containing substances such as Fe (iron), Al (aluminum), Mg (magnesium), and Ca (calcium) (decrease in gastrointestinal absorption of antibiotic, which reduces antimicrobial effect); and metronidazole and warfarin (decreased warfarin metabolism causing increased anticoagulation effect).

The issue of cost of antimicrobial therapy for patients regardless of age is always an important consideration in the management of infections. The cost of parenteral administration of antibiotics includes not only the price of drug purchase but also costs for preparation and administration (drug reconstitution, intravenous administration materials, pharmacy labor), monitoring drug levels, and laboratory tests for adverse reactions. Clearly, antibiotics that have favorable pharmacokinetics permitting once–or twice–a–day dosing would reduce costs of parenteral administration and improve drug compliance when antibiotics are taken orally. Because older patients are often prescribed many different medications, drug compliance is a serious issue. Reducing the frequency of dosing would assist in better adherence to prescriptions and improve therapeutic outcomes *(7)*. Transitioning antimicrobial therapy from parenteral administration to oral treatment impacts greatly on hospitalization costs. This is particularly important for the geriatric population because the elderly account for the vast majority of health care costs, especially those related to hospitalization *(8)*. With select antibiotics having comparable serum levels when administered parenterally or orally (e.g., ciprofloxacin), patients can be discharged earlier from acute care facilities and managed as outpatients without adversely impacting on the success of therapy. Additionally, more older patients with infections can be treated on an ambulatory basis with the availability of several effective oral antibiotics *(9)*.

2. APPROACH TO ANTIMICROBIAL THERAPY

Given the special and unique problems and challenges involved with older patients with potential infectious diseases, a somewhat different approach is needed to appropriately manage infections in the elderly than that which is practiced traditionally for the general or younger population.

With many diseases and illnesses presenting atypically in the elderly, it is often difficult to rely on classic or typical symptoms and signs to make a diagnosis of infection. As described in Chapter 3, fever may be minimal or absent in older infected patients and cognitive impairment or nonspecific complaints may be the initial manifestations of a septic process. Thus, it is imperative that clinicians always consider an infectious disease process whenever an older patient presents with an acute or subacute change in functional capacity, health status, or well–being that cannot be explained by other causes. Once an infectious disease is considered as a primary diagnosis, it is essential to quickly determine the site(s) of infection by history, physical examination, underlying illness, and residential setting (home, hospital, long–term care facility). During the preliminary assessment, it is also important to quickly obtain initial laboratory tests that will assist in diagnosing the primary source of infection, clinical status of the patient, and whether care can be delivered as an outpatient or inpatient (e.g., complete blood count, urinalysis with culture, chest radiograph, oxygenation status, renal function, and so on). In seriously ill patients, unnecessary and time–consuming diagnostic tests should be avoided at the outset and reserved for a time when the clinical status of the patient has stabilized. For all patients requiring acute hospital care, at least two sets of blood cultures should be obtained.

If hospitalization is deemed to be necessary for managing the infection, most elderly patients will be best managed with initiation of empiric antimicrobial therapy until culture and other laboratory data indicate a specific microbial etiology. Once it is decided that empiric antimicrobial therapy will be initiated, a broad-spectrum antibiotic should be selected. For most elderly patients with septic complications, the β-lactam class of antibiotics, i.e., penicillins, cephalosporins, carbapenems, monobactams, and β-lactam/β-lactamase inhibitor combinations, and fluoroquinolones are especially useful in treating infections in the elderly because of the broad spectrum of activity (Gram–positive, Gram–negative, anaerobic), favorable pharmacokinetics (once- or twice-daily administration, penetration into most body fluids and tissues), monitoring of serum concentrations is not necessary, relative safety, and availability of both parenteral and oral preparations of several of the drugs *(10)*.

After microbiological data become available, indicating a specific causative pathogen(s), appropriate changes in the empiric antibiotic regimen should be made. Ideally, a more narrow–spectrum antibiotic that is effective against the offending pathogen, nontoxic, easy to administer, and available in oral preparation should be prescribed. Generally, an aminoglycoside antibiotic is not prescribed for elderly patients because of its inherent ototoxicity and nephrotoxicity *(11)*. However, aminoglycosides should be considered in elderly patients with serious *Pseudomonas aeruginosa* infections (usually in combination with another antipseudomonal agent), life–threatening enterococcal infections (in combination with ampicillin or vancomycin for synergistic activity), septic shock of unknown cause (as part of a combined antibiotic regimen), and infections caused by organisms susceptible only to this drug *(10)*. Under these circumstances, the risk of death related to septic complications outweigh the risks of aminoglycoside toxicities.

As with all patients, careful monitoring for adverse effects must be done on a daily basis when administering parenteral antibiotics. Special attention should be directed to potential drug interactions because of the high number of medications elderly patients usually receive. When indicated, laboratory testing may be required to assess adverse effects (e.g., renal function tests). Newly developed cognitive impairment (confusion, altered sensorium) or worsening of underlying mental disorder (e.g., mild dementia) during antibiotic treatment should prompt a reassessment of the infection under therapy, search for another infection (superinfection), or evaluation of potential drug side effects. In addition, the clinician should consider noninfectious complications as the cause of a change in status in hospitalized elderly patients with infections, e.g., pulmonary embolus, cardiac dysrhythmias, heart failure, uncontrolled diabetes mellitus, and the like.

When the clinical status of the patient has improved, parenteral therapy should be changed to oral antibiotics. It should be noted that elderly patients are more likely to have slower or delayed responses to antimicrobial therapy than younger patients with similar infections. Moreover, although there may be objective evidence of effective treatment of an underlying infection (e.g., negative cultures, improving radiographs), elderly patients, especially those who are frail and with multiple chronic underlying disorders, may not show an improvement in their overall functional status. That is, despite improvement in the infection, the patient is not functionally improved—the patient is unable return to the same premorbid functional level, such as the ability to independently care for him or herself, walk without assistance or not depend on others to dress, eat, bathe, or use the bathroom. Under these circumstances, a comprehensive assessment of the patient's overall clinical status including cardiac, pulmonary, renal, hepatic and metabolic, and hematological systems, as well as review of all medications should be implemented. If no abnormalities are uncovered, then the patient may be safely discharged to a lower level of care (e.g., home) with adequate home support and increasing levels of physical rehabilitation as deemed safe and appropriate.

3. SELECT ANTIMICROBIAL AGENTS

3.1 β Lactams

The beta–lactam antibiotics remain one of the most frequently prescribed antibiotics for the treatment of infections in elderly patients. As stated earlier, these drugs have a broad spectrum, favorable pharmacokinetics, and a good safety record, and they do not require measurement of serum concentrations. Although most β-lactams are excreted by the kidney, there is very little risk of serious toxicities when standard doses are administered in patients with mild to moderate renal failure.

Penicillins have a limited role in treating infections in elderly patients. Although *S. pneumoniae* is a common pathogen infecting older patients, there is an increasing frequency of penicillin-resistant *S. pneumoniae* isolated in the elderly *(12)*. Thus, penicillin is no longer recommended as the initial drug of choice for older patients with serious *S. pneumoniae* infections, in whom the drug sensitivity data are not available. Penicillin and ampicillin are still the drugs of choice for infections caused by some other organisms commonly found in the elderly, i.e., *L. monocytogenes, S. bovis,* and viridans group streptococci. With an increasing incidence of methicillin-resistant *Staphylococcus aureus* (MRSA), the role of semisynthetic antistaphylococcal penicillins in treating staphylococcal infections has diminished. MRSA has been frequently isolated from hospitalized patients and now is often found in residents of long–term care facilities *(13)*.

Cephalosporins offer the greatest diversity and choices for antimicrobial therapy of any class of antibiotics. Currently, there are four "generations" of cephalosporins *(14)*. Of the first-generation cephalosporins, cefazolin has been the preferred drug for surgical prophylaxis, particularly for orthopedic cases such as repairing of hip fractures in the elderly *(15)*. Cefuroxime, a second-generation cephalosporin, has been an effective agent in treating mild to moderate pneumonia in elderly patients caused by drug-susceptible organisms. Cefoxitin and cefotetan, which are also second-generation cephalosporins, have good spectrum of activity against anaerobic bacteria including *Bacteroides* spp. and are useful for treating mixed anaerobic and aerobic infections such as infected pressure ulcers and uncomplicated intraabdominal infection *(16)*. Third-generation cephalosporins have gained wide popularity in treating a variety of infections in elderly patients. Ceftriaxone may be prescribed for treatment of community- or nursing home-acquired pneumonia and bacterial meningitis (in combination with ampicillin); ceftazidime, because of its superior Gram–negative spectrum, is indicated for treatment of nosocomial pneumonia, febrile neutropenic patient, and gram–negative meningitis caused by *P. aeruginosa* *(14)*. Cefepime is currently the only commercially available fourth-generation cephalosporin at the time of this writing. It has enhanced anti-Gram–negative activity including *P. aeruginosa* and also possesses moderately good activity against *S. aureus* *(14)*. The role of cefepime in treating infections in geriatric patients has yet to be determined.

β-Lactam and *β-lactamase inhibitor* combinations, i.e., ticarcillin–clavulanate, ampicillin–sulbactam, piperacillin–tazobactam, and amoxicillin–clavulanate, have similar spectra of activity as do third–generation cephalosporins but with improved antibacterial action against anaerobic organisms. Excluding amoxicillin–clavulanate, an oral preparation, β lactam/β-lactamase inhibitors are often prescribed for seriously ill elderly patients with nosocomial pneumonia, intraabdominal infections, urinary tract infection, and skin and soft tissue infections *(17)*.

Aztreonam is the only monobactam on the market and its spectrum of activity is limited to facultative and aerobic Gram–negative bacilli including *P. aeruginosa*, which is comparable to that of ceftazidime. It has been successfully used to treat a variety of infections in the elderly including urinary tract infection, sepsis, intraabdominal infections (in combination with another agent effective against anaerobes), and pneumonia caused by susceptible Gram–negative bacilli *(18,19)*.

Carbapenems represent the newest β–lactams used for treating infections. Imipenem–cilastatin and meropenem are currently the two carbenems that are commercially available. These drugs have an antibacterial spectrum that includes Gram–positive cocci, Gram–negative bacilli (including *P. aeruginosa*) and anaerobes. However, they are inactive against MRSA, vancomycin–resistant enterococci and some other less commonly isolated gram–negative bacilli (e.g., *Stenotrophomonas maltophilia*). Generally, these agents are reserved for infections involving drug–resistant organisms or in patients with life–threatening infections in whom other antibiotics cannot be used because of potential adverse effects. Meropenem has been administered to elderly patients with serious infections with good therapeutic outcome and relatively few side effects *(20)*. Meropenem, in contrast to imipenem–cilastatin, does not enhance seizure potential and thus is preferred over carbapenem in elderly patients with seizure activity or central nervous system infections.

3.2. Fluoroquinolones

Fluoroquinolones (also called quinolones) are the other class of antibiotics that have similar favorable characteristics as β lactams for use in treating infections in the elderly. The earliest marketed quinolones possessed primarily excellent activity against Gram–negative bacilli including *P. aeruginosa* with moderate activity against Gram–positive cocci and were available in an oral preparation. This permitted earlier transition from parenteral therapy for Gram–negative bacillary infections to oral treatment and thus reduced hospitalization days. Also, the need to hospitalize a clinically stable patient for anti–Gram–negative therapy was reduced with the advent of oral quinolones. The early quinolones included ciprofloxacin, ofloxacin, lomefloxacin, norfloxacin, and enoxacin *(21)*. Presently, ciprofloxacin is the most widely used of these earlier quinolones because of its superior activity against *P. aeruginosa* (and it remains the most active against *P. aeruginosa* of all quinolones marketed today), availability in both a parenteral and oral preparation, and its excellent bioavailability after oral administration. There have been numerous pharmacokinetic and clinical trial studies of these earlier quinolones in the elderly, which have been reviewed recently *(22)*. These drugs have been proven to be effective and relatively safe in treating elderly patients with serious Gram–negative infections.

More recently, a newer generation of quinolones have been emerging. These quinolones have greater activity against Gram–positive cocci than the older quinolones with comparable Gram–negative activity. In addition, they have improved activity against such pathogens as *Mycoplasma* spp., *Chlamydia* spp., and *Legionella* spp.*(23,24)*. The currently commercially available newer quinolones include levofloxacin, sparfloxacin, moxifloxacin, grepafloxacin (Grepafloxacin was removed from the market in October, 1999, because of seven unexpected deaths and other cardiovascular events.), and trovafloxacin (trovafloxacin has also excellent anti-anaerobic activity but its indications for clinical use have been restricted because of its unexpected high incidence of associated liver toxicity*)*. With these newer quinolones having such broad antibacterial activity including *S. pneumoniae* as well as *Legionella*, *Mycoplasma,* and *Chlamydia*, there has been increased prescribing of these agents for the treatment of lower respiratory tract infections *(25–27)*. Some preliminary data indicate that these quinolones may become the first line of therapy for community-acquired pneumonia *(28)*. However, in a recent study in Canada, there was an increased prevalence of reduced susceptibility of *S. pneumoniae* to these newer forms of quinolones, particularly in isolates from persons aged 65 yr and older vs. those aged 15–64 yr (2.6% vs. 1%) *(29)*. With increased prescribing of quinolones, selective pressures from these drugs will inevitably result in growing numbers and percentages of quinolone-resistant bacteria. Thus, it remains unclear the role of quinolones in the routine management of infections in the elderly.

3.3. Macrolides

Erythromycin, clarithromycin, and azithromycin are the currently available macrolides. Macrolides have a limited role in the overall management of infections in the elderly. Because of erythromycin's substantial frequency of gastrointestinal intolerance and side effects, clarithromycin and azithromycin are now the most commonly prescribed macrolides. Macrolides have activity against most strains of streptococci, methicillin–sensitive *S. aureus, Mycoplasma* spp, *Chlamydia* spp., and *Legionella* spp. *(30)*. With regards to infections in elderly patients, these drugs would be an initial consideration in the management of community-acquired pneumonia either alone or in combination with a second drug (e.g., β-lactam, quinolone) depending on the severity of illness and potential respiratory pathogens.

3.4. Other Agents

Vancomycin is being prescribed with increased regularity by clinicians because of the emergence of MRSA, ampicillin-resistant enterococci, and penicillin-cephalosporin-resistant *S. pneumoniae*. Its use in elderly patients has been primarily in treating MRSA infections, infections caused by multidrug-resistant *S. pneumoniae*, prosthetic device infections as part of empiric therapy, and *Clostridium difficile* colitis when metronidazole is contraindicated or ineffective *(31)*. Unfortunately, the high level of vancomycin administration has led to vancomycin-resistant enterococci (VRE), with VRE now appearing in long-term care facilities *(12)*.

Trimethoprim-sulfamethoxazole is often prescribed for elderly patients with uncomplicated urinary tract infections *(32)*. It has been recommended for treatment of chronic bacterial prostatitis, but more recently, quinolones have supplanted trimethoprim-sulfamethoxazole for this infection *(22,23)*.

Metronidazole is an agent active against anaerobic bacteria and select anaerobic parasites *(34)*. Infections involving anaerobic bacteria are relatively common in elderly patients (e.g., intraabdominal sepsis, infected pressure ulcers, diabetic foot ulcers, and aspiration pneumonia). In these infections, metronidazole is recommended usually in combination with another agent that is effective against Gram–negative bacilli and/or Gram–positive cocci *(35)*. In addition, metronidazole should be prescribed for older patients with *C. difficile* colitis and in those with a pyogenic brain abscess as part of a combination therapeutic regimen until specific microbiology of the abscess is determined.

Antiviral agents that are especially relevant to older patients include amantadine, rimantadine, acyclovir, famciclovir, and valcyclovir. Amantadine and rimantadine are effective in reducing the severity and duration of influenza A (but not B) illness if administered within 48 h of illness onset. These agents are recommended for all residents, regardless whether they received influenza vaccine during the previous fall, with an institutional outbreak (e.g., nursing facilities) of proven influenza A. The medications should be continued for at least 2 wk or until approximately one wk after the end of the outbreak *(36)*. Recently, zanamivir and oseltamivir, new antiviral agents effective against both influenza A and B, have become available for clinical use *(37)*. However, adequate data are unavailable at this time to determine their efficacy and safety in the elderly. Acyclovir, famciclovir, and valcylcovir are antiviral drugs that are effective in the reduction of pain of acute herpes zoster if given within the first 72 h of the onset of illness *(37)*. There is also some evidence that early antiviral therapy may diminish the overall duration of chronic pain associated with herpes zoster, which is commonly seen in elderly patients.

Antituberculous drug therapy for tuberculosis in the elderly is well described in Chapter 7. The primary drugs of choice for treating most cases of active tuberculosis (tuberculous diseases) in elderly patients will be isoniazid and rifampin because the vast majority of this infection will be caused by isoniazid– and rifampin–sensitive *Mycobacterium tuberculosis (38)*. Elderly patients should also receive isoniazid for treating tuberculous infection (chemoprophylaxis for inactive disease) when the appropriate indications are present.

Treatment of important fungal infections in the elderly has been reviewed in Chapter 18. The most frequently prescribed *antifungal agents* for serious fungal infections in elderly patients will be amphotericin B and fluconazole. Because of the toxicity of amphotericin B and the efficacy and availability of fluconazole in both parenteral and oral preparation, the latter drug is being prescribed with greater frequency in older patients.

4. ANTIMICROBIAL THERAPY IN AN AMBULATORY SETTING

With an increasing emphasis on outpatient and ambulatory management of diseases, it is not surprising that more physicians are treating older patients with infections outside an inpatient setting. The most common infections of elderly patients that are encountered in an ambulatory setting are acute pharyngitis, sinusitis, bronchitis, cellulitis, infected pressure ulcers, and urinary tract infection *(8,39)*. In addition, most cases of tuberculous disease and infection will be managed in an outpatient clinic or office, and infections requiring hospitalization will most often complete treatment at home. The most frequently prescribed oral antibiotics will be amoxicillin–clavulanate (streptococci, staphylococci, anaerobes, select Gram–negative bacilli), dicloxacillin (*S. aureus*), cefuroxime axetil (streptococci, *Haemophilus influenzae*, select Gram–negative bacilli), clindamycin (streptococci, staphylococci, anaerobes), macrolides (streptococci, staphylococci, *Mycoplasma, Chlamydia, Legionella*), trimethoprim– sulfamethoxazole (streptococci, Gram–negative bacilli), quinolones (Gram–negative bacilli), and metronidazole (anaerobes). Physicians should become familiar with the pharmacology, dosing, duration, and adverse effects of these agents because they will become a common therapeutic armamentarium for managing elderly infected patients.

5. ANTIMICROBIAL AGENTS IN LONG–TERM CARE SETTINGS

The problem of diagnosis and treatment of infections in long–term care settings especially nursing facilities (nursing homes) has been extensively reviewed (40–42). (See also Chapter 20.) The vast majority of serious infections in a long–term care setting will be urinary tract infections, lower respiratory infection (primarily pneumonia), and skin and soft–tissue infections (infected pressure ulcers). In addition, gastrointestinal infections including gastroenteritis, diverticulitis, and cholecystitis are not uncommonly diagnosed in elderly residents in nursing facilities.

The approach to antimicrobial therapy in this setting will largely depend on whether the resident requires acute hospitalization because of clinical instability and/or need for parenteral antimicrobial therapy. In some residents with serious infection, they may be clinically stable but may require parenteral antibiotics (i.e., unable to take oral medications or oral preparation of appropriate antibiotic is not available or inadequate for successful outcome). These patients can be managed in the long-term care facility provided there are (1) 24-h-7-d acute nursing care, (2) immediate availability of a physician or physician extender (nurse practitioner, physician assistant), (3) easy access to necessary radiological and laboratory testing, and (4) equipment and supplies for acute care management including intravenous therapy. Antibiotics that would be especially useful for parenteral therapy in such a setting include the long–acting cephalosporins (e.g., ceftriaxone) and quinolones. As stated earlier, their broad spectrum, once or twice a day dosing, relative safety, and lack of the need for measuring drug levels make these class of drugs a reasonable choice for managing infections in elderly residents of long-term care facilities as part of empiric therapy. However, whenever possible, specific directed therapy based on microbiological findings should be initiated. Indiscriminate use of such broad–spectrum antibiotics will invariably lead to multidrug–resistant organisms, which is already a growing problem in long–term care facilities (12) (see Chapter 21).

REFERENCES

1. Yoshikawa, T.T. (1990) Antimicrobial therapy for the elderly patient. *J. Am. Geriatr. Soc.* **38**, 1353–1372.
2. McCue, J.D. (1992) Antimicrobial therapy. *Clin. Geriatr. Med.* **8(4)**, 925–945.
3. Yoshikawa, T.T. and Norman, D.C. (eds.) (1994) *Antimicrobial Therapy in the Elderly Patient*, Marcel Dekker, New York.
4. Rho, J.P. and Wong, F.S. (1998) Principles of prescribing medications, in *Practical Ambulatory Geriatrics* (Yoshikawa, T.T., Cobbs, E. L., and Brummel-Smith, K., eds.), Year-Book Mosby, St. Louis, MO, pp. 19–25.
5. Schwartz, J.B. (1999) Clinical pharmacology, in *Principles of Geriatric Medicine and Gerontology,* 4th ed. (Hazzard, W.R., Blass, J.P., Ettinger, W.H., Jr., et al. eds.), McGraw–Hill, New York, pp. 303–331.
6. Nilsson–Ehle, I. and Ljungberg, B. (1994) Pharmacology of antimicrobial agents with aging, in *Antimicrobial Therapy in the Elderly Patient* (Yoshikawa, T.T. and Norman, D.C., eds.), Marcel Dekker, New York, pp. 33–45.
7. Rho, J.P. and Yoshikawa, T.T. (1995) The cost of inappropriate use of anti-infective agents in older patients. *Drugs Aging* **6**(4), 263–267.
8. McGinnis, J.M. (1988) The Tithonus syndrome: health and aging in America, in *Health Promotion and Disease Prevention in the Elderly* (Chernoff, R. and Lipschitz, D.A., eds.), Raven Press, New York, pp. 1–15.
9. Yoshikawa, T.T. (1991) Ambulatory management of common infection in elderly patients. *Infect. Med.* **8**, 37–43.
10. Rajagopalan, S. and Yoshikawa, T.T. (1999) Antibiotic selection in the elderly patient. *Antibiot. Clin.* **3**(3), 51–56.
11. Rybak, M.J., Abate, B.J., Kang, S.L., et al. (1999) Prospective evaluation of the effect of an aminoglycoside dosing regimen on rates of observed nephrotoxicity and ototoxicity. *Antimicrob. Agents Chemother.* **43**(7), 1549–1555.
12. Yoshikawa, T.T. (1998) VRE, MRSA, PRP, and DRGNB in LTCF: lessons to be learned from this alphabet. *J. Am. Geriatr. Soc.* **46**, 241–243.
13. Bradley, S.F. (1992) Methicillin–resistant *Staphylococcus aureus* infection. *Clin. Geriatr. Med.* **8(4),** 853–868.
14. Marshall, W.F. and Blair, J.E. (1999) The cephalosporins. *Mayo Clin. Proc.* **74**,187–195.
15. Gorbach, S.L. (1989) The role of cephalosporins in surgical prophylaxis. *J. Antimicrob. Chemother.* **23**, 61–70.
16. McCue, J.D. and Tessier, E.G. (1994) Cephalosporins, in *Antimicrobial Therapy in the Elderly Patient* (Yoshikawa, T.T. and Norman, D.C., eds.), Marcel Dekker, New York, pp. 99–123.
17. Rho, J.P., Takemoto, F.C.S., An A., et al. (1994) Beta–lactamase inhibitors, in *Antimicrobial Therapy in the Elderly Patient* (Yoshikawa, T.T. and Norman, D.C., eds.), Marcel Dekker, Inc., New York, pp. 151–167.

18. Deger, F., Douchamps, J. Freschi, E. et al (1988) Aztreonam in the treatment of serious gram–negative infections in the elderly. *Internatl. J. Clin. Pharmacol. Ther. Toxicol.* **26**, 22–26
19. Knockaert, D.C., Dejaeger, E., Nester, L., et al (1991) Aztreonam–flucloxacillin double beta–lactam treatment as empirical therapy of serious infections in very elderly patients. *Age Ageing* **20**, 135–139.
20. Jaspers, C.A., Kieft, H., Speelberg, B., et al. (1998) Meropenem versus cefuroxime plus gentamicin for treatment of serious infections in elderly patients. *Antimicrob. Agents Chemother.* **42(5)**, 1233–1238.
21. Borchering, S.M., Stevens, R., Nicholas, R.A., et al (1996) Quinolones: a practical review of clinical uses, dosing considerations, and drug interactions. *J. Fam. Pract.* **42(1)**, 69–78.
22. Guay, D.R.P. (1994) Quinolones, in *Antimicrobial Therapy in the Elderly Patient* (Yoshikawa, T.T., and Norman, D.C., eds.), Marcel Dekkelr, New York, pp. 235–310.
23. Ridgeway, G.L., Salman, H., Dencer, C., et al. (1997) The in–vitro activity of grepafloxacin against *Chlamydia* spp., *Mycoplasma* spp.*, Ureaplasma urealyticum* and *Legionella* spp. *J. Antimicrob. Chemother.* **40(suppl. A)**, 31–34.
24. Wiedemann, B. and Heisig, P. (1997) Antibacterial activity of grepafloxacin. *J. Antimicrob. Chemother.* **40(suppl. A.)**, 19–25
25. File, T.M., Jr., Segret, J., Dunbar, L., et al. (1997) A multicenter, randomized study comparing the efficacy and safety of intravenous and/or oral levofloxacin versus ceftriaxone and/or cefuroxime axetil in treatment of adults with community–acquired pneumonia. *Antimicrob. Agents Chemother.* **41**, 1965–1972.
26. File, T.M., Jr. (1997) Management of community–acquired pneumonia. Challenges, controversies and new therapeutic options. *Infect. Dis. Clin. Pract.* **21(2)**, 9–12.
27. Geddes, A.M. (1997) Grepafloxacin—focus on respiratory infections. *J. Antimcrob. Chemother.* **40(suppl. A)**, 1–4.
28. Marrie, T.J. (1999) Clinical strategies for managing pneumonia in the elderly. *Clin. Geriatr.* August (suppl.), 6–10.
29. Chen, D.K., McGeer, A., de Azavedo, J.C., et al. (1999) Decreased susceptibility of *Streptococcus pneumoniae* to fluoroquinolones in Canada. *N. Engl. J. Med.* **341**, 233–239.
30. Alvarez-Elcoro, S. and Enzler, M.J. (1999) The macrolides: erythromycin, clarithromycin and azithromycin. *Mayo Clin. Proc.* **74**, 613–634.
31. Cunha, B.A. and Klein, N.C. (1994) Vancomycin, in *Antimicrobial Therapy in the Elderly Patient* (Yoshikawa, T.T. and Norman, D.C., eds.), Marcel Dekker, New York, pp. 311–321.
32. Wood, C.A. and Abrutyn E. (1998) Urinary tract infection in older adults. *Clin. Geriatr. Med.* **14(2)**, 267–283.
33. Childs, S.J. (1994) Ciprofloxacin in treatment of chronic bacterial prostatitis. *Urology* **35** (suppl.), 15–18.
34. Samuelson, J. (1999) Why metronidazole is active against both bacteria and parasites. *Antimicrob. Agents Chemother.* **43(7)**, 1533–1541.
35. Shriner, K.A. and Mathisen, G.E. (1994) Metronidazole, in *Antimicrobial Therapy in the Elderly Patient* (Yoshikawa, T.T. and Norman, D.C., eds.), Marcel Dekker, New York, pp. 367–378.
36. Centers for Disease Control and Prevention (1999) Prevention and control of influenza. Recommendations of the Advisory Committee on Immunization Practices. *M.M.W.R.* **48(No. RR–4)**, 1–28.
37. Centers for Disease Control and Prevention (1999) Neurominidase inhibitors for treatment of influenza A and infections. *M.M.M.R.* **48(No. RR-14)**, 1–9.
38. Rajagopalan, S. and Yoshikawa, T.T. (1999) Tuberculosis, in *Principles of Geriatric Medicine and Gerontology*, fourth edition (Hazzard, W.R., Blass, J.P., Ettinger, W.H., Jr., et al, eds.), McGraw–Hill, New York, pp. 737–744.

39. Yoshikawa, T.T. (1994) Antimicrobial therapy in the ambulatory setting, in *Antimicrobial Therapy in the Elderly Patient* (Yoshikawa, T.T. and Norman, D.C., eds.), Marcel Dekker, New York, pp. 479–484.
40. Verghese, A. and Berk, S.L. (eds.) (1990) *Infections in Nursing Homes and Long-Term Facilities*, Karger, Basel, Switzerland.
41. Williams, E.A. and Berk, S.L. (1994) The use of antimicrobials in nursing home, in *Antimicrobial Therapy in the Elderly Patient* (Yoshikawa, T.T. and Norman, D.C., eds.), Marcel Dekker, New York, pp. 485–504.
42. Yoshikawa, T.T. and Norman, D.C. (1996) Approach to fever and infection in the nursing home. *J. Am. Geriatr. Soc.* **44**, 74–82.

II
Specific Infections

5
Sepsis

Jirayos Chintanadilok and Bradley S. Bender

1. EPIDEMIOLOGY AND CLINICAL RELEVANCE

1.1. Definitions

Sepsis is the clinical syndrome denoting systemic inflammatory response to an infection. There is some confusion over the use of the terms "bacteremia" and "septicemia." Most studies in the United States used the term bacteremia to denote a positive blood culture with evidence of infection. Septicemia was used to denote a state of microbial invasion from a portal of entry into the bloodstream that causes signs of illness. Sepsis syndrome was initially described by Bone et al. to identify a population of patients at risk for adult respiratory distress syndrome (ARDS) and death *(1)*.

In 1991, the American College of Chest Physicians/Society of Critical Care Medicine (ACCP/SCCM) developed a classification system for patients with severe infection and its sequelae to help standardize research protocols and allow comparisons with results of clinical trials. Use of the terms septicemia and septic syndrome was discouraged because they were ambiguous and often used inappropriately to imply bacteremia *(2)*. Standardized terms were developed and defined. Bacteremia is defined as the presence of viable bacteria in the blood. Infection is defined as the inflammatory response to the microorganisms of the invasion of normally sterile host tissues by those organisms. The systemic inflammatory response syndrome (SIRS) is used to denote the physiological response to inflammation/infection and the criteria are given in Table 1, which also defines four stages of increasing severity of sepsis. Sepsis is defined as SIRS plus evidence of infection (e.g., positive microbial culture).

There is evidence of a clinical progression of the SIRS from sepsis to severe sepsis and to septic shock showing that the ACCP classification is a hierarchical continuum of increased inflammatory response to infection. For example, Rangel–Frausto and co-workers *(3)* showed that 44–71% of patients in any category had progressed from a previous state of biologic response syndrome and the rest either progressed through more than two stages within a 24-h period or skipped a stage. Also, bacteremia rates, end-organ failure rates, and mortality increased with each subsequent stage of SIR.

Sepsis studies use standard guidelines to decrease recruitment time and increase the ability to generalize the study findings to the practice community *(4)*. Most of the sepsis studies in the elderly were done before 1991, so that bacteremia was used as for the

From: *Infectious Disease in the Aging*
Edited by: Thomas T. Yoshikawa and Dean C. Norman
© Humana Press Inc., Totowa, NJ

Table 1
Definitions for Sepsis and Organ Failure[a]

Systemic inflammatory response syndrome (SIRS)	Four stages of sepsis
Two or more of the following conditions: 1. Temperature >38°C or <36°C 2. Heart rate >90 beats p min 3. Respiratory rate >20 beats p min PaCO$_2$ or <32 mmHg 4. WBC >12,000/mm^3, <4,000/mm^3, or >10% band forms	**Severe sepsis**: sepsis associated with organ dysfunction, hypoperfusion, hypotension. Hypoperfusion and perfusion abnormalities may include, but are not limited to, lactic acidosis, oliguria, or an acute alteration in mental status. **Sepsis-induced hypotension:** a systolic blood pressure <90 mmHg or a reduction of >40 mmHg from baseline in the absence of other causes for hypotension. **Septic Shock**: sepsis-induced hypotension despite adequate fluid resuscitation along with the presence of perfusion abnormalities that may include, but are not limited to, lactic acidosis, oliguria, or an acute alteration in mental status. Patients who are receiving inotropic or vasopressor agents may not be hypotensive at the time that perfusion abnormalities are measured. **Multiple organ dysfunction syndrome (MODS)**: presence of altered organ function in an acutely ill patient such that homeostasis cannot be maintained without intervention.

[a]Adapted from Ref. *2*; PaCO$_2$ = arterial partial pressure of carbon dioxide; WBC = white blood cell.

early phase of sepsis and septicemia denoted a severe infection. This chapter preserves these terms as their originals and also implies them as parts of sepsis.

1.2. Epidemiology

In the United States, sepsis was diagnosed in approximately 2.5 million patients in the period 1979–1987, and accounted for $5–10 billion in annual health care expenditures *(5,6)*. Overall, the incidence of sepsis is 2–2.6 cases per 100 admissions and is higher in the elderly and patients with multiple comorbidities *(7,8,9)*.

Sepsis has a mortality sevenfold higher than other general medical conditions *(10)*. It affects up to 25% of all intensive care unit patients and is the most common cause of death in the noncoronary intensive care unit *(11)*. Sepsis was ranked third among infectious diseases as a cause of death, following respiratory tract infections and HIV/AIDS. The overall mortality rate of sepsis varies between 18% and 33%, increasing to 40%–80% in patients with septic shock *(12)*.

The mortality of bacteremia in the elderly varies from 15–40% (*see* Table 2). A prospective study by Knaus *(9)* found that the 28-d mortality of sepsis increased with age from 26–33% in the persons under 65 yr, compared with 35–42% in the persons aged 65 and older. The higher mortality is observed mostly in older subjects with non-fatal underlying illnesses *(15)*. This point emphasizes that old age alone is not a poor indicator of ultimate outcome.

From 1980–1992, the death rate from sepsis increased 83% from 4.32 per 100,000 population to 7.7 per 100,000 population. The recent incidence and mortality of sepsis in the elderly are not available from the national databases. However, the death certificate data from 1980 and 1992 showed that there was a 25% increase in the rate of infectious disease deaths, and the persons aged 65 yr and older had the highest death rate *(13)*. Two possible explanations for this increase could be increasing awareness of physicians and the real increasing risk of sepsis. The mortality rate from the death certificate data could be overestimated because there were comorbidities independent of the occurrence of sepsis in about 50% of all septic patients, and severe underlying diseases could be found in up to 95% *(10,14)*. The severity of the sepsis and the degree of related organ dysfunction makes comparison between the studies difficult, so it is not surprising that some studies show that mortality rate of sepsis in the elderly is unchanged *(10,15,16)*.

2. CLINICAL MANIFESTATIONS

2.1. Pathophysiology

Sepsis results from infection with a variety of microbes, especially Gram-negative and Gram-positive bacteria and fungi; clinical studies have documented that clinical symptoms are essentially identical with all organisms *(17)*. The process of sepsis begins with the proliferation of microorganisms at a nidus of infection. The organisms can invade the bloodstream directly or release inflammatory mediators into the bloodstream. These mediators are composed of both structural components of the organisms such as teichoic acid and endotoxin, and synthetic products such as exotoxins, which cause a systemic proinflammatory reaction by stimulating the release of endogenous mediators such as tumor necrosis factor (TNF-α)-alpha; interleukins (IL)-1,2,4,6,8; platelet-activating factor; eicosanoids; α-interferon, granulocyte–macrophage colony-stimulating factor; endothelial-derived releasing factor; endothelin-1; and complement. Normally, the body regulates itself by counteracting the proinflammatory stage by production of such factors as interleukin-10 and -11, soluble TNF-α receptors, and IL-1 receptor antagonists. If the equilibrium is lost, however, these mediators can cause systemic damage, including endothelial damage, microvascular dysfunction, and impaired tissue oxygenation and organ injury *(18)*.

Aging has a profound effect on immune function. Immune senescence is characterized by a dysregulation of the immune system, especially in the balance of Th1 and Th2 helper cells that potentially make elderly persons more susceptible to bacterial and virus infections than younger adults. There is, however, no consistent correlation of cytokine production with the severity of the sepsis. The phagocytes (neutrophils, monocytes, and macrophages) have subtle abnormalities that can be detected only by quite sophisticated testing, and thus these minor defects most likely have little impact on

Table 2
Factors Contributing to the Severity of Sepsis in Elderly Patients[a]

Aging changes in various organ systems	Effect of sepsis on various organ systems	Clinical outcome and manifestations
Neurological		
Atherosclerotic plaques, aneurysms, thrombi, and compromised cerebral perfusion	Direct bacterial invasion	Septic encephalopathy
Neuronal organelles subtle changes with unclear clinical signifigance	Endotoxin effects on the brain	Polyneuropathy
Higher incidence of dementia, stroke, Parkinsons disease	Inadequate or altered cerebral perfusion	Susceptible to delirium
	Altered plasma or CNS levels of amino acids	Altered mental status, simple fatigue, or unexplained fall as initial presentations
	Altered brain metabolism	
Cardiovascular		
Hypertrophy, fibrosis, and atherosclerosis	Redistribution of intravascular fluid volume and increase capillary pressure	Hypotension
Diastolic dysfunction	Depressed LV preload by decreased venous return	Less tachycardia in sepsis
Diminished response to adrenergic stimulation	Depressed ventricular contractility by myocardial depressant substances	Drop in CO and increased risk of pulmonary edema
Loss of chronotropic reserve compensation	Early: vasodilatation and decrease systemic vascular resistance	Difficult fluid management and may lead to more invasive monitoring, which can increase in iatrogenic complications
	Late: contracted plasma volume	
Pulmonary		
Decreased VC , no change in TLC	Depressed respiratory muscle contractile performance	Acute lung injury
Increased RV and FRC	Endothelial injury in pulmonary vessel	ARDS 25–42% of patients with sepsis
Decreased chest wall compliance and respiratory muscle strength	Interstitial and alveolar edema and hemorrhage	Less hypoxia but more tachypnea
Decreased PaO$_2$ and increased ventilation–perfusion mismatch both at rest and during exercise		Decreased ventilatory reserve in response to higher oxygen demand causing rapid cardiopulmonary derangement
Decreased ventilatory responses to hypoxia or hypercapnia		Increased frequency of mechanical ventilation
		Difficult to wean off ventilator
		Increase nosocomial pneumonia

Organ system		
Renal		
Atrophy of cortex and medulla and increase in connective tissue and fibrosis	Ischemic acute tubular necrosis	Increased risk of drug-induced nephrotoxicity, e.g., gentamicin, β-lactam, sulfa, amphotericin B
Decrease in GFR	Rhabdomyolysis	Acute renal failure and increased mortality
Impaired ability to dilute and concentrate urine	Veno-occlusive disease	Electrolyte imbalance especially Na, K, Ca, Mg, and P
Incontinence predisposes to UTI		Indwelling catheterization may mask symptoms and increase risk of nosocomial infection
Gastrointestinal tract		
Esophagus: achalasia, diverticula, decrease peristalsis, increase reflux	Increased intestinal permeability and predispose to develop MODS	Impaired gastrointestinal motility
Stomach: atrophic gastritis, gastric achlorhydria	Impaired gut barrier function, allowing translocation of bacteria and endotoxin into the systemic circulation and extending the septic response	Increase aspiration
Intestine: mucosal atrophy, diverticulosis, polyps, diarrhea and constipation		Gut ischemia, ulcer, bleeding
		Gastric achlorhydria increase susceptibility to intestinal infections
Hepatobiliary tract		
Deficiency in the inducible mixed oxidase microsomal enzymes	Adrenergic receptor dysfunction	Elevation of liver enzymes
Cholelithiasis	Early: increased glycogenolysis and gluconeogenesis	Hyperbilirubinemia
		Drug-induced hepatoxicity
Pancreas		
No change in exocrine function	Late: decreased gluconeogenesis	Hyperglycemia
	Increased glucose-independent fat oxidation	Hypoglycemia in cirrhosis patients
	Decreased albumin, prealbumin, transferrin	Prolonged effect of liver-excreted drugs, e.g., benzodiazepines
		Acalculous cholecystitis
Hematologic		
Immune dysregulation	Demarginalization of neutrophils by catecholamines	Leukopenia may be a poor prognostic sign
Subtle abnormalities of the phagocytes (neutrophils, monocytes, and macrophages)	Cytokine-induced release of immature neutrophils from bone marrow	Most have leukocytosis
Anemia of chronic disease	Shortened red blood cell survival	Anemia
	Increased platelet destruction	Thrombocytopenia
		DIC

[a] Refs. 82–92

Abbreviations: CNS = central nervous systems, LV = left ventricular, CO = cardiac output, VC = vital capacity, TLC = total lung capacity, RV= residual volume, FRC = functional residual capacity, PaO2 = partial arterial oxygen pressure, ARDS = adult respiratory distress syndrome, GFR = glomerular filtration rate, UTI = urinary tract infection, MODS = multiple organ dysfunction syndrome, Na = sodium, K = potassium, Ca = calcium, Mg = magnesium, P = phosphorus, DIC = disseminated intravascular coagulation.

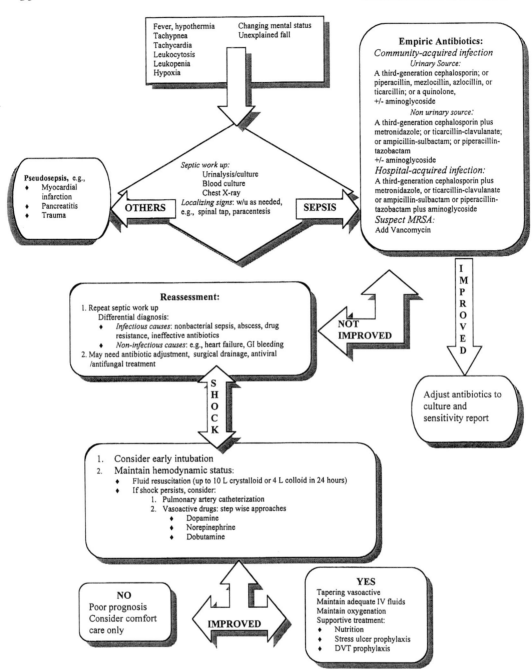

Fig. 1. Management of sepsis in the elderly: MRSA = methicillin-resistant *Staphylococcus aureus*. GI = gastrointestinal; L = liters; W/U = workup; DVT = deep vein thrombosis; IV = intravenous

age-related severity of sepsis. For example, after in vitro lipopolysaccharide (LPS)-induced activation of leukocytes of elderly persons, there were higher amounts of IL-1, IL-6, IL-8, and TNF-α than in younger persons *(20)*. Furthermore, a small prospective study of the influence of age on circulating adhesion molecules in critically ill patients showed that elderly patients had higher levels of the soluble adhesion molecules, but the clinical significance of this finding is unclear *(19)*.

The foregoing age-related changes in immune function probably play only a small role in the severity of sepsis. A major contributing factor to the higher frequency and mortality of sepsis in older patients, however, is the large number of anatomic and physiologic changes that occur with age *(see* Table 1). These include changes in neurological, cardiovascular, pulmonary, and renal systems.

Infections may not only result from many of the coexisting diseases of aging but also may exacerbate other illnesses. Thus, it is not unusual to see a patient with congestive heart failure and a recent stroke develop an aspiration pneumonia, then sepsis, and further cardiac decompensation.

2.2. Symptoms and Signs

An overview of the manifestations of sepsis in the elderly is given in Fig. 1. There are no pathognomonic symptoms or signs of bacteremia in the elderly. The triad of tachycardia, rigors, and hypotension, as the classical manifestations of sepsis, are also rare in most studies. In a prospective study, Chassagne and colleagues *(21)* compared the presentations of bacteremia in young and elderly patients and noted that elderly patients had fewer symptoms and signs than younger infected patients. Elderly persons may have atypical presentation of bacteremia, e.g., lower body temperatures (even hypothermia), change in functional capabilities, simple fatigue, unexplained recurrent falls (up to 30% of a geriatric unit admission), and altered mental status (observed in 30-50% of cases) *(22–26)*. The atypical presentation in elderly patients may delay diagnosis, and septic shock may be the first clue that the patient is infected. A clinical indication of a source of infection can be identified in up to 75% of bacteremic elderly patients *(21)*. A summary of several studies on the clinical presentation of bacteremia in the elderly is shown in Table 3. Many of these studies have emphasized the occurrence of altered mental status, abdominal symptoms, and that fever is not a universal finding.

Fever, increased erythrocyte sedimentation rate, and a clinical indication of the source of infection, were found at least 70% of bacteremic elderly patients *(21)*. The febrile response in the elderly is different from the younger persons. Lower body temperatures with infection are more common in elderly persons and are correlated with higher mortality *(16,24,26,28-30)*. Kreger and colleagues *(31)* noted that transient hypothermia at the onset of bacteremia was not associated with increased fatality, but failure to mount a febrile response >99.6°F (37.6°C) within 24 h was. Body temperatures are normally maintained over a relatively narrow range, and older persons have basal temperatures that are about 0.3–0.5°C lower than in younger persons *(32)*. A retrospective study of infections in nursing home residents by Castle and co-workers found that 47% had temperature less than 101°F (38.3°C) *(33)*. Many of these patients had an adequate change in temperature from baseline (a change in temperature of more than 2.4°F) but failed to achieve a significant temperature (>101°F) because of a low baseline value *(33)*. Possible mechanisms for lower body temperature have not been completely elucidated but may be due to both a reduced capacity for thermogenesis and increased heat loss following infection *(34); see* also Chapter 3.

Table 3
Clinical Presentation of Bacteremia and Sepsis in Older Persons

Clinical/Reference	Madden 1981 (41) Septicemia in the elderly	Windsor 1983 (23) Bacteremia in a geriatric unit	Rudman 1988 (40) Nursing home Bacteremia	Meyers 1989 (40) Bloodstream infection in the elderly	Whitelaw 1992 (44) CA[a] Bacteremia in the elderly
Study method and population	Retrospective 44 patients[b] Geriatric unit	Retrospective 50 patients Geriatric unit	Retrospective 42 episodes Nursing home	Retrospective 100 episodes Hospital	Prospective 121 patients Hospital
Fever	88%	60%	95%	T>101°F = 65% T99–101°F = 25%	47%
Altered mental status	16%	36%	43% lethargy 2% delirium 1% seizure	52%	21%
Nausea and vomiting	40%	NA[c]	25%	NA	30%
Rigors	28%	NA	25%	34%	35%
Abdominal pain	28%	Included vomiting and diarrhea 14%	17%	NA	NA

Source	NA High ratio of common bile duct stone (15%)	GU 50% Pneumonia 22% Joint 10% Cellulitis 8% Biliary 8% Endocarditis 4% Pressure sore 4% Unknown 20%	GU 60% Pneumonia 7% Skin/soft tissue 7% Surgical wound 5% Bone/joint 2% Unknoan 22%	GU 27% Pneumonia 12% Intra-abdominal 16% Intravascular devices 9% Skin/soft tissue 6% Indeterminate 21% Endocarditis 3% Graft 3% Multiple 3%	GU 32% Pneumonia 18% Unknown 26%
Mortality	33%	24%	21%	40%	38%

[a]CA = community acquired; GU = genitourinary
[b]Total of 4; data given 26 patients with Gram-negative bacteremia.
[c]NA = Not available.

There are other differences in the presentation of sepsis between elderly and younger persons. The incidence of tachycardia and hypoxemia was significantly lower and the incidence of increased respiration, elevated plasma lactate, and altered mentation significantly higher in the patients >75 yr of age with Gram-negative sepsis as compared with patients <75 yr old *(35)*. Leukocytosis (greater than 10,000/mm³) is seen about 70% *(21,23,29,40)*. Leukopenia is rare (less than 10%) and the incidence does not differ from younger persons *(21)*.

Elderly patients are prone to have associated clinical problems that can mislead the physician into making an incorrect diagnosis. For example, the history from a patient with dementia may be unreliable. As with other diseases of the elderly, physicians must coordinate the complexities of multiple, interacting diseases often present in the elderly. Particular expertise is required to discriminate important and relevant clinical problems in an initial evaluation.

2.3. Source and Microbial Causes

The genitourinary tract is the most common source of bacteremia in older persons, accounting for 20–50% of cases. Other sources include the respiratory tract, the gastrointestinal tract, and endovascular devices. Esposito noted that 10–20% of bacteremias were due to biliary tract infection and should be considered as a feature unique to aged patients presenting with community-acquired bacteremia *(36)*.

Because the urinary tract is the most frequently identified site of infection in older persons, it is not surprising that Gram-negative bacteria account for most cases of bacteremia in this age group. *Escherichia coli* is the most common Gram-negative organism, accounting for between 14% and 44% of isolates *(15,16,21–23,29)*. *Klebsiella*, *Providencia*, and *Proteus* are also commonly isolated.

The bacterial etiology of sepsis appears to be changing with rising number of cases of Gram-positive bacteremia. This has been related to changing demographics, new antibiotics, immunosuppressive agents, and invasive technology in the treatment of inflammatory, infectious, and neoplastic diseases *(37)*. Patients from long-term facilities in particular have a higher incidence of Gram-positive bacteremia *(39)*, and *Staphylococcus aureus* is the most frequently recovered organism *(23,39)*. *Streptococcus pneumoniae* is more common than *S. aureus* in community-dwelling elders who were admitted from the emergency room *(38)*. Other Gram-positive organisms frequently found include *Enterococcus* spp, and viridans group streptococci (23,40–42).

When polymicrobial sepsis occurs in the elderly, the most likely sources are the urinary and respiratory tracts, frequently associated with indwelling catheters and aspiration, respectively *(38)*. There are no published studies on the epidemiology of the sepsis in the elderly related to emerging pathogens such as *Legionella*, human immunodeficiency virus, and *Haemophilus influenzae*.

Elderly patients also have an increased risk of nosocomial infection and sepsis. The daily bacteremia rates of hospitalized patients were 0.59% in patients over age 60 and 0.40% in younger patients (a relative risk of 1.49) *(43)*. *E. coli* was the most common isolate in older persons with hospital-acquired bacteremia, most of which were associated with a urinary or abdominal focus. Staphylococci species, especially *S. aureus*, were the second most common isolates, mainly associated with intravenous access or surgical wound infection *(16,29)*.

3. DIAGNOSTIC TESTS

Microbiologic studies should be performed promptly when sepsis is suspected and before starting antibiotics (*see* Fig.1). All patients should have blood cultures obtained from two different sites as well as cultures and smears (e.g., Gram stain) of relevant body fluids (sputum, urine, cerebrospinal/peritoneal/pleural fluid) and exudates (abscesses, transcutaneous drain, loculated fluids). Other diagnostic tests may be required and obtained later if the diagnosis remains unclear.

Approximately half the patients with severe sepsis have positive blood cultures at the time of diagnosis *(2)*. Broad-spectrum antibiotics are frequently initiated pending culture and sensitivity, but physicians seem to be reluctant to change the antibiotic regimen when culture results return *(45)*.

The yield from sputum examination is lower in the elderly when compared with the younger patients due to inadequate cough or cooperation in the patients with impaired cognition. Adequate specimens have fewer than 10 squamous epithelial cells and more than 25 polymorphonuclear cells per low-power (100×) field. Only one third of sputum specimens from the elderly patients meet these cytologic criteria *(46)*.

The most common source of sepsis in older persons is the urinary tract. Urinary tract infections are discussed more completely in Chapter 10.

Chest X-rays are usually obtained in the initial evaluation of most septic patients. Elderly patients may have an underlying illness, especially heart failure, malignancy, or chronic lung disease that may make radiologic interpretation more difficult. Older persons are also more prone to have dehydration, which, theoretically could blunt the initial radiographic appearance, but this has not been confirmed in animal and human studies *(47,48)*.

Patients with sepsis and acute respiratory distress syndrome (ARDS) may have a normal chest radiograph despite abnormal blood gases early in the disease, but the majority will develop radiograph abnormalities within 24 h. The rate of progression to ARDS is variable. There is no relationship between the amount of infiltration and gas exchange or survival at any time point, but a worsening or persistently opacified chest radiograph suggests a poor prognosis. If there are new findings after 5 d, a superimposed process, e.g., nosocomial pneumonia, fluid overload, atelectasis, barotrauma, or sepsis, should be suspected. Effects of advancing age on ARDS is unknown.

In the elderly septic patient with an acute abdomen, flat and erect plain radiographs are an appropriate first diagnostic step because of their low cost, portability, rapidity, and high yield. They can identify free air collections in the intraperitoneal or retroperitoneal space and also radio-opaque stones in the hepatobiliary tract as well as genitourinary tract. To search for an occult source of infection, ultrasonography and computed tomographic (CT) scan have higher yields. The CT scan is superior to the ultrasonogram for detection of an intraabdominal abscess, which carries a mortality of 30% for surgically treated abdominal abscess, and 80–90% for cases without surgical drainage *(49)*. (*See also* Chapter 9.)

Currently, the diagnosis of sepsis requires combination of clinical signs of systemic inflammation and evidence of infection. Elderly persons with sepsis may present with minimal or subtle findings of infection, however, and diagnosis can be delayed. Because many of the inflammatory cells and mediators have been identi-

fied, future studies and clinical management will likely focus on using these mediators as both diagnostic and prognostic markers for sepsis. Because of the relative
ease with which they can be obtained, peripheral blood markers are likely to become
clinically useful diagnostic and prognostic markers. In a recent study in febrile patients with community-acquired infection, a high serum ratio of IL-10 to TNF-α was
associated with poor outcome, but age, sex, and duration of fever were not *(50)*.

4. TREATMENT

The two most important aspects of the initial management in the patient suspected of
sepsis are prompt initiation of antibiotics and fluid and hemodynamic resuscitation.
Pseudosepsis or conditions that mimic sepsis, e.g., myocardial infarction, adrenal insufficiency, gastrointestional hemorrhage, pulmonary emboli, and acute pancreatitis,
should be excluded to avoid unnecessary use of antibiotics *(51)* (*see* Fig.1). Older patients still benefit from having their management occur in an intensive care unit (ICU).
For example, a retrospective study by Lundberg and colleagues *(52)* showed that the
mortality of septic shock was higher (70%) in patients treated on a hospital ward as
compared with patients treated in an ICU (39%), despite the fact that the ICU patients
were older and more ill.

Even though older patients have higher mortality rates than their younger counterparts, factors other than age, such as the presence of multiorgan system failure, are
more important in predicting outcome *(53)*. For example, a prospective study by
Deulofeu and colleagues *(54)* noted that age alone did not influence the outcome of
bacteremia, and the main prognostic factors were shock, impaired functional status,
immunodeficiency, acquisition of infection in the hospital, and absence of fever on
admission. Therefore, treatment in elderly patients is generally similar as in younger
patients. Because of the age-related decline in the general physiological reserve and
more comorbid conditions, care has to be even more individually adjusted.

4.1. Antimicrobial Therapy

The outcome of sepsis is improved with early diagnosis and initiation of antibiotics.
Inadequate and delayed antibiotic treatment can lead to higher mortality rate *(55,56)*.
Empiric antibiotic therapy is based on the site of infection and the usual resident flora
of the involved organ. Because a large variety of pathogens is possible, broad-spectrum coverage is mandatory (*see* Fig.1). A third-generation cephalosporin, imipenem/
cilastin, ticarcillin/clavulanate, or antibiotic combinations such as a penicillin or cephalosporin with an aminoglycoside, aztreonam, or parenteral quinolone are probably
equally efficacious in most patients *(34)*. Empiric therapy with vancomycin and an
aminoglycoside is effective against most aerobic pathogens including methicillin-resistant staphylococci species and resistant Gram-negative organisms. However, this
regimen is potentially nephrotoxic, especially in older patients with already compromised renal function, and fails to treat anaerobic infections. Sepsis caused by anaerobic
organisms is particularly common in intraabdominal sepsis and aspiration pneumonia.
When the culture and sensitivity results are available, the initial regimen should be
changed based on the laboratory results and the patient's response to initial therapy.

Once culture and sensitivity data become available, monotherapy may be considered if organisms are susceptible; multiple antibiotics do not necessarily cure patients

more quickly or effectively. A retrospective study showed that patients older than age 70 with Gram-negative bacteremia given multiple antibiotics had a signficantly higher mortality rate (30%) than those given one antibiotic (13%), but this may have been owing to a selection bias with sicker patients receiving more antibiotics *(15)*. Double-drug therapy is generally perceived to be more effective in the treatment of serious *Pseudomonas aeruginosa* infections, febrile neutropenic patients, and possibly the treatment of intraabdominal infections *(57)*. Further principles of antibiotic therapy in the elderly are discussed in Chapter 4.

4.2. Hemodynamic Support

The goals of hemodynamic support in sepsis are to restore and maintain an adequate tissue perfusion pressure (mean arterial pressure greater than 60 mmHg), decrease heart rate, maintain adequate renal perfusion (urine output greater than 0.5 mL/kg/h), and improve mental status. In its early stage, sepsis causes tachycardia and peripheral vasodilatation, as well as myocardial depression and ventricular dilatation despite normal or increased cardiac output. Stroke work and ejection fraction are decreased. These outcomes lead to a reduction in the effective intravascular volume and circulatory instability. If volume resuscitation is not adequate, multiple organ failure and death can result despite control of the infection. Aggressive volume resuscitation is the best initial treatment. Hypotension can be usually reversed with fluid administration up to 10 L of crystalloid or 4 L of colloid in the first 24 h *(58)*. However, aggressive fluid replacement must be carefully monitored in elderly patients, especially those with coexisting cardiac and/or renal disease (see next paragraph). No conclusive data have shown which type of resuscitation fluid has the best impact on outcome.

Pulmonary artery catheters may be helpful to determine the optimum ventricular filling pressures and cardiac output in such settings as ARDS, cardiac and/or renal dysfunction, or hypotension unresponsive to fluid administration. The characteristic hemodynamic changes in sepsis are high cardiac output and low systemic vascular resistance. Elderly patients frequently have poor cardiac compliance, which can be compromised by pulmonary edema after aggressive fluid resuscitation. Even though pulmonary artery catheter placement in patients with sepsis/septic shock has not been proven to improve the clinical outcome and may even increase in mortality and cost *(59)*, it is generally agreed that it is appropriate in patients with septic shock who have not responded to initial fluid resuscitation and low-dose inotropic/vasoconstrictor therapy or have significant underlying comorbidities affecting hemodynamic status.

Sepsis causes a hypermetabolic state with increased oxygen consumption resulting in tissue hypoxia. Studies in adults up to age 80 suggest that a mean arterial pressure of 70–80 mmHg and/or cardiac index of 2.8 L/min/m^2 is required to maintain adequate tissue oxygenation. An older practice was to deliver therapy to induce supranormal hemodynamic variables (cardiac index more than 4.5 L/min/m^2, oxygen delivery greater than 600 mL/min/m^2, and systemic vascular resistance index of 1100 to 1300 dyne·s/cm^3·m^2), but more recent randomized trials have not found this to be effective in lowering mortality *(60,61)*.

If fluid resuscitation alone can not restore mean arterial pressure to adequate level, a vasoactive agent should be given (*see* Fig.1). Dopamine is the most commonly used first-line agent. It is usually given in a low dose (<2 µg/kg/min; activates dopaminergic vasodilatory receptors) for renal or gastrointestinal protection, although this not been demonstrated to be beneficial in critically ill patients because the increase in blood flow to the renal and splanchnic regions may be due to increase in cardiac output alone *(62)*. In higher doses (5–10 µg/kg/min), dopamine activates β adrenergic receptors; at doses above 10 µg/kg/min, especially over 20 µg/kg/min, alpha adrenergic (vasoconstricting) receptors are activated. Older patients with coronary artery disease may not be able to tolerate this $β_1$-adrenergic receptor-mediated cardiac stimulation due to increased myocardial oxygen demand and decreased coronary artery blood flow. In patients with severe shock that requires the higher doses of dopamine (>10µg/kg/min), norepinephrine should be added or therapy switched to this agent. Norepinephrine is a potent α adrenergic agonist with moderate $β_1$ and minimal $β_2$ adrenergic activity. It increases the systemic vascular resistance, which may reverse the vasodilatation effects of sepsis. Because of this effect, some clinicians use norepinephrine early in the treatment of septic shock *(63)*. Dobutamine is a selective $β_1$ adrenergic agent without α agonist activity and should be used to support the myocardium and maintain an adequate oxygen supply to the tissues if shock is persistent *(64)*. Dopexamine, a new agent that combines β adrenergic and dopaminergic effects, may be a useful alternative to increase splanchnic blood flow. Epinephrine is usually used as a last resort because of its tachyarrhythmic effect and decrease in splanchnic perfusion.

Experimental treatments for septic shock include phosphodiesterase inhibitors, calcium agonists, and nitric oxide inhibitors. No definitive recommendations can be made regarding the use of these agents due to inconclusive published data *(65)*.

Sepsis can increase the ventilatory load by increasing oxygen demand from poor tissue extraction and increasing catabolism. It also compromises the ventilatory supply by impairing gas exchange and respiratory muscle function. Because elderly patients have less cardiopulmonary reserve, intubation should be considered if there is an early sign of respiratory failure or poor tissue perfusion. Adequate oxygenation should be monitored carefully to maintain saturation of oxygen at >95%.

In seriously ill patients, old age alone is not an appropriate criterion to make a decision to withhold life-sustaining treatment. Unfortunately, physicians typically underestimate older patients' preferences for life-extending care. A recent study showed that although there was an age-associated decrease in the desire of older persons for life-extending care (from 61% of those under age 50 yr to 27% of those over age 80 yr), physicians thought that octagenerians wanted life-extending care in only 14% of the cases. Moreover, for patients who wanted life-extending care, in 79% of the cases of octagenerians, the treating physician thought that the patient did not want this therapy. Probably because of these views, the rate of decision to withhold ventilator support increased 15% with each decade of age over 50 yr *(66)*.

Although anemia can decrease oxygen delivery, there is little improvement in oxygen consumption following blood transfusion in patients with sepsis *(67)*.

Nutritional support can increase lymphocyte counts and serum albumin, which are used as surrogate markers of immune competency *(68)*. The route of feeding must be individualized, but the enteral route is preferred to maintain gut function and avoid complications from catheter-induced infection. Gastric tube feeding may decrease the risk of bleeding from a stress ulcer but may increase the risk of aspiration pneumonia *(69)*.

Sepsis can lead to stress ulcers with higher risk in the patients with mechanical ventilation. Appropriate cytoprotective agents are indicated to prevent stress ulcers, such as using a continuous parenteral histamine 2 blocker drug, unless the patient develops side effects of nephritis, thrombocytopenia, and confusion *(70)*. Sucralfate might be a better choice as a cytoprotective agent because of the lower incidence of late-onset pneumonia *(71)*.

5. PREVENTION AND IMMUNOTHERAPIES

Indwelling catheters should be removed as soon as clinically feasible. Elderly persons are more prone to aspiration pneumonia, which is the leading cause of death due to hospital-acquired infections. Selective decontamination of the digestive tract is not recommended by the Centers for Disease Control and Prevention *(72)*. Simple procedures such as elevation of the head, using sucralfate, and early detection in at-risk patients (chronic lung disease, changing mental status, nasogastric tube, reintubation) are preferred. Old age probably does not increase the risk of intravenous catheter-associated infection, but these occur more frequently in the elderly due to the age-associated increased use of these devices. Appropriate skin care, e.g., using chlorhexidine antiseptic, and probable antibiotic-coated intravascular devices, may decrease the incidence. Hand washing after examining each patient is a simple preventive method that is commonly ignored.

Sepsis is characterized by an imbalance in proinflammatory and anti-inflammatory cytokines. TNF-α and IL-1 are the principal mediators causing most manifestations of sepsis and shock. In animal studies, anti-TNF α antibody and IL-1 receptor antagonists can protect septic animals from death *(73,74)*. Clinical trials, however, have had mixed results. Two multicenter phase II/III trials in patients with sepsis were held evaluating a monoclonal antibody to TNF-α (antiBAY x1351). The North American Sepsis Trial I (NORASEPT 1) showed that septic patients without shock had no benefit from treatment with this monoclonal antibody and in septic patients with shock, the 3-d mortality rate was decreased but not the 28-d mortality. In the International Sepsis Trial (INTERSEPT), the circulating TNF-α levels and the development of organ failure were decreased with the use of the monoclonal antibody, but there was no reduction in the 28-d mortality. Recently, a double-blind, randomized control phase III trial, NORASEPT II, that was conducted in 105 hospitals with 1879 patients, did not find any survival benefit from TNF α blockade *(75–77)*.

Studies on endotoxin blockade have also yielded disappointing results. Clinical studies of two antibodies to the lipid A fraction of lipopolysaccharide and the core region of endotoxin yielded conflicting results. Although the first study showed some clinical benefit in patients not in shock *(78)*, a second randomized large controlled clinical study of a monoclonal antibody to endotoxin found no improvement in survival, although a modest benefit in resolution of organ dysfunction was shown *(79)*.

Despite some early enthusiasm for the use of corticosteroids in patients with septic shock, a meta-analysis has shown that corticosteroids are not beneficial *(80)*. A study on the use of ibuprofen showed that it decreased fever but not survival *(81)*.

A variety of other agents, e.g., interferon-γ, N-acetylcysteine, antithrombin III, naloxone, pentoxifylline, and hemofiltration, have been tested in patients with sepsis, but the results are disappointing. The immune response to infection is quite complicated so that it is unlikely that a single agent will prove beneficial. It is clear that the mortality of sepsis is not improved dramatically despite more intensive therapy. The greater frequency of underlying comorbid conditions in study subjects that included more elderly with chronic illness, immunosuppressive patients, and new innovative and invasive treatment may have contributed to the lack of improvement in survival. There are no published studies focusing on older patients. Whether septic elderly patients would respond differently from younger remains to be answered.

REFERENCES

1. Bone, R.C., Fisher, C.J., Clemmer, T.P., et al. (1989) Sepsis syndrome: a valid clinical entity. *Crit. Care Med.* **17,** 389–393.
2. Bone, R.C., Balk, R.A., Cerra, F.B., et al. (1992) American College of Chest Physicians/ Society of Critical Care Medicine Consensus Conference: definitions for sepsis and multiple-organ failure and guidelines for the use of innovative therapies in sepsis. *Chest* **101,** 1644–1655.
3. Rangel-Frausto, M.S., Pittet, D., Costigan, M., et al. (1996) The natural history of the systemic inflammatory response syndrome (SIRS). A prospective study. JAMA *273,* 117–123.
4. Bernard, R.B. (1997) Issues in the design of clinical trials for sepsis. Cytokines and pulmonary infection. Part 2; the role of cytokines in systemic and pulmonary medicine. ATS Continuing Education Monograph Series (Pratter, M.R., ed.), American Thoracic Society New York, pp 1–6.
5. Centers for Disease Control and Prevention. Increase in national hospital discharge survey rates for septicemia, United States 1979–1987. (1990) *M.M.W.R.* **39,** 31–34.
6. CDC National Center for Health Statistics. Mortality patterns—United States, 1990. (1993) *Monthly Vital Stat. Rep.* **41,** 45.
7. Sands, K.E., Bates, D.W., Lanken, P.N,. et al. (1997) Epidemiology of sepsis syndrome in 8 academic medical centers. JAMA **278,** 234–240.
8. Brun-Buisson, C., Doyon, F., Carlet, J., et al. (1995) Incidence, risk factors, and outcome of severe sepsis and septic shock in adults. A multicenter prospective study in intensive care units. *JAMA 274,* 968–974.
9. Knaus, W.A., Harrell, F.E., Fisher, C.J., et al. (1993) The clinical evaluation of new drugs for sepsis. A prospective study design based on survival analysis. *JAMA* **270,** 1233–1241.
10. Geerdes, H.F., Ziegler, D., Lode H., et al. (1992) Septicemia in 980 patients at a university hospital in Berlin: prospective studies during 4 selected years between 1979 and 1989. *Clin. Infect. Dis.* **15,** 991–1002.
11. Niederman, M.S. and Fein, A.M. (1990) Sepsis syndrome, the adult respiratory distress syndrome, and nosocomial pneumonia: a common clinical sequence. *Clin. Chest Med.* **11,** 663–665.
12. Friedman, G., Silva, E., and Vincent, J.L. (1998) Has the mortality of septic shock changed with time? *Crit. Care Med.* **26,** 2078–2086.
13. Pinner, R.W., Tutsch, S.M., Simonsen, L., et al. (1996) Trends in infectious diseases mortality in the United States *JAMA* **275,** 189–193.
14. Winn, T., Tayback, M., and Israel, E. (1991) Mortality due to septicemia in the elderly: factors accounting for a rapid rise. *Maryland Med. J.* **40,** 803–807.
15. McCue, J.D. (1987) Gram-negative bacillary bacteremia in the elderly: incidence, ecology, etiology and mortality. *J. Am. Geriatr. Soc.* **35,** 213–218.
16. Sonnenblick, M., Carmon, M., Rudenski, B., et al. (1990) Septicemia in the elderly: incidence, etiology and prognostic factors. *Isr. J. Med. Sci.* **26,** 195–199.
17. Parker, M.M. and Parrillo, J.E. (1983) Septic shock. Hemodynamics and pathogenesis. *JAMA* **250,** 3324–3327.

18. Bone, R.C. (1991) The pathogenesis of sepsis. *Ann. Intern. Med.* **115,** 457 –469.
19. Boldt, J., Muller, M., Heesen, M., et al. (1997) Does age influence circulating adhesion molecules in the critically ill? *Crit. Care Med.* **25,** 95–100.
20. Rink, L., Cakman, I., and Kirchner, H. (1998) Altered cytokine production in the elderly. *Mech. Ageing Dev.* **102(2–3)**, 199–209.
21. Chassagne, P., Perol, M.B., Trivalle, C., et al. (1996) Is presentation of bacteremia in the elderly the same as in younger patients. *Am. J. Med.* **100,** 65–70.
22. Van Dijk, J.M., Rosin, A.J., and Rudenski, B. (1982) in the elderly. *Practitioner* **226,** 1439–1443.
23. Windsor, A.C.M. (1983) Bacteraemia in a geriatric unit. *Gerontology* **29,** 125–130.
24. Finkelstein, M.S., Petkun, W.M., Freedman, M.L., et al. (1983) Pneumococcal bacteremia in adults: Age-dependent differences in presentation and in outcome. *J. Am. Geriatr. Soc.* **31,** 19–27.
25. Gleckman, R. and Hibert, D. (1982) Afebrile bacteremia. A phenomenon in geriatric patients. *JAMA* **248,** 1478–1481.
26. Miller, D., Yoshikawa, T., Castle, S.C., et al. (1991) Effect of age on fever response to recombinant tumor necrosis factor alpha in a murine model. *J. Gerontol.* **46,** M176–179.
27. Norman, D.C. and Yoshikawa, T.T. (1983) Intraabdominal infections in the elderly. *J. Am. Geriatr. Soc.* **31,** 677–684.
28. Weinstein, M.P., Towns, M.L., Quartey, S.M., et al. (1997) The clinical significance of positive blood cultures in the 1990s: a prospective comprehensive evaluation of the microbiology, epidemiology, and outcome of bacteremia and fungemia in adults. *Clin. Infect. Dis.* **24,** 584–602.
29. Gransden, W.R. (1994) Septicemia in the newborn and elderly. *J. Antimicrob. Chemother.* **34(Suppl. A),** 101–119.
30. Muder, R.R., Brennen, C., Wagener, M.M., et al (1992) Bacteremia in a long-term-care facility: five-year prospective study of 163 consecutive episodes. *Clin. Infect. Dis.* **14,** 647–654.
31. Kreger, B.E., Craven, D.E., Carling, P.C., et al. (1980) Gram-negative bacteremia. III. Reassessment of etiology, epidemiology and ecology in 612 patients. *Am. J. Med.* **68,** 332–343.
32. Howell, T.H. (1948) Normal temperatures in old age. *Lancet* **1,** 517–520.
33. Castle, S.C., Norman, D.C., Yeh, M., et al. (1991) Fever response in elderly nursing home residents. Are the older truly colder? *J. Am. Geriatr. Soc.* **39,** 853 –857.
34. Bender, B. (1992) Sepsis. *Clin. Geriatr. Med.* **8,** 913–924.
35. Iberti, T.J., Bone, R.C., Fein, A., et al. (1993) Are the criteria used to determine sepsis applicable for patients >75 years of age? *Crit. Care Med.* **21,** S130.
36. Esposito, A.L.M., Gleckman, R.A., Cram, S. et al. (1980) Community-acquired bacteremia in the elderly: analysis of one hundred consecutive episodes. *J. Am. Geriatr. Soc.* **28,** 315–319.
37. Centers for Disease Control and Prevention. (1990) Increase in national hospital discharge survey rates for septicemia: United States, 1979–1987. (1990) *M.M.W.R.* **39,** 31–34.
38. Leibovici, L., Pitlik, S.D., Konisberger, H., et al. (1993) Bloodstream infections in patients older than eighty years. *Age Ageing* **22,** 431–442.
39. Setia, U., Serventi, I., and Lorenz, P. (1984) Bacteremia in a long-term care facility. *Arch. Intern. Med.* **144,** 1633–1635.
40. Meyers, B.R., Sherman, E., Mendelson, M.H., et al. (1989) Bloodstream infections in the elderly. *Am. J. Med.* **86,** 379–386.
41. Madden, J.W., Croker, J.R., and Beynon, C.P.J. (1981) Septicemia in the elderly. *Postgrad. Med. J.* **57,** 502–509.
42. Rudman, D., Hontanosas, A., Cohen, Z., et al. (1988) Clinical correlates of bacteremia in a Veterans Administration extended care facility. *J. Am. Geriatr. Soc.* **36,** 726–732.

43. Saviteer, S.M., Samsa, G.P., and Rutala, W.A. (1998) Nosocomial infections in the elderly. Increased risk per hospital day. *Am. J. Med.* **84**, 661–666.

44. Whitelaw, D.A., Rayner, B.L., and Willcox, P.A. (1992) Community-acquired bacteremia in the elderly: A prospective study of 121 cases. *J. Am. Geriatr. Soc.* **40**, 996–1000.

45. Arbo, M.D.J. and Snydman, D.R. (1994) Influence of blood culture results on antibiotic choice in the treatment of bacteremia. *Arch. Intern. Med.* **154**, 2641–2644.

46. Levy, M., Dremer, F., and Brion, N. (1998) Community-acquired pneumonia: importance of initial noninvasive bacteriologic investigations. *Chest* **92**, 43–48.

47. Caldwell, A., Glauser, F.L., Smith, W.R., et al. (1975) The effects of dehydration on the radiologic and pathologic appearance of experimental canine segmental pneumonia. *Am. Rev. Respir. Dis.* **112**, 651–656.

48. Hall, F.M., Simon, B. (1987) Occult pneumonia associated with dehydration: myth or reality. *Am. J. Roentgenol.* **148**, 853–854.

49. Mueller, P.R. and Simeonne, J.F. (1983) Intraabdominal abcesses diagnosis by sonography and computed tomography. *Radiol. Clin. North Am.* **21**, 425–448.

50. Van Dissel, J.T., van Langevelde, P., Westendorp, R.G., et al. (1998) Anti-inflammatory cytokine profile and mortality in febrile patients. *Lancet* **28**, 950–953.

51. Cunha, B.A. (1992) Sepsis and its mimics. *Intern. Med.* **13**, 48–52.

52. Lundberg, J.S., Perl, T.M., Wiblin, T., et al. (1998) Septic shock: An analysis of outcomes for patients with onset on hospital wards versus intensive care units. *Crit. Care Med.* **26**, 1020–1024.

53. Diep, D., Tran, A., Johan, B., et al. (1990) Age, chronic disease, sepsis, organ system failure, and mortality in a medical intensive care unit. *Crit. Care Med.* **18**, 474–479.

54. Deulofeu, F., Cervello., B, Capell, S., et al. (1998) Predictors of mortality in patients with bacteremia: The importance of functional status. *J. Am. Geriatr. Soc.* **46**, 14–18.

55. Leibovici, L., Paul, M., Poznanski, O., et al. (1997) Monotherapy versus beta-lactam aminoglycoside combination treatment for gram-negative bacteremia: a prospective, observational study. *Antimicrob. Agents Chemother.* **41**, 1127–1138.

56. Kollef, M.H., Sherman, G., Ward, S., et al. (1999) Inadequate antimicrobial treatment of infections:A risk factor for hospital mortality among critically ill patients. *Chest* **115**, 462–474.

57. Cunha, BA. (1995) Antibiotic treatment of sepsis. *Med. Clin. North Am.* **79**, 551–558.

58. Ognibene, F.P. (1996) Hemodynamic support during sepsis. *Clin. Chest Med.* **17**, 279–287.

59. Connors, A.F. Jr, Speroff, T., Dawson, N.V., et al (1998) The effectiveness of right heart catheterization in the initial care of critically ill patients. JAMA **18**, 889–897.

60. Parker, M.M. and Peruzzi, W. (1997) Pulmonary artery catheters in sepsis/septic shock. *New Horiz.* **5**, 228–232.

61. Alia, I., Esteban, A., Gordo, F., et al. (1999) A randomized and controlled trial of the effect of treatment aimed at maximizing oxygen delivery in patients with severe sepsis or septic shock. *Chest* **115**, 453–461.

62. Maynard, N.D., Bihari, D.J., Dalton, R.N., et al. (1995) Increasing splanchnic blood flow in the critically ill. *Chest* **108**, 1648–1654.

63. Meadows, D., Edwards, J.D., Wilkins, R.G., et al. (1998) Reversal of intractable septic shock with norepinephrine therapy. *Crit. Care Med.* **16**, 663–666.

64. Vincent, J.L., Roman, A., and Kahn, R.J. (1990) Dobutamine administration in septic shock: addition to a standard protocol. *Crit. Care Med.* **18**, 689–693.

65. Rudis, M.I., Basha, M.A., and Zarowitz, B.J. (1996) Is it time to reposition vasopressors and inotropes in sepsis? *Crit. Care Med.* **24**, 525–537.

66. Hamel, M.B., Teno, J.M., Goldman, L., et al. (1999) Patient age and decisions to withhold life-sustaining treatments from seriously ill, hospitalized adults. SUPPORT Investigators. Study to understand prognoses and preferences for outcomes and risks of treatment. *Ann. Intern. Med.* **130**, 116–125.

67. Marik, P.E. and Sibbald, W.J. (1993) Effect of stored-blood transfusion on oxygen delivery in patients with sepsis. *JAMA* **269,** 3024–3029.
68. Mullin, T.J. and Kirkpatrick, J.R. (1981) The effect of nutritional support on immune competency in patients suffering form trauma, sepsis, or malignant disease. *Surgery* **90,** 610–615.
69. Navab, F., Steingrub, J.(1995) Stress ulcer: is routine prophylaxis necessary? *Am. J. Gastroenterol.* **90,** 708–712.
70. Cook, D., Guyatt, G., and Marshall, J. (1998) A comparison between sucralfate and ranitidine for the prevention of upper gastrointestinal bleeding in patients requiring mechanical ventilation. Canadian Critical Care Trials. *N. Engl. J. Med.* **398,** 791–807.
71. Prod'hom, G., Leuenberger, P., Koerfer, J., et al. (1997) Nosocomial pneumonia in mechanically ventilated patients receiving antacid, ranitidine, or sucralfate as prophylaxis for stress ulcer. *Ann. Intern. Med.* **120,** 653–662.
72. Centers for Disease Control and Prevention. (1997) Guideline for prevention of nosocomial pneumonia. *M.M.W.R.* **46(RR-1),** 1–79.
73. Walsh, C.J., Sugerman, H.J., Mullen, P.G., et al. (1992) Monoclonal antibody to tumor necrosis factor alpha attenuates cardiopulmonary dysfunction in porcine Gram-negative sepsis. *Arch. Surg.* **127,** 138–144.
74. Fisher, C.J. Jr., Opal, S.M., Lowry, S.F, et al. (1994) Role of IL-1 and the therapeutic potential of IL-1 receptor antagonist in sepsis. *Circ. Shock* **44,** 1–8.
75. Abraham, E., Wunderink, R., Silverman, H., et al. (1995) Efficacy and safety of monoclonal antibody to human tumor necrosis factor alpha in patients with sepsis syndrome: a randomized, controlled, double-blind, multicenter clinical trial. *JAMA* **273,** 934–941.
76. Cohen, J. and Carlet, J. (1996) INTERSEPT: an international, multicenter, placebo-controlled trial of monoclonal antibody to human tumor necrosis factor-alpha in patients with sepsis. *Crit. Care Med.* **24,** 1431–1440.
77. Abraham, E., Anzueto, A., Gutierrez, G., et al. (1998) Double-blind randomised controlled trial of monoclonal antibody to human tumour necrosis factor in treatment of septic shock. NORASEPT II Study Group. *Lancet* **28,** 929–933.
78. Greenman, R.L., Schein, R.M.H, and Martin, M.A. (1991) A controlled clinical trial of E5 murine monoclonal IgM antibody to endotoxin in the treatment of gram-negative sepsis. *JAMA* **266,** 1097–1102.
79. Bone, R.C., Balk, R.A., and Fein, A.M. (1995) A second randomized large controlled clinical study of E 5, a monoclonal antibody to endotoxin, multicenter, randomized, controlled trial. *Crit. Care Med.* **23,** 994–1006.
80. Lefering, R. and Neugebauer, E.A.M.(1995) Steroid controversy in sepsis and septic shock: a meta-analysis. *Crit. Care Med.* **23,** 1294–1303.
81. Haupt, M.T., Jastremski, M.S., Clemmer, T.P., et al. (1991) Effects of ibuprofen in patients with severe sepsis: a randomized double-blind, multicenter study. *Crit. Care Med.* **19,** 1339–1347
82. King, D.W., Pushparaj, N., and O'Toole, K. (1992) Morbidity and mortality in the aged. *Hosp. Pract.* **17(2),** 97–109.
83. Bolton, C.F., Young, G.B., and Zochodne, D.W. (1993) The neurological complications of sepsis. *Ann. Neurol.* **33,** 94–100.
84. Schlag, G., Krosl, P., and Redl, H. (1988) Cardiopulmonary response of the elderly to traumatic and septic shock. Prog. Clin. Biol. Res. **264,** 233–242.
85. Chan, E.D. and Welsh, C.H. (1998) Geriatric respiratory medicine. *Chest* **114,** 1704–1733.
86. Dematte, J.E., Barnard, M.L., and Sznajder, J.I. (1997) Acute respiratory failure in sepsis, in *Sepsis and Multiorgan Failure* (Fein, A.M., ed.), Williams & Wilkins, MD, pp.155–167.
87. Hussain, S.N. (1998) Respiratory muscle dysfunction in sepsis. *Mol. Cell Biochem.* **179,** 125–134.

88. Xu, D., Lu, Q., Guillory, D., et al. (1993) Mechanisms of endotoxin-induced intestinal injury in a hyperdynamic model of sepsis. *J. Trauma* **34,** 676–683.
89. Van Lanschot, J.J.B., Mealy, K., and Wilmore, D.W. (1990) The effects of tumor necrosis factor on intestinal structure and metabolism. *Ann. Surg.* **212,** 663–670.
90. Doig, C.J., Sutherland, L.R., Snadham, J.D., et al. (1998) Increased intestinal permeability is associated with the development of multiple organ dysfunction syndrome in critically ill ICU patients. *Am. J. Respir. Crit. Care Med.* **158,** 444.
91. Matuschak, G.M. (1997) Liver dysfunction in sepsis, in *Sepsis and Multiorgan Failure* (Fein, A.M., ed.), Williams & Wilkins, MD, pp. 168–180.
92. Neveu, H., Kleinknecht D., Brivet F., et al. (1996) Prognostic factors in acute renal failure due to sepsis. Results of a prospective multicenter study. The French study group on acute renal failure. *Nephrol. Dial. Transplant* **11,** 293–299.

6

Bronchitis and Pneumonia

Thomas J. Marrie

1. BRONCHITIS

1.1. Clinical Relevance

Several advances have occurred in our knowledge of the natural history and management of bronchitis. The first step has been a classification of patients with chronic bronchitis into four groups (*see* Table 1) *(1)*. Chronic bronchitis is a syndrome defined by cough and production of sputum on most days for at least 3 months a year for 2 consecutive years *(2)*. It is often complicated by airway obstruction leading to the commonly used term chronic obstructive pulmonary disease (COPD).

Acute bronchitis and acute exacerbation of chronic bronchitis account for about 14 million physician visits each year in the United States, making these conditions among the most common illnesses encountered by family physicians *(3)*. Not only is there considerable morbidity from chronic bronchitis, there is also substantial mortality, as chronic obstructive lung disease is the fourth leading cause of death in the United States *(4)*.

1.2. Diagnostic Tests

Despite the common nature of chronic bronchitis, there has been, and continues to be, considerable controversy about its management. Bacterial infection is but one factor in the production of inflammation in chronic bronchitis, but according to Ball it is fundamental to the vicious circle hypothesis leading to a pattern of repetitive infective exacerbations *(5)*. *Haemophilus influenzae* seems to be the most important pathogen in chronic bronchitis. *Streptococcus pneumoniae* and *Moraxella catarrhalis* are also important. It is noteworthy that there is a correlation between the severity of lung disease as indicated by a forced expiratory volume in 1 s (FEV1) value and the bacterial species recovered during exacerbations of chronic bronchitis. Eller and colleagues *(6)* found that in patients with an FEV1 of ≥50% of predicted that about 10% of patients had Enterobacteriaceae or *Pseudomonas* species isolated from purulent respiratory secretions, and 40% of those who had an FEV1 of <35% of predicted had these bacteria isolated.

From: *Infectious Disease in the Aging*
Edited by: Thomas T. Yoshikawa and Dean C. Norman
© Humana Press Inc., Totowa, NJ

Table 1
Classification of Patients with Chronic Bronchitis

Group	Definition
1	Previously healthy patient with postviral tracheobronchitis
2	Simple chronic bronchitis
3	Chronic bronchitis plus airflow obstruction and/or other medical problems such as diabetes mellitus, heart failure, and/or elderly
4	Chronic bronchial sepsis; daily purulent sputum production (these patients usually have bronchiectasis on computed tomographic examination of the lungs)

1.3. Therapy

1.3.1. Role of Antibiotics

For some time it was unclear which population of patients with bronchitis would benefit from antibiotic therapy. It is the clear impression of infectious diseases consultants that antibiotics are overused in the management of patients with bronchitis. A meta-analysis of randomized trials of antibiotics in exacerbations of COPD found a small, but statistically significant, improvement due to antibiotic therapy *(7)*. These investigators found 239 trials published between 1955 and 1994, but only 9 trials met their criteria for inclusion in the analysis. They also noted a summary change in peak expiratory flow rate of 10.75 L/min (95% CI, 4.96– 16.54 L/min) in favor of the antibiotic-treated group. A concept that is now being used in trials of antibiotic therapy for acute exacerbations of chronic bronchitis is time to next relapse *(8,9)*. In a randomized double-blind trial clinical, resolution was noted in 89/99 (90%) of those treated with ciprofloxacin compared with 82% (75/91) of clarithromycin recipients*(8)*. The median infection–free interval was 142 d for ciprofloxacin recipients and 51 d for clarithromycin recipients (P =0.15). Bacteriological eradication rates were superior for ciprofloxacin–treated patients 91% vs 77% (P = 0.01). In a similar trial of cefuroxime axetil vs ciprofloxacin, the clinical resolution rates were similar at 93% and 90%; bacteriologic eradication rates were higher for ciprofloxacin-treated patients 96% vs 82%, (P <.01). Median infection free interval was 178 d for cefuroxime recipients and 146 d for ciprofloxacin-treated patients (P = 0.37) *(9)*. Given the widespread use of antibiotics to treat bronchitis, several groups have developed guidelines for the treatment of this condition *(3)*. A consensus has now developed that group 1 patients *(see* Table 1) have acute bronchitis that is usually due to viral infection and do not need antibiotic treatment *(3)*; group 2 patients have mild to moderate impairment of lung function (FEV1 $\geq$50%) and have less than four exacerbations per year. Treatment with a β-lactam antibiotic is recommended for this group, as the usual infecting pathogens are *H. influenzae, S. pneumoniae,* and *M. catarrhalis.* It is important to remember that about 30% of *H. influenzae* isolates, and 90% *of M. catarrhalis* isolates produce β-lactamases and are resistant to ampicillin. Amoxicillin-clavulanic acid as well as second-generation cephalosporins are effective. Group 3 patients are older than group 1 or group 2 patients and have an FEV1 <50% of predicted and or comorbidities such as diabetes mellitus, congestive heart failure, chronic renal failure and the like. They may also experience four or more exacerbations per year. The same organisms as for group 2 patients are involved here as well. The recommendations for antibiotic therapy include amoxicillin-clavulanic acid, a second-generation cephalosporin, or a fluoroquinolone. Group 4 patients have frequent exacebations and tend to have a chronic progressive course. Many of these patients have underlying bronchiectasis. In addition to the foregoing listed pathogens, Enterobacteriaceae or *Pseudomonas* species may be isolated. A fluoroquinolone with activity against *Pseudomonas* is probably the best therapeutic choice. Ciprofloxacin is still the most active quinolone against *P. aeruginosa*.

1.3.2. Prognosis

There are many other aspects to the management of patients with chronic obstructive lung disease other than antibiotic therapy *(10)*, which will not be discussed here. Seneff and colleagues *(11)* studied 362 patients with acute exacerbation of COPD who required admission to an intensive care unit (ICU). The in-hospital mortality was 24%. For the 165 patients who were 65 yr of age and older the in-hospital mortality rate was 30%; it was 41% at 90 d; 47% at 180 d, and 59% at 1 yr. Variables associated with in-hospital mortality (by multivariate analysis) included age, severity of respiratory and nonrespiratory organ dysfunction and hospital length of stay before ICU admission. Development of nonrespiratory organ dysfunction was the major predictor of hospital mortality—60% of the total explanatory power, and 180-day outcomes—54% of explanatory power. This study is in sharp contrast to the one by Torres and colleagues *(12)* in which 124 patients with chronic obstructive lung disease (COLD) and community-acquired pneumonia (CAP) who required admission to ICU had an 8% mortality.

1.4. Prevention

The best treatment for chronic bronchitis is primary prevention—no smoking programs in schools and clean-air programs in communities would reduce the burden of COPD. Failing this primary preventive strategy, secondary prevention with yearly influenza vaccination and a single pneumococcal vaccine (repeated once in 6 years for select circumstances) does reduce the number of cases of pneumonia and hospital admissions.

2. PNEUMONIA

2.1. Clinical Relevance

2.1.1. Epidemiology

Pneumonia is a common and often serious illness. It is the sixth-leading cause of death in the United States. About 600,000 persons are hospitalized with pneumonia each year, and there are 64 million days of restricted activity due to this illness *(13,14)*. Unmeasured to date is caregiver burden associated with pneumonia. Recovery is prolonged in the elderly (especially the frail elderly), and these patients may require up to 2 months to return to their baseline state of function.

The rate of pneumonia is highest at the extremes of age. In a population-based study in a Finnish town, Koivula and co-workers *(15)* found that 14/1000 persons/yr > 60 years of age developed pneumonia. Seventy-five percent of these cases of pneumonia were community acquired. In this study, independent risk factors for CAP were: alcoholism, relative risk (RR) 9; asthma, RR 4.2; immunosuppression, RR 1.9; age >70 vs. age 60–69 yr, RR 1.5.

For specific etiologies of pneumonia the risk factors may differ from those for pneumonia as a whole. Thus dementia, seizures, congestive heart failure, cerebrovascular disease and COLD were risk factors for pneumococcal pneumonia *(16)*. Among human immunodeficiency virus-(HIV) infected patients the rate of pneumococcal pneumonia is 41.8 times higher than those in the same age group who are not HIV infected *(17)*. Risk factors for Legionnaires' disease include male gender, tobacco smoking, diabetes mellitus, hematologic malignancy, cancer, end- stage renal disease, and HIV infection *(18)*.

There have been major changes in both the host and microorganisms that are reflected in changes in the epidemiology of pneumonia. Penicillin-resistant *S. pneumoniae* (PRSP) is now a common in North American communities. Many of the PRSP isolates are resistant to three or more antibiotic classes (multidrug resistance). In a recent study, 14% of bacteremic *S. pneumoniae* isolates were resistant to penicillin, 12% to ceftazidime, and 24% were resistant to trimethoprim-sulfamethoxazole *(19)*. In the study by Butler and colleagues *(19)*, 740 *S. pneumoniae* isolates from sterile sites were collected during 1993–1994. Twenty-five percent of the isolates were resistant to more than one antibiotic; 3.5% were resistant to erythromycin, and 5% were resistant to clarithromycin (19). This is probably a harbinger for the future, in that in Madrid in 1992, 15.2% of *S. pneumoniae* isolates were resistant to erythromycin *(20)*. Fortunately, it is possible to predict who is likely to have pneumonia due to PRSP. Previous use of β-lactam antibiotics, alcoholism, non-invasive disease, age <5 or ≥65 yr and immunosuppression are risk factors for PRSP pneumonia *(21,22)*. Host factors that have had a major impact on the epidemiology of pneumonia are increased in immunosuppressed individuals living in the community and are markedly increased in the advanced elder years (>80 years of age). Clustering of these individuals in retirement villages or nursing home has led to a new entity— nursing home-acquired pneumonia (NHAP).

There is a seasonal variation in the rate of pneumonia. Both attack rates and mortality rates are highest in the winter months *(23)*. This is likely due to an interaction between influenzae viruses and *S. pneumoniae*. In a squirrel monkey model, infection with influenza A virus prior to *S. pneumoniae* inoculation led to a 75% mortality rate vs. no mortality for infection with influenzae virus alone *(24)*.

2.1.2. Etiology

Although there are well over 100 microbal agents that can cause pneumonia, only a few cause most of the cases of pneumonia. There are changes in the rank order of the causes of pneumonia according to the severity of illness (usually reflected in the site of care decision—home, hospital ward, hospital intensive care unit, or nursing home). Patients with CAP who are treated on an ambulatory basis are much younger than those who are treated in hospital. *Mycoplasma pneumoniae* is the most commonly identified etiological agent in this setting accounting for 24% of the cases (25–28). *S. pneumoniae* is probably underdiagnosed in outpatients, as a diagnostic workup is rarely done. In published data, *S. pneumoniae* account for about 5% of the cases of ambulatory pneumonia; in reality the number is probably closer to 50%. A compilation of data from 9 comprehensive studies of the etiology of CAP among 5225 patients requiring hospitalization identified *S. pneumoniae* as the etiological agent in 17.7% of cases (29–37). However, if one focuses on the 3 studies that used serological methods in addition to blood and sputum culture to identify *S. pneumoniae,* then this microorganism accounted for up to 50% of the cases of CAP *(29,30,35)*. The etiology of NHAP is not well established since these studies have relied almost entirely on the results of sputum culture. The problem is distinguishing colonization from infection especially when aerobic Gram-negative bacilli such as *Escherichia coli, Klebsiella* spp., *Proteus* spp., *Enterobacter* spp., *Pseudomonas aeruginosa*, and so on are identified. Colonization of the oropharyngeal mucosa with aerobic Gram-negative bacilli increases with increasing age and is especially common among residents of nursing homes *(38)*. *S. pneumoniae* is the most commonly identified agent in patients with nursing home-acquired pneumonia (NHAP). In 6 studies reporting on 471 patients with NHAP *S. pneumoniae* accounted for 12.9% of the cases, followed by *H. influenzae*, 6.4%; *S. aureus*, 6.4% *M. catarrhalis*, 4.4%; and aerobic Gram-negative bacilli, 13.1% *(34,39–43)*.

2.2 Clinical Manifestations

Pneumonia is an infection involving the alveoli and bronchioles. Pathologically it is characterized by increased weight and replacement of the normal lung sponginess by induration (consolidation). This induration may involve most or all of a lobe (or multiple lobes) or it may be patchy and localized around bronchi, i.e., bronchopneumonia. Microscopic examination can show dense alveolar infiltration with polymorphonuclear leukocytes as is found in patients with pneumonia due to bacterial agents or interstititial inflammation as is usually seen in viral pneumonia.

Clinically pneumonia is typically characterized by a variety of symptoms and signs. Cough that may produce purulent, mucopurulent, or "rusty" sputum is common; fever, chills, and pleuritic chest pain are other manifestations. Extrapulmonary symptoms such as nausea, vomiting, or diarrhea may occur. There is a spectrum of physical findings on chest examination, the most common of which is rales ("crackles") heard over the involved lung segment. Other findings that may be present include dullness to percussion, increased tactile and vocal fremitus, bronchial breathing, and a pleural friction rub. However, in many older patients, especially those who are frail and debilitated, typical respiratory manifestations may not be found. Such findings as cognitive impairment (delirium), decline in physical functional capacity, anorexia, weakness, or falls may be the initial or only symptoms or signs of pneumonia. Fever is often absent *(44,45)*. A new opacity on chest radiographic examination is necessary to substantiate a clinical diagnosis of pneumonia.

2.3. Diagnostic Tests

The chance of determining a causative pathogen for pneumonia is approximately 60% in all age groups *(46)*. The elderly have a lower diagnostic yield compared with younger patients with CAP (45% vs 70% in one study) *(44)*. The inability to cough or provide quality sputum as well as oral and pharyngeal contamination of the specimen

Table 2
Key Decisions in the Management of CAP

- Site of care
- Diagnostic workup
- Empiric antimicrobal therapy
- Switch from intravenous to oral antibiotic therapy
- Discharge decision
- Followup

limit the usefulness of sputa as a diagnostic test for pneumonia in the elderly. Nevertheless, if quality sputa can be obtained, a Gram stain of the specimen can be examined to provide guidance on initial antimicrobal therapy. Blood culture (two sets) should be obtained in all elderly pneumonia patients who require hospitalization or intravenous therapy. Serological studies and tests for antigens in urine have been helpful in diagnosing certain types of pneumonia (e.g., *Mycoplasma pneumoniae*, *Chlamydia* spp., *Legionella* spp., viruses) *(34)*. However, the information is obtained 3–4 weeks after initial clinical diagnosis. A chest roentgenograph and complete blood count, especially white blood cell count with differential count, should be obtained in every patient suspected of pneumonia *(46)*.

2.4. Treatment

Table 2 gives the key decisions that have to be made to successfully treat CAP.

2.4.1. Site of Care

The site of care is dictated by the severity of the pneumonia. This decision can be helped by using a severity of illness score. Fine and co-workers *(47)* developed a pneumonia specific severity of illness score. There are 20 different items (three demographic features, five comorbidity features, five physical examination findings, and seven laboratory data items). Points are assigned to each feature and summed. Patients are placed into one of five risk classes. Those in risk classes I–III are at low risk, <1% for mortality, whereas those in class IV had a 9% mortality, and class V patients had a 27% mortality rate. In general, patients in classes I–III could be treated at home whereas those in classes IV and V should hospitalized. The potential of this system is demonstrated by a study by Atlas and colleagues *(48)*. These investigators prospectively enrolled 166 low-risk patients with pneumonia presenting to an emergency department. Physicians were given the pneumonia severity index score and offered enhanced visiting nursing services and the antibiotic clarithromycin. Two groups of controls were used—147 consecutive retrospective controls identified during the prior year and 208 patients from the study hospital who participated in the Pneumonia Patient Outcomes Research Team (PORT) cohort study. The percentage of patients initially treated as outpatients increased from 42% in the control period to 57% in the intervention period (36% relative increase; $P=0.01$). More outpatients failed outpatient therapy in the intervention period compared with the control period: 9% vs 0%, respectively. However, because these were historical controls, the conclusions from this study are weakened. Marrie and co-workers *(49)* enrolled 20 Canadian teaching and community hospitals into a study of a critical pathway for the management of CAP. Ten hospitals were randomized to the intervention arm (critical pathway) and 10 to conventional management. Hospitals were matched for teaching or community hospital status and for historic length of stay for patients with CAP. One teaching hospital in the intervention arm withdrew after randomization and was not replaced. Levofloxacin was the antibiotic used in the intervention arm, whereas antimicrobial therapy for patients in the conventional arm was at the discretion of the attending physician. The pneumonia–specific severity of illness score was used to assist with the site of care decision. An intent to treat analysis was performed on data from 1753 patients enrolled in the study. At the intervention hospitals the admission rate was lower for low-risk (classes I–III) patients, (31% vs 49% for conventional management; P = 0.013) or to use the terminology of Atlas and colleagues (48) 69% in the intervention arm were sent home vs. 41% in the conventional management arm. Follow–up of these patients revealed that there was no difference in the failure rates of outpatient therapy, i.e., about 6% of patients in both groups required admission.

2.4.2. Guidelines for Admission to Intensive Care Unit

The American Thoracic Society guidelines for the management of CAP gave criteria for severe pneumonia that could be used to help with the decision to admit a patient to an intensive care unit (ICU) *(50)*. Ewig and co-workers *(51)* calculated the sensitivity, specificity, and positive and negative predict values of these criteria utilizing data from a prospective study of 422 consecutive patients with CAP, 64 of whom were admitted to an ICU. They found that no single criterion was of sufficient sensitivity to use alone. For example, a respiratory rate of >30 breaths per minute had a sensitivity of 64% and a specificity of 57%. Requirement for mechanical ventilation had a sensitivity of 58% and a specificity of 100%. Sensitivity and specificity values for other parameters were the following: septic shock, 38% and 100%; renal failure, 30% and 96%; systolic blood pressure <90 mmHg, 12% and 99%; diastolic blood pressure <60 mm Hg 15% and 95%; progressive pulmonary infiltrates, 28% and 92%; bilateral infiltrates, 41% and 86%; and multilobe infiltrates, 52% and 80%. Ewig and co-workers concluded that the definition of severe pneumonia using one of the American Thoracic Society criteria had a sensitivity of 32%, a specificity of 98%, a positive predictive value of 24%, and a negative predictive value of 99%. These authors developed new criteria for severe pneumonia, which include the three following parameters: arterial partial pressure of oxygen/inspired fraction of oxygen (PaO$_2$/FI0$_2$) <250; multilobe infiltrates; and systolic blood pressure of 90 mmHg or less plus septic shock or mechanical ventilation. These three criteria together had a sensitivity of 78%, a specificity of 94%, and a positive predictive value of 75%.

2.4.3. Empiric Antibiotic Therapy

The Infectious Diseases Society of America has published guidelines for the empiric therapy of CAP *(52)* *(see* Table 3). The recent introduction of fluoroquinolones with enhanced activity against *S. pneumoniae* and activity against most of the pathogens that cause CAP is an advance in the treatment of CAP. However, there are many unanswered questions regarding these new drugs: Which one is best? Should they be used only for patients requiring hospitalization? Will widespread use of the new fluoroquinolones for the treatment of ambulatory pneumonia

Table 3
Antibiotic Therapy (First and Second Choices) of Community-Acquired
Pneumonia When Etiology is Unknown *(52)*

A. Patient to be treated on an ambulatory basis
   1. Macrolide (erythromycin 500 mg q 6h po × 10 d, clarithromycin 500 mg bid po × 10 days or azithromycin 500 mg po once then 250 mg/day po × 4 days)
   2. Doxycycline 100 mg bid po × 10 days. If risk factors for penicillin or macrolide-resistant *Streptococcus pneumoniae* present, consider a fluoroquinolone with enhanced activity against *S. pneumoniae*[a]
B. Patient to be treated in hospital ward
   1. Fluoroquinolone with enhanced activity against *S. pneumoniae*; e.g., levofloxacin, sparfloxacin, trovafloxacin or grepafloxacin[b]. (Levofloxacin 500 mg/d iv; trovafloxacin 200 mg/d iv; grepafloxacin[b] 600 mg/d po, sparfloxacin 400 mg × 1 dose then 200 mg/d po). If creatinine clearance <50 mL/min, reduce levofloxacin dose to 250 mg/d
   2. Cefuroxime 750 mg q8h iv or ceftriaxone 1 g/d iv or cefotaxime 2 g q h iv plus azithromycin 500 mg/d.
C. Patient to be treated in an intensive care unit
   1. Azithromycin 1 g iv then 500 mg/d iv plus ceftriaxone 1 g q 12 h iv or cefotaxime 2 g 8 h iv (ceftazidime and an aminoglycoside if *Pseudomonas aeruginosa* is suspected)
   2. Fluoroquinolone with enhanced activity against *S. pneumoniae* (not recommended as first choice because of lack of clinical trial data in the ICU setting)
D. Patient to be treated in a nursing home
   1. Amoxicillin - clavulanic acid 500 mg q 8 h po
   2. Fluroquinolone with enhanced activity against *S. pneumoniae*
E. Aspiration pneumonia
   1. Large-volume aspiration:Previous healthy individual—no antibiotic therapy
   2. Small-volume aspiration
      (a) Pneumonia (poor dental hygiene) and anaerobic infection suspected—clindamycin 2400–3600 mg/d iv in divided doses or penicillin 2–4 million units/d iv in divided doses
      (b) Pneumonia in a nursing home or in elderly subject at home—amoxicillin-clavulinic acid plus fluoroquinolone

---

Abbreviations: bid, twice a day; po, oral; q, every; iv, intravenous; ICU, intensive care unit.
[a] Levofloxacin, sparfloxacin.
[b] Removed from market.

lead to the emergence of resistance among *S. pneumoniae*? The new fluoroquinolones are levofloxacin, sparfloxacin, moxifloxacin, grepafloxacin and trovafloxacin (trovafloxacin, at the time of this writing, has restricted indications because of reported cases of liver failure, and grepaflexacin has been removed from use because of prolonged QT interval resulting in torsade de pointes). There are others in the clinical trial stage (e.g., gatifloxacin). Some of the salient characteristics of these agents are summarized in Table 4. The advantages of the new fluoroquinolones are excellent bioavailability, so that even hospitalized non-ICU patients can be treated orally if they can eat and drink, and their activity against the spectrum of agents that cause CAP, hence only one antibiotic is necessary for the empiric treatment of CAP.

Table 4
Salient Features of New Fluoroquinolones Compared With Ciprofloxacin

	Cipro	Levo	Grepa	Gati	Trova	Moxi
S. pneumoniae MIC[a]						
Penicillin sensitive (µg/mL)	2	1	0.25	0.5	0.12	0.12
Penicillin resistant (µg/mL)	2	1	0.25	N/A	0.12	0.12
P. aeruginosa MIC 90 (µg/mL)	4	16	>4	8	8	8
Percent bioavailability	70	99	72	approx 100%	88	90%
$T\frac{1}{2}$ (h)	4.0	6.7	11.4	7.1	11.0	11.0
Dosage adjustment						
Renal dysfunction	Yes	Yes	No	Yes	No	No
Hepatic dysfunction	No	No	Yes	No	Yes	No
Intravenous formulation available	Yes	Yes	No	Yes (alatrovafloxacin)	Yes (in development)	Yes
Usual oral dose to treat pneumonia	500 mg bid	500 mg qd	600 mg qd	200 mg qd	200 mg qd	400 mg qd
C_{max} (µg/mL) at dose given above	2.2	5.3	1.41	1.71	1.1	3.1
AUC (mg × h/L)	10	48	19.7	14.5	27	30.8

[a] MIC = minimum inhibitory concentration; Cipro = ciprofloxacin; Levo = levofloxacin; Grepa = grepafloxacin; Gati = gatifloxacin; Trova = trovafloxacin; Moxi = moxifloxacin; qd = daily; bid = twice daily; $T\frac{1}{2}$ = drug half life; C_{max} = peak serum or plasma concentration; AUC = area under the concentration vs time curve

2.4.4. Duration of Intravenous Antibiotic Therapy

In a series of studies, Ramirez and colleagues have defined criteria for switch from intravenous to oral antibiotics for treatment of patients with CAP *(52,53)*. Criteria for switch to oral antibiotics include the following: (1) two normal temperature readings over 16 h in previously febrile patients, (2) white blood cell count returning toward normal, (3) subjective improvement in cough, and (4) subjective improvement in shortness of breath. Using these criteria 33 patients randomized to ceftizoxime therapy met switch criteria, in 2.76 d vs 3.17 d for those randomized to receive ceftriaxone *(52)*. Seventy-four of the 75 evaluable patients were cured at 3–5 wk follow-up. Similar results were obtained in another study by this group in which patients were initially treated with ceftriaxone and, when criteria were met, patients were given clarithryomycin therapy orally. Ninety-six patients were enrolled in this study, and 59 were evaluable at 30-d follow-up. All 59 were cured *(53)*. The presence of bacteremia or identification of high-risk pathogens such as *S. aureus* or *P. aeruginosa* are not contraindications for switch therapy *(54)*. Patients who are clinically improving with empiric third-generation cephalosporin therapy are switched to oral third-generation cephalosporins, whereas patients who are receiving β-lactam/β-lactamase inhibitor agents are switched to oral β lactam/β-lactamase inhibitors. If intravenous therapy is with a β-lactam antbiotic and erythromycin, oral therapy is with a new macrolide *(54)*.

2.4.5. Give Antibiotics as Soon as Possible

Meehan and co-workers *(55)* carried out a retrospective multicenter cohort study of those ≥65 yr of age presenting to emergency rooms with CAP using Medicare National Claims History File from October 1, 1994 through September 30, 1995. Just over 75% of patients received antibiotics within 8 h of presenting at the emergency room. A significant lower 30-d mortality rate was observed for those who received antibiotic therapy within 8 h of presentation.

2.4.6. Discharge Decision

Halm and colleagues *(56)* defined how long it took to achieve stability in patients hospitalized with CAP. The median time to stability was 2 d for heart rate <100 beats/min and systolic blood pressure > 90 mmHg. Three days were required to achieve stability if the following parameters were used: respiratory rate ≤24 breaths/min, oxygen saturation >90%, and temperature <37.2°C (<99°F). Once stability was achieved, clinical deterioration requiring admission to a critical care unit or telemetry monitoring occurred in less than 1% of patients. Patients in the study by Halm and co-workers frequently remained in hospital after reaching stability. In a recent study (Marrie and colleagues unpublished observations, 1999), it was found that immobility was a significant factor in prolonging hospital stay in the elderly with pneumonia.

2.4.7. Follow-up

All elderly patients with CAP should have a follow-up chest radiograph to verify that the pneumonia has resolved. Pneumonia distal to an obstructed bronchus is one of the presentations of cancer of the lung; in about 50% of these patients the diagnosis of cancer is made at the time of presentation. In the remainder, the main clue to the underlying disease is the failure of the pneumonia to resolve. Time to resolution of pneumonia is influenced by the patient's age and presence of underlying chronic obstructive pulmonary disease. The follow-up chest radiograph is best performed 10–12 wk after the diagnosis of pneumonia. If complete resolution has not occurred, further investigation to exclude an obstructed bronchus is necessary.

REFERENCES

1. Wilson, R. and Wilson, C.B. (1997) Defining subsets of patients with chronic bronchitis. *Chest* **112,** 303S–309S.
2. Medical Research Council (1965) Definition and classification of chronic bronchitis for clinical and epidemiological purposes. *Lancet* **1**, 775–779.
3. Grossman, R.F. (1997) Guidelines for the treatment of acute exacerbations of chronic bronchitis. *Chest* **112,** 310S–313S.
4. US Bureau of the Census (1994) Statistical abstract of the United States, 114th edition, US Bureau of the Census, Washington DC: p. 95.
5. Ball, P. (1998) Infective pathogenesis and outcomes in chronic bronchitis. *Curr. Opin. Pulm. Med.* **2**, 161–165.
6. Eller, J., Ede, A., Schaberg, T., et al (1998). Infective exacerbations of chronic bronchitis. Relation between bacterial etiology and lung function. *Chest* **113**, 1542–1548.
7. Saint, S., Bent, S., Vittinghoff, E., et al. (1995). Antibiotics in chronic obstructive pulmonary disease exacerbatons. *JAMA* **273**, 957–960.
8. Chodosh, S., Schreurs, A., Siami, G., et al., and the Bronchitis Study Group (1998) Efficacy of oral ciprofloxacin vs. clarithromycin for treatment of acute bacterial exacerbations of chronic bronchitis. *Clin. Infect. Dis.* **27**, 730–738.
9. Chodosh, S., McCarty, J., Farkas, S., et al., and the Bronchitis Study Group (1998) Randomized, double-blind study of ciprofloxacin and cefuroxime axetil for treatment of acute bacterial exacerbations of chronic bronchitis. *Clin. Infect. Dis.* **27,** 722–729
10. Canadian Thoracic Society Workshop Group (1992) Guidelines for the assessment and management of chronic obstructive pulmonary disease. *Can. Med. Assoc. J.* **147**, 420–428.
11. Seneff, M.G., Wagner, D.P., Wagner, R.P., et al. (1995) Hospital and 1-year survival of patients admitted to intensive care units with acute exacerbations of chronic obstructive pulmonary disease. *JAMA* **274**, 1852–1857.
12. Torres, A., Dorca, J., Zalacain, R., et al. (1996) Community-acquired pneumonia in chronic obstructive pulmonary disease. A Spanish multicenter study. *Am. J. Respir. Crit. Care Med.* **154**, 1456–1461.
13. Dixon, R.E. (1985) Economic costs of respiratory tract infections in the United States. *Am. J. Med.* **78**, 45–51.
14. National Center for Health Statistics (1992) National hospital discharge survey: annual summary, 1990. *Vital Health Stat.* **13**, 1–225.
15. Koivula, I., Stenn, M., and Makela, P.H. (1994). Risk factors for pneumonia in the elderly. *Am. J. Med.* **96**, 313–320.
16. Lipsky, B.A., Boyko, E.J., Inui, T.S., et al. (1986) Risk factors for acquiring pneumococcal infections. *Arch. Intern. Med.* **146,** 2179–2185.
17. Plouffe J.F., Breiman R.E., and Facklam, R.R., for the Franklin County Pneumonia Study Group. (1996) Bacteremia with *Streptococcus pneumoniae*. Implications for therapy and prevention. *JAMA* **275**, 194–198.
18. Marston B.J, Lipman, H.B. and Breiman, R.F. (1994) Surveillance for Legionnaires' disease. Risk factors for morbidity and mortality. *Arch. Intern. Med.* **154**, 2417–2422.
19. Butler, J.C., Hofmann, J., Cretron, M.S., et al. (1996) The continued emergence of drug-resistant *Streptococcus pneumoniae* in the United States: an update from the Centers for Disease Control and Prevention's surveillance system. *J. Infect. Dis.* **74**, 986–993.

20. Moreno, S., Garcia-Leoni M.E., Cercenado, E., et al. (1995) Infections caused by erythro-mycin-resistant *Streptococcus pneumoniae*. Incidence, risk factors, and response to therapy in a prospective study. *Clin. Infect. Dis.* **20**, 1195–1200.

21. Clavo-Sanchez, A.J., Giron-Gonzalez, J.A., Lopez-Prieto, D., et al. (1997) Multivari-ate analysis of risk factors for infection due to penicillin-resistant and multidrug-resis-tant *Streptococcus pneumoniae*: A multicenter study. *Clin. Infect. Dis.* **24**, 1052–1059.

22. Nava, J.M., Bella, F., Garau, J., et al. (1994) Predictive factors for invasive disease due to penicillin-resistant *Streptococcus pneumoniae*: a population-based study. *Clin. Infect. Dis.*19, 884–890.

23. Flournoy, D.J., Stalling, F.H., and Catron, T.L. (1983) Seasonal and monthly variation of *Streptococcus pneumoniae* and other pathogens in bacteremia (1961–1981) *Ecol. of Dis.* **2**, 157–160.

24. Berendt, R.F., Long, G.G., and Walker, J.S. (1975) Influenza alone and in sequence with pneumonia due to *Streptococcus pneumoniae* in the squirrel monkey. *J. Infect. Dis.* **132**, 689–693.

25. Berntsson, E., Lagergard, T., Strannegard, O., et al. (1986) Etiology of community-acquired pneumonia in outpatients. *Europ. J. Clin. Microbiol.* **5**, 446–447.

26. Marrie, T.J, Peeling, R.W., Fine, M.J., et al. (1996) Ambulatory patients with commu-nity-acquired pneumonia. The frequency of atypical agents and clinical course. *Am. J. Med.* **101**, 508–515.

27. Erard, P.H., Moser, F., Wenger, A., et al. (1991) Prospective study on community-acquired pneumonia diagnosed and followed up by private practitioner. Abstracts of the 1991 Interscience Conference on Antimicrobal Agents and Chemotherapy. *Am. Soc. for Microbiol.* **108,** 56A.

28. Langille, D.B., Yates, L., and Marrie,T.J. (1993). Serological investigation of pneu-monia as it presents to the physicians office. *Can. J. Infect. Dis.* **4**, 328–332.

29. Porath, A., Schlaeffer, F., and Liberman, D. (1997). The epidemiology of community-acquired pneumonia among hospitalized patients. *J. Infect.* **34**, 41–48.

30. Burman, L.A., Trollfors, B., Andersen, B., et al. (1993). Diagnosis of pneumonia by cultures, bacterial and viral antigen detection tests, and serology with special refer-ence to antibodies against pneumococcal antigen. *J. Infect. Dis.* **163**, 1087–1093.

31. Boht, R., van Furth, R., and van den Broek, P.J. (1995) Aetiology of community-ac-quired pneumonia: a prospective study among adults requiring admission to hospital. *Thorax* **50,** 543–547.

32. Mundy, L.M., Aurwaeter, P.G., Oldach, D., et al. (1995) Community-acquired pneu-monia: impact of immune status. *Am. J. Respir. Crit. Care Med.* **152**, 1309–1315.

33. Marston, B.J., Plouffe, J.F., File, T.M., Jr., et al. (1997) Incidence of community-ac-quired pneumonia requiring hospitalization. Results of a population-based active sur-veillance study in Ohio. *Arch. Intern. Med.* **157**, 1709–1817.

34. Marrie, T.J., Durant, H., and Yates, L. (1989) Community-acquired pneumonia requir-ing hospitalization. *Rev. Infect. Dis.* **11**, 586–599.

35. Kauppinen, M.T., Herva, E., Kujala, P., et al. (1995) The etiology of community-ac-quired pneumonia among hospitalized patients during a *Chlamydia pneumoniae* epi-demic in Finland. *J. Infect. Dis.* **172**, 1330–1335.

36. Levy, M., Dromer, F., Brion, N., et al. (1998) Community-acquired pneumonia. Im-portance of initial noninvasive bacteriologic and radiographic investigations. *Chest* **93**, 43–48.

37. Fang, G. D., Fine, M., Orleff, J., et al. (1990) New and emerging etiologies for com-munity-acquired pneumonia with implications for therapy. *Medicine* **69**, 307–316.

38. Valenti, W.M., Trudell, R.G., and Bentley, D.W. (1978) Factors predisposing to oropharyngeal colonization with gram negative bacilli in the aged. *N. Engl. J. Med.* **298**, 1108–1111.

39. Garb, J.L, Brown R.B, Garb, J., et al. (1978) Differences in etiology of pneumonias in nursing home and community patients. *JAMA* **240**, 2169–2172

40. Orr, P.H., Peeling, R.W., Fast, M., et al. (1996) Serological study of responses to selected pathogens causing respiratory tract infection in the institutionalized elderly. *Clin. Infect. Dis.* **23,** 1240–1248.

41. Phillips, S.L. and Branaman-Phillips, J. (1993). The use of intramuscular cefoperazone versus intramuscular ceftriaxone in patients with nursing home acquired pneumonia. *J. Am. Geriatr. Soc.* **41**, 1071–1074.

42. Drinka, P.J., Gauerke, C., Voeks, S., et al. (1994) Pneumonia in a nursing home. *J. Gen. Intern. Med.* 9, 650–652

43. Chow, C.W., Senathiragah, N., Rawji, M., et al. (1994) Interim report on drug utilization review of community-acquired and nosocomial pneumonia: clinical bacteriological and radiological spectrum. *Can. J. Infect. Dis.* **5(Suppl. C),** 20C–27C.

44. Marrie, T.J., Haldone, E.F., Faulkner, R.S., et al. (1985) Community-acquired pneumonia requiring hospitalization. Is it different in the elderly? *J. Am. Geriatr. Soc.* **33**, 671–680.

45. Fein, A.M. (1994) Pneumonia in the elderly. Special diagnostic and therapeutic considerations. *Med. Clin. North Am.* **78**, 1015–1033.

46. Granton, J.T. and Grossman, R.F. (1993) Community-acquired pneumonia in the elderly patient. Clinical features, epidemiology, and treatment. *Clin. Chest. Med.* **14**, 537–552.

47. Fine, M.J., Auble, T.E., Yealy, D.M., et al. (1997) A prediction rule to identify low-risk patients with community-acquired pneumonia. *N. Engl. J. Med.* **336**, 243–250.

48. Atlas, S.J., Benzer, T.I., Borowsky, L.H., et al. (1998) Safely increasing the proportion of patients with community-acquired pneumonia treated as outpatients. *Arch. Intern. Med.* **158**, 1350–1356.

49. Marrie, T., Lau, C., Feagan, B., et al. (1998) A randomized controlled trial of a critical pathway for the management of community-acquired pneumonia. 6th International Quinolone Meeting, Nov. 16–18, Denver, CO.

50. Niederman, M.S., Best, J.B., Campbell, G.D., et al. (1993) Guidelines for the initial management of adults with community-acquired pneumonia: diagnosis, assessment of severity and initial antimicrobial therapy. *Am. Rev. Respir. Dis.* **148**, 1418–1426.

51. Ewig, S., Ruiz, M., Mensa, J., et al. (1988) Severe community-acquired pneumonia. Assessment of severity criteria. *Am. J. Respir. Crit. Care Med.* **158**, 1102–1108.

52. Ramirez, J.A., Srinath, L., Ahkee, S., et al. (1995) Early switch from intravenous to oral cephalosporins in the treatment of hospitalized patients with community-acquired pneumonia. *Arch. Intern. Med.* **155**, 1273–1276.

53. Ramirez, J.A. and Ahkee, S. (1997) Early switch from intravenous antimicrobial to oral clarithromycin in patients with community-acquired pneumonia. *Infect. Med.* **14**, 319–323.

54. Ramirez, J.A. (1995) Switch therapy in adult patients with pneumonia. *Clin. Pulm. Med.* **2**, 327–333.

55. Meehan, T.P., Fine, M.J., Krumholz, H.M. et al. (1997) Quality of care, process and outcomes in elderly patients with pneumonia. *JAMA* **278**, 2080.

56. Halm, E.A., Fine, M.J., Marrie, T.J., et al (1998) Time to clinical stability in patients hospitalized with community-acquired pneumonia. Implications for practice guidelines. *JAMA* **279,** 1452–1457.

Shobita Rajagopalan

1. CLINICAL RELEVANCE

Tuberculosis (TB), in the United States has changed significantly during the past decade. Since 1993, TB morbidity has steadily declined, and the disease has focused on well-defined risk groups, geographic areas, and certain vulnerable segments of our society. The elderly represent the largest reservoir of TB infection, especially in developed nations *(1)*. Clinical features of TB in older adults can be nonspecific and confused with concomitant age-related illnesses. Biological changes associated with aging, underlying acute or chronic diseases, and malnutrition can disrupt integumental barriers, impair microbial clearance mechanisms, and contribute to the expected age-associated decline in cellular immune responses to infecting agents such as *Mycobacterium tuberculosis* (*Mtb*) *(2)*. The subtle clinical manifestations of TB in the elderly can often make the diagnosis problematic, resulting in increased morbidity and mortality; this treatable infection may unfortunately be recognized postmortem. The increased incidence of adverse drug reactions associated with aging can also make the treatment of TB in older adults more challenging *(3)*. In addition, it is important to provide optimal treatment of associated chronic diseases, minimize invasive procedures, limit polypharmacy, and ensure adequate nutrition. The institutionalized elderly represent an especially vulnerable subgroup of the geriatric cohort that are both at high risk for reactivation of latent TB as well as susceptible to new TB infection *(4)*.

2. GLOBAL EPIDEMIOLOGY

Worldwide, an estimated 8 million cases and 2 million deaths have been attributed to TB in 1998 *(1)*. TB remains the world's leading cause of death among all infectious diseases. An approximate third of the world's population (1.7 billion persons) is infected with *Mtb* (TB infection is defined as harboring *Mtb* without evidence of active infection, and TB disease is active infection without *Mtb* based on clinical and laboratory findings). In the U.S., the resurgence of TB from 1985–1992 had been associated with the human immunodeficiency virus (HIV) epidemic, immigration from TB endemic countries, TB transmission in congregate settings, (e.g., prisons, long-term care

From: *Infectious Disease in the Aging*
Edited by: Thomas T. Yoshikawa and Dean C. Norman
© Humana Press Inc., Totowa, NJ

facilities, and hospitals) deterioration of the infrastructure for TB control services, and the emergence of difficult-to-treat cases of multiple drug-resistant (MDR)-TB *(5)*. Since that time, there has been a tremendous decline of TB cases, reaching a record low of 18,361 cases in 1998, with a case rate of 6.8/1000,000, and an overall decline of 31% (Centers for Disease Control and Prevention [CDC] unpublished data 1998), attributed largely to effective TB control programs that emphasize prompt identification of cases, initiation of appropriate therapy, and monitoring of therapy completion *(6)*.

The recent success of TB control in the U.S. has been negated by the burden of TB among foreign-born persons (i.e., individuals from Asia, Africa, or Latin America, in whom TB rates are 5–30 times higher than U.S. rates) residing in this country *(7)*. During 1992–1997, the number of TB cases across both sexes and all age groups among U.S.-born persons declined 38%, while the number of cases among foreign-born persons in the U.S. increased by 6%. Although the TB case rates for foreign-born persons have remained at least four to five times higher than for U.S.-born persons, the number of U.S. cases occurring in foreign-born persons (the birth countries with highest number of such cases are represented by Mexico, the Philippines, and Vietnam), has increased steadily since the mid 1980s, reaching 42% in 1998 (CDC unpublished data, 1998). Developed nations, i.e., the U.S., Canada, Europe, Australia, New Zealand, and Japan, report an estimated 380 million persons infected with *Mtb*; about 80% of infected persons in Europe are 50 yr of age or older *(1)*.

Increase in TB notification rates from England and Wales since 1987 for all ethnic groups have been especially significant in the elderly; from 1987–1989 the increase was 6% for all ages combined, but 13% in females and 16% in males over the age of 75 yr *(8)*. Although a significant percentage (80%–90%) of TB in the elderly occurs in community dwellers, there is a two to three times higher incidence of active TB in nursing home residents compared with their counterparts living in noninstitutionalized settings *(9)*. The knowledge regarding the enhanced efficiency of TB transmission within closed environments such as prisons, nursing homes, chronic disease facilities, and shelters for the homeless has raised concerns about TB infection and disease in the institutionalized elderly *(10)*.

3. PATHOGENESIS AND IMMUNOLOGIC ASPECTS

The principal portal of entry of the tubercle bacilli as well as the major organ of disease is the lung. Inhaled tubercle bacilli are deposited in the basal segments of the lower lobe, middle lobe, lingula, or anterior segments of the upper lobe, the so-called primary infection segments. Alveolar macrophages that are nonspecifically activated (natural immunity) engulf the inhaled bacilli and are transported to regional lymph nodes. Infected macrophages produce chemokines that result in recruitment of additional macrophages and circulating monocytes, which in turn secrete significant amounts of proteolytic enzymes, generating an exudative lesion *(11)*. Activated mononuclear phagocytes (MP) also secrete tumor necrosis factor, which incite granuloma formation. Eventually, T cells activated by chemokines in the draining lymph nodes as well as natural killer (NK) cells are attracted to the site of inflammation with subsequent production of interferon-gamma, which in turn activates tuberculostatic macrophage functions. At this stage (acquired immunity), the onset of cell-mediated immunity and delayed type hypersensitivity responses, which occur after approximately

3 wk of initial infection, are associated with a positive dermal reactivity to standard-dose tuberculin antigen. The characteristic tubercle granuloma or the Ghon complex ultimately develops consisting of organized collections of epithelioid cells, lymphocytes, and capillaries; tubercle bacilli are confined and their growth restrained within lesions showing caseous necrosis, surrounding fibrosis, and ultimate healing *(12)*. Reactivation (secondary or postprimary) TB is associated with uncontrolled cell destruction by cytolytic T cells, NK cells, and activated MP cells, which promote granuloma liquefaction and rupture into the bronchoalveolar and vascular systems promoting widespread microbial dissemination.

Containment of the TB infection results in an asymptomatic and noninfectious state with a positive tuberculin skin test reaction (TB infection); the viable tubercle bacilli remain dormant indefinitely with intact host immune integrity. Factors that compromise host immunity, e.g., HIV infection, aging, illicit drug use, alcoholism, poor nutrition, and certain chronic diseases, may result in reactivation of latent TB infection (TB disease). The increased frequency of TB seen in aging may be explained in large part by the impairment of cell-mediated immunity, which results from senescence (demonstrated in murine models) as well as age-associated diseases (diabetes mellitus, malignancy), renal impairment, malnutrition, and immunosuppressive agents *(13)*.

Approximately 90% of TB disease cases in the elderly are due to reactivation of primary infection *(9)*. TB infection without disease may occur in 30%–50% of individuals in elderly nursing facility residents as demonstrated by positive tuberculin skin tests. Rarely, previously infected older persons may eventually eliminate the viable tubercle bacilli and revert to a tuberculin negative state; nevertheless, these persons are at risk for new infection (reinfection) with *Mtb*. Thus older persons potentially at risk for TB consist of individuals never exposed to *Mtb*, those with latent and dormant primary infection that may reactivate, and others who are no longer infected and consequently at risk for reinfection.

4. UNIQUE CLINICAL CONSIDERATIONS

TB in older patients is represents a diagnostic dilemma for many clinicians. The vast majority (75%) of elderly persons infected with *Mtb* manifest active disease in their lungs *(1,14)*.

In addition, disseminated or miliary TB, tuberculous meningitis, and skeletal TB increase in frequency with advancing age. However, many older patients with TB disease may not exhibit the classic features of TB, i.e., cough, hemoptysis, fever, night sweats, and weight loss. TB in this population may present clinically with changes in functional capacity (e.g., activities of daily living), chronic fatigue, cognitive impairment, decreased appetite, or unexplained low-grade fever. An undefinable etiology for nonspecific symptoms and signs over a period of weeks to months must alert clinicians to the possibility of unrecognized TB *(15)*.

4.1. Pulmonary TB

Pulmonary TB is by far the commonest form of TB in the elderly population *(9)*. Although aging patients with pulmonary TB can present with typical respiratory as well as systemic symptoms, i.e., sputum production, hemoptysis, fever, night sweats, weight loss, or anorexia, a significant number of such patients may exhibit minimal pulmonary symptoms. The radiographic manifestations and variations of pulmonary TB in older persons are briefly described in the *Subheading 5*.

4.2. Miliary TB

Miliary or disseminated TB often occurs in aging patients; many cases are diagnosed at autopsy. Miliary TB in the elderly may manifest in one of two atypical forms: the chronic hematogenous form and the non-reactive form. In the chronic hematogenous variety, there are recurrent episodes of low-grade *Mtb* bacillemia manifesting as a protracted illness often without fever, localizing symptoms or signs *(9,16)*. The classical radiographic evidence of miliary mottling on the chest radiograph may be not be present. The nonreactive form of miliary TB is common in elderly and immunocompromised hosts *(17)*. Overwhelming infection results in numerous caseous lesions harboring enormous numbers of replicating tubercle bacilli and minimal neutrophil infiltrate with no granulomatous reaction. Clinical features include fever, weight loss, and hepatosplenomegaly without other focal signs; this form of TB should be considered in the differential diagnosis of "fever of unknown origin."

4.3. Tuberculous Meningitis

Tuberculous meningitis in the elderly occurs as a consequence of reactivation of a primary dormant focus or as a part of miliary seeding of infection. Older patients, not unlike their younger counterparts, present with a subacute onset of fever, headache, and confusion with simultaneous or preceding systemic symptoms of weakness, anorexia, and fatigue. Some older patients can also present with unexplained dementia or obtundation without fever or nuchal rigidity; in such patients it is imperative to maintain a high index of suspicion for tuberculous meningitis until proven otherwise *(18)*. Tuberculous meningitis is associated with an exceedingly high mortality in the elderly; neurologic sequelae or deficits are common in survivors (19).

4.4. Skeletal TB

Skeletal involvement with *Mtb* infection in the elderly, commonly affects the spine *(20)*. The thoracic and lumbar spines are commonly involved; cervical disease is rare. Paravertebral abscesses or "cold abscesses" are often associated with spinal infection *(21)*. Primary symptoms of spinal TB consist of pain over the involved vertebrae; neurological deficits and sinus tracts may occur with more advanced disease. Low-grade fever, weight loss, fatigue, and anorexia maybe present. Tuberculous arthritis tends to commonly involve the large weight-bearing joints; however, in the elderly, peripheral joints, i.e., the knees, wrists, ankles, and the metatarso-phalangeal joints may be involved *(22)*. Pain and swelling of the involved joints and loss of range of motion can sometimes occur. Because older patients often have degenerative joint disease or other arthritides, the diagnosis of coexisting tuberculous arthritis may be overlooked.

4.5 Genitourinary TB

Despite the fact that genitourinary (GU) TB is seen in a significant number of elderly persons, this form of TB disease largely occurs in persons in their third, fourth, and fifth decades of life *(23)*. The kidney is the major site of involvement with as many as 20% to 30% of patients being asymptomatic *(24)*. GU TB can also involve the ureters, bladder, prostate, epididymis, and seminal vesicles. Presenting symptoms may include dysuria, frequency, flank pain, and hematuria. The diagnosis must be considered in the presence of an abnormal urinary sediment, pyuria without bacteruria, or hematuria. Significant disease may result in pelvic or scrotal masses, and draining sinuses; systemic manifestations (fever, anorexia, weight loss) may be absent.

4.6. Other Sites

Similar to younger patients, TB in older adults can involve virtually any organ in the body. In elderly patients, TB disease involving the lymph nodes, pleura, liver, gall bladder, small and large bowel, pericardium, middle ear, and carpal tunnel have been described *(25)*.

5. DIAGNOSTIC TESTS

The tuberculin skin test remains the screening intervention of choice, despite its potential for false-negative results. Negative tuberculin skin tests on initial application have been noted in up to 25% of proven cases of active TB *(9)*. A negative reaction to tuberculin increases with age and may be partly explained due to anergy. Moreover, the "booster effect" of skin-test reactivity to antigen increases in prevalence in the elderly population *(26)*. Thus, it is essential that all older persons who receive a tuberculin skin test [using the standard Mantoux method with 5 tuberculin units of Tween-stabilized purified protein derivative (PPD), and results read in 48–72 h] be retested within two wk of a negative response (induration of less than 10 mm) to ensure recognition of a potentially false-negative reaction. Application of the second tuberculin skin test should ideally be accompanied by common dermal control antigens (e.g., candida, mumps) to determine the presence of cutaneous anergy. A positive booster effect—and therefore a positive tuberculin skin test—is a skin test reaction of 10 mm or more and an increase in induration of 6 mm or more over the first skin test reaction *(27)*. A positive PPD skin test after the initial placement, by the booster effect, or by conversion, or if the patient has clinical manifestations suggestive of TB, warrant a chest radiograph because 75% of all TB cases in the elderly occur in the respiratory tract. Most pulmonary TB cases in elderly patients represent reactivation disease; 10–20% of cases are as a consequence of primary infection or reinfection. Although reactivation TB classically involves the upper lobes of the lung (apical and posterior segments), several studies have shown that many elderly TB patients manifest their pulmonary infection in either middle or lower lung lobes *(14)*. Thus, clinicians should exercise caution when interpreting radiographic diagnoses of TB in older patients because of the atypical location of the infection in the lung fields.

Sputum examination for *Mtb* by smear and culture is indicated in all patients with pulmonary symptoms and/or have radiographic changes compatible with TB and who have not been treated with anti-TB therapy. Elderly persons unable to expectorate sputum should be considered for a more aggressive diagnostic intervention. Flexible fiberoptic bronchoscopy to obtain bronchial washings and bronchial biopsy is a feasible and valuable option to diagnose TB in persons aged 65 years and older *(9)*.

For suspected pulmonary TB, three fresh consecutive morning sputum specimens are recommended for routine mycobacteriologic studies that include an initial smear and culture for *Mtb* *(28)*. There are two basic acid-fast staining techniques: carbolfuchsin and fluorochrome. Both the Ziehl–Neelson (heating) and Kinyoun (phenol) methods utilize carbolfuchsin and stain the organism red against a blue or green counterstain (e.g., methylene blue). Auramine–rhodamine dye applies the fluorochrome method in which the mycobacterial cells appear golden-yellow against a dark background. Routine mycobacterial culture methods, e.g., Lowenstein–Jensen (L-J) medium, that require up to 6 wk for the growth of *Mtb* have been replaced by more rapid techniques that utilize radiometric systems, specific DNA probes and the polymerase chain reaction (PCR) *(29)*. At the National Jewish Center for Immunology and Respiratory Diseases in Denver, CO, four types of mycobacterial culture media are used: (1) 7H12 broth for radiometric detection of growth in the BACTEC TB 460 system. The growth of *Mtb* in this medium can be detected in 1–2 wk. (2) Inoculation of Middlebrook-Cohn 7H10 or 7H11 agar provides the opportunity to examine colonial morphology and detect mixed cultures if the specimen contains more than one species. (3) 7H11 selective media containing antibiotics to inhibit growth of nonmycobacterial contaminants can also be inoculated. (4) Inoculation on the egg-based L-J slant serves as a backup for rare *Mtb* isolates that may not grow on the other three media.

Nucleic acid amplification (NAA) tests such as PCR and other methods for amplifying DNA and RNA may facilitate rapid detection of *Mtb*. An NAA test for *Mtb* complex (Amplified *Mtb* Direct Test or MTD [Gen-Probe, San Diego, CA] was recently approved by the Food and Drug Administration for use on processed clinical specimens in conjunction with culture for respiratory specimens that are positive on smear *(29)*. The MTD test uses transcription-mediated amplification to detect *Mtb*-complex ribosomal RNA; based on the product label, the test sensitivity in clinical trials was 95.6%, and the specificity was 100%. Several other NAA tests are under commercial development, including the Roche Amplicor test, a PCR test that amplifies mycobacterial DNA.

The rapid diagnosis of TB is especially important in the high-risk elderly population, as well as HIV-infected persons and patients with MDR-TB. Novel developments in mycobacteriology laboratory technology can be divided into three major groups—automated systems for isolation of mycobacteria in liquid media, application of the same system for rapid drug susceptibility testing, and development of new amplification methods for mycobacterial speciation and detection of drug resistance.

Histological examination of tissue from various sites such as the liver, lymph nodes, bone marrow, pleura or synovium that show the characteristic tissue reaction (caseous necrosis with granuloma formation) is also useful for the diagnosis of TB disease.6.

TREATMENT AND PREVENTION

The CDC in conjunction with the American Thoracic Society in 1994 modified its TB treatment recommendations because of the rise of MDR-TB cases (*see* Table 1) *(30)*. However, the CDC also recommends that if the frequency of isoniazid resistance is 4% or less in a given community or if the population in question has a low risk for drug resistance, the empiric four-drug regimen is not necessary. Although there has been much concern over the emergence of drug-resistant isolates of *Mtb* and the complex issue of TB in HIV-infected persons, the vast majority of cases of TB in the elderly in the U.S. is fortunately caused by drug-sensitive strains of *Mtb*. TB in older persons is an easily treatable and preventable infection and a highly curable disease. As

Table 1
Treatment Regimens and Tuberculosis[a]

Drugs	Frequency
Option 1	
Isoniazid, rifampin, pyrazinamide and ethambutol or streptomycin for 8 wk[b] followed by	Daily
isoniazid and rifampin for 16 wk (for susceptible strains)	Daily or 2–3 times weekly[c]
Option 2	
Isoniazid, rifampin, pyrazinamide and ethambutol or streptomycin[b] for 2 weeks	Daily
followed by the same drugs for 6 weeks[b]	Twice weekly[c]
then isoniazid and rifampin for 16 wk	Twice weekly[c]
Option 3	
Isoniazid, rifampin, pyrazinamide and ethambutol or streptomycin for 24 wk[b]	Three times weekly[c]

[a] From Refs. *30* and *31*.
[b] In areas where primary isoniazid resistance is less than 4%, omit fourth drug; streptomycin is not recommended for the elderly.
[c] Intermittent dosing should be directly observed.

evidenced by several studies most cases of active TB in the elderly result from reactivation of a latent infection. These individuals presumably acquired the infecting organism during the time prior to the availability of effective antituberculous chemotherapy. Hence, unless the older patient is from a country with a high prevalence of drug-resistant *Mtb*, had previously been inadequately treated with *Mtb* chemotherapy, or had acquired the infection from a known MDR-TB contact, the overwhelming number of TB cases in the elderly will be highly susceptible to isoniazid and rifampin. Hence, once TB is suspected, appropriate diagnostic tools have been utilized, and reasonable caution exercised to ensure low probability of *Mtb* drug resistance, antituberculous chemotherapy with standard doses of isoniazid (300 mg/d) and rifampin (600 mg/d) can be instituted *(10)*. An effective alternative for older patients is a regimen commencing with isoniazid (300 mg/d), rifampin (600 mg/d), and pyrazinamide (30 mg/kg/d up to 2 g) for 2 mo, followed by 4 mo of isoniazid and rifampin. This 6-mo regimen is sufficient for disease at any site, with the exception of tuberculous meningitis, for which treatment with isoniazid and rifampin should be continued for one full yr. Some authorities also recommend that miliary and bone and joint disease be treated for one full year. Although the more intensive, shorter duration, antituberculous drug regimens can generally minimize treatment non compliance and development of drug resistance, particularly when administered by directly observed therapy (DOT), the potential for drug toxicity limits its use in older patients.

Elderly persons are at greater risk for hepatic toxicity from isoniazid; however, this risk is relatively low in frequency and mild in severity. It is recommended that clinical assessments as well as baseline liver function tests be performed prior to the initiation of isoniazid and rifampin (and pyrazinamide) therapy to older persons; periodic laboratory monitoring seems a prudent practice particularly in the frail old who may not be able to communicate warning symptoms of drug toxicities. A rise in the serum aminotransferase (SGOT) level to five times above normal or clinical evidence of hepatitis necessitates the prompt discontinuation of isoniazid (as well as other hepatotoxic drugs); these drugs may subsequently be resumed at lower doses and gradually increased to full doses as tolerated. Relapse with drug rechallenge will require trial of an alternative regimen.

Heightened awareness of MDR-TB has prompted public health agencies to institute strict TB identification, isolation, treatment, and prevention guidelines *(31)*. The TB infection control program in most acute care as well as long-term care facilities should consist of three types of control measures: administrative actions (i.e., prompt detection of suspected cases, isolation of infectious patients, and rapid institution of appropriate treatment), engineering controls (negative-pressure ventilation rooms, high efficiency particulate air [HEPA] filtration, and ultraviolet germicidal irradiation, and personal respiratory protection requirements (masks). While instituting such infection control measures in elderly TB patients, clinicians should be cognizant of the presence of concomitant chronic conditions and functional disabilities that often require more assistance and care, as well as the importance of minimizing prolonged isolation or physical incarceration.

Treatment of TB infection (previously referred to as prophylaxis) with isoniazid (300 mg/d) for a minimum of 6 mo is currently recommended for older persons infected with *Mtb* (as evidenced by a positive tuberculin test) and associated high-risk conditions, as well as persons with tuberculin skin test conversions (*see* Table 2) *(31)*. A 12-mo regimen of isoniazid is recommended for persons with chest radiographic evidence of prior untreated TB infection and in persons coinfected with HIV.

Tuberculin skin testing is recommended using the two-step technique for all older persons admitted to nursing homes; comprehensive geriatric assessment and complete physical examination of the elderly should also ideally incorporate tuberculin screening in their protocol. For health care professionals, staff, and administrators of facilities providing care to the elderly, the following is a brief summary of the Advisory Committee for Elimination of TB's published recommendations *(32)*.

6.1. Surveillance

1. All new residents on admission and all employees should receive a two-step tuberculin test.
2. All persons with a tuberculin skin test reaction of 10 mm or more of induration should receive a chest radiograph to identify current or past tuberculous disease.
3. Skin-test-negative employees or volunteers having contact (of 10 or more hours per week) with patients should periodically have repeat skin tests, the frequency depending on the risk of tuberculous infection at that facility.

Table 2
Criteria for Positive Tuberculin Skin Reaction[a]

Skin test criteria (mm induration)	Population at risk
≥5 mm	Persons with known or suspected HIV infection[b]
	Close contacts of person(s) with infectious tuberculosis[b]
	Persons with chest radiographs consistent with tuberculosis (e.g., fibrotic changes)[b]
≥10 mm	Recent converters (≥10 mm with ≥6 mm increase within 2 yr; ≥15 mm for those age ≥ 35 yr)[b]
	Intravenous drug uses known to be HIV seronegative[b]
	Persons with certain risk factors; silicosis; gastrectomy;-Jejunoileal bypass; >10% below ideal body weight; chronic renal failure; diabetes mellitus; corticosteroid and other immunosuppressive therapy; hematologic and other malignancies (alcoholics are also considered high risk)[b]
	Foreign-born from country with high tuberculosis prevalence[c]
	Medically underserved low-income populations (homeless, African-Americans, Hispanics, Native Americans)
	Residents of long-term care facilities (nursing home, correctional institutions)[c]
	None of the above factors ≥ 15 mm[c]

[a] Reference *(31)*.
[b] Chemoprophylaxis recommended for all persons regardless of age.
[c] Chemoprophylaxis recommended for persons less then 35 yr.
HIV = human immunodeficiency virus.

4. Repeat skin tests should be performed for tuberculin-negative persons after any suspected exposure to a documented case of active TB.
5. Staff and patients with TB infection or disease should be assessed for HIV infection.

6.2. Containment

Persons with confirmed or suspected infectious TB do not require isolation precautions providing the following conditions are met:

1. Chemotherapy is begun promptly at the time of confirmation or suspicion of diagnosis.
2. Current and recent contacts are evaluated and given appropriate therapy.
3. New contacts can be prevented for a 1-2 wk period.

In the event that these conditions cannot be fulfilled, and in case of homelessness, suspected or known history of noncompliance, MDR-TB, and illicit drug use, the local health department (that should be informed of all suspected or proven TB cases) facilitates methods to achieve appropriate respiratory isolation.

REFERENCES

1. World Health Organization (1999) The world health report. Making a difference. *World Health Org.* **3**, 310–320.

2. Bender, B.S., Nagel, J.E., and Adler, W.H. (1986) Absolute peripheral lymphocyte count and subsequent mortality in elderly males: The Baltimore Longitudinal Study of Aging. *J. Am. Geriatr. Soc.* **34**, 649–654.

3. Girling, D.J. (1982) Adverse effects of antituberculous drugs. *Drugs* **23**, 56–74.

4. Centers for Disease Control and Prevention (1990) Prevention and control of tuberculosis in facilities providing long-term care to the elderly. *M.M.W.R.* **39/RR-10,** 7–20.

5. Centers for Disease Control and Prevention (1999) Tuberculosis elimination revisited: obstacles, opportunities, and renewed commitment. Advisory Council for the Elimination of Tuberculosis. *M.M.W.R.* **48/RR-9**, 1–14.

6. McKenna, M.T., Mccray, E., Jones, J.L., et al. (1998) The fall after the rise: tuberculosis in the United States, 1991 through 1994. *Am. J. Public Health* **88**, 1059–1063.

7. Zubert, P.L.F., McKenna, M.T., Binkin, N.J., et al. (1997) Long-term risk of tuberculosis among foreign-born persons in the United States. *JAMA* **278**, 304–307.

8. Davies, P.D.O. (1994) Tuberculosis in the elderly. *J. Anticrob. Chemother.* **34(Suppl. A),** 93–100.

9. Yoshikawa, T.T. (1992) Tuberculosis in aging adults. *J. Am. Geriatr. Soc.* **40**, 178–187

10. Stead, W., Lofgren, J., Warren, E., et al. (1985) Tuberculosis as an endemic and nosocomial infection among the elderly in nursing homes. *N. Eng. J. Med.* **312**, 1483–1487.

11. Chaparas, S.D. (1982) Immunity in tuberculosis. *Bull. W.H.O.* **60**, 447–462.

12. Bloom, B.R. (1994) *Tuberculosis in Pathogenesis, Protection and Control: Immune Mechanisms of Protection,* American Society for Microbiology Press, Washington, DC, pp. 389–415.

13. Orme, I.M. (1987) Aging and immunity to tuberculosis: increased susceptibility of old mice reflects a decreased capacity to generate mediator T lymphocytes. *J. Immunol.* **138**, 4414–4418.

14. Morris, C.D.W. (1989) The radiography, haematology and bronchoscopy of pulmonary tuberculosis in the aged. *Q. J. Med.* **71,** 529–536

15. Yoshikawa, T.T. and Norman, D.C. (1987*) Infectious Diseases and Diagnosis and Treatment. Aging and Clinical Practice,* Igaku-Shoin, New York, pp. 127–139.

16. Sahn, S.A. and Neff, T.A. (1974) Miliary tuberculosis. *Am. J. Med.* **56**, 495–505.

17. Saltman, R.L. and Peterson, P.K. (1987) Immunodeficiency of the elderly. *Rev. Infect. Dis.* **9**, 1127–1139.

18. Nagami, P. and Yoshikawa, T.T. (1983) Tuberculosis in the geriatric patient. *J. Am. Geriatr. Soc.* **31**, 356–363.

19. Molavi, A. and LeFrock, J.L. (1985) Tuberculous meningitis. *Med. Clin. North Am.* **69,** 315–331.

20. Tuli, S.M. (1975) Results of treatment of spinal tuberculosis by "middle path" regime. *J. Bone Joint Surg.* (British Volume) **57**, 13–23.

21. Paus, B. (1977) The changed pattern of bone and joint tuberculosis in Norway. *Acta Orthop. Scand.* **48**, 277–279.

22. Evanchick, C.C., Davis, D.E., and Harrington, T.M. (1986) Tuberculosis of peripheral joints: an often missed diagnosis. *J. Rheum.* **13**, 187–189.

23. Quinn W. (1984) Genitourinary tuberculosis: a study of 1117 cases over a period of 34 years. *Br. J. Urol.* **56**, 449–455.

24. Alvarez, S. and McCabe, W. (1984) Extrapulmonary tuberculosis revisisted: A review of experience at Boston City and other hospitals. *Medicine* **63**, 25–55.

25. Lai, K.K., Stottmeier, K.D., Sherman, I.H., et al. (1984) Mycobacterial cervical lymphadenopathy. Relation of etiologic agents to age. *JAMA* **251**, 1286–1288.

26. Nash, D.R. and Douglass, J.E. (1980) Anergy in active pulmonary tuberculosis. A comparison between positive and negative reactors and an evaluation of 5 TU and 250 TU skin test doses. *Chest* **77**, 32–35.

27. Thompson, N.J., Glassroth, J.L., Snider, D.E., Jr., et al. (1979) The booster phenomenon in serial tuberculin screening. *Am. Rev. Respir. Dis.* **119**, 587–597.
28. Dutt, A.K., Moers, D., and Stead, W.W. (1989) Smear and culture negative pulmonary tuberculosis: four month short course chemotherapy. *Am. Rev. Resp. Dis.* **139**, 867–870.
29. Centers for Disease Control and Prevention (1996) Nuclei acid amplification tests for tuberculosis. *M.M.W.R.* **45**, 950–952.
30. American Thoracic Society (1994) Treatment and prevention of tuberculosis in adults and children. *Am. J. Resp. Crit. Care Med.* **149**, 1359–1374.
31. Centers for Disease Control and Prevention (1990) Screening for tuberculosis and tuberculosis infection in high-risk populations. Recommendations of the Advisory Committee for Elimination of Tuberculosis *M.M.W.R.* **39**/*RR-8*, 1–7.
32. Centers for Disease Control and Prevention (1990) Prevention and control of tuberculosis in facilities providing long-term care to the elderly. Recommendations of the Advisory Committee for Elimination of Tuberculosis *M.M.W.R.* **39**/RR-10, 7–20.

8

Infective Endocarditis

Margaret S. Terpenning

1. EPIDEMIOLOGY AND CLINICAL RELEVANCE

Infective endocarditis is an infection of the heart valves or the endothelium of the heart with any of a variety of bacteria, fungi, rickettsiae, or other agents. Infective endocarditis has a worldwide distribution with 10,000–20,000 new cases per year in the United States *(1)*. This disease has been known virtually since the beginning of the history of internal medicine and was referred to in detail by Sir William Osler, who did the writing concerning clinical criteria for its diagnosis *(2)*. Because the vast majority of infective endocarditis cases are caused by bacteria, the discussion will focus primarily on bacterial endocarditis.

The entity bacterial endocarditis involves certain pathogens more frequently than others. The major pathogens identified are the streptococci, and in particular the streptococci with a green pattern of hemolysis (alpha hemolysis) known as viridans group streptococci. Another very prominent pathogen in bacterial endocarditis is *Staphylococcus aureus* and, in more recent years, *S. epidermidis (3,4)*. There are some pathogens that are entirely unique to bacterial endocarditis and therefore the isolation of these pathogens strongly reinforces the possibility that the diagnosis is infective endocarditis. These pathogens are referred to as HACEK organisms, which is an acronym of their actual species names, described in Subheading 3. In addition to these pathogens, Gram-negative bacilli are capable of causing bacterial endocarditis, as are a variety of other organisms that are described in other reports *(4–7)*.

In the development of infective endocarditis, there are many important sources. It is possible for human beings to acquire infective endocarditis from virtually any source of bacteremia, fungemia, or spread of other organisms within the blood. Bacteremia of oral origin is particularly important and has been of growing importance in the elderly in the 1990s *(8)*. In addition, the organisms of oral origin, which include oral streptococci, are often particularly well-adapted to infect cardiac valves *(9)*. The adaptation of these oral organisms to produce such problems may be evolving. Streptococci are the predominant organism in infective endocarditis in many studies *(3–5)*. In addition, it is possible to develop infective endocarditis from invasion of the skin by *S. aureus* and *S. epidermidis*. These organisms are a very prominent source of infective endocarditis in

From: *Infectious Disease in the Aging*
Edited by: Thomas T. Yoshikawa and Dean C. Norman
© Humana Press Inc., Totowa, NJ

the elderly and, indeed, in all age groups *(4)*. In addition, anything that disrupts the integrity of the skin barrier can increase the risk of infective endocarditis. This includes intravenous drug abuse, and many medical procedures that occur as part of hospitalization. It is possible for infective endocarditis to develop also from urinary tract procedures or gastrointestinal procedures with characteristic organisms, including Gram-negative bacilli and enterococci *(3)*.

In recent years, the frequent practice of replacing natural (native) cardiac valves with prosthetic valves has resulted in an ever-growing new group of people at special risk for infective endocarditis. Prosthetic valves have a high propensity to become infected with *S. epidermidis* or enterococci. An increasing proportion of the elderly possess a prosthetic heart valve and therefore are at special risk from enterococcal or *S. epidermidis* endocarditis *(4)*. (*See also* Chapter 17.)

Of relevance to the elderly, therefore, are the following major risk factors and sources of infective endocarditis: (1) dental procedures as more elderly retain their teeth; (2) breaks in skin integrity associated with intravenous therapy or hospital procedures; (3) a variety of other in-hospital procedures including gastrointestinal or urologic procedures; (4) the increased number of older people possessing a prosthetic heart valve versus a native heart valve; and (5) increased survival of persons possessing old valvular damage or congenital valve disease (4).

2. CLINICAL MANIFESTATIONS

Infective endocarditis, as it presents in the elderly population, can be extremely diverse in its clinical manifestations. Although initially these clinical manifestations can be extremely minimal or absent and seemingly unimportant, the physician must constantly be on the alert or infective endocarditis will elude diagnosis. The difficulty of diagnosis of infective endocarditis in the elderly has been noted many times before *(4)*. The elderly patient may have nonspecific symptoms such as lethargy, nausea, or vertigo. The older patient may lack fever, leading the physician away from an infectious diagnosis. Diagnostic findings for infective endocarditis may include all of the following: (1) the patient may have had a predisposing heart condition; (2) the patient may or may not have had a fever greater than 38°C (100.4°F); (3) although rare in the elderly, there may be a history of intravenous drug abuse; (4) the patient may have any of a variety of vascular phenomena of infective endocarditis, which are actually much less common in recent years, such as Janeway lesions or Osler's nodes; (5) there may be Roth spots in the eyes; (6) there may be septic infarcts at any of a variety of other locations in the body including the spleen or the extremities; (7) there may be embolic aneurysms developing in the brain or at other locations in the vasculature or stroke may be a manifestation, one of the most important and most frequently overlooked clinical findings; (8) there may be glomerulonephritis; (9) the blood cultures may be positive multiple times or only a single time for the organism responsible; and (10) in recent years it has been possible to perform echocardiography, which has become an important part of the diagnostic process and criteria.

3. DIAGNOSTIC TESTS

As a result of these multiple clinical manifestations of infective endocarditis, a variety of criteria for the diagnosis have come to be recognized. An important consideration is the nature of the blood cultures. Blood cultures may be positive a single time, or positive twice; usually they are positive more than twice, indeed three, four, or five times for the causative organism. Clinical criteria for infective endocarditis have, therefore, recognized the importance of intermittently positive blood cultures or persistently positive blood cultures. In addition, the presence of the viridans streptococci, the HACEK organisms (*Haemophilus* spp., *Actinobacillus actinomycetemcomitans*, *Cardiobacterium hominis*, *Eikenella* spp., and *Kingella kingae*) or other characteristic endocarditis organisms, is important in the interpretation of the blood cultures. The HACEK group of organisms often grow slowly in culture, and it is thus important to retain and examine these cultures for at least 1 wk.

In the interpretation of the echocardiography results, transesophageal echocardiography (TEE) provides the strongest evidence now and is superior to transthoracic echocardiography (TTE) in supporting the diagnosis of infective endocarditis. There now are criteria based on echocardiography that establish how suspicious for endocarditis the findings are *(10)*. The strongest findings on echocardiography are: (1) an oscillating mass in the path of a blood jet, (2) evidence of an abscess present in the endocardium, and (3) the new dehiscence of a valve, in particular a prosthetic valve. Thus, the final diagnostic criteria for infective endocarditis is new valvular regurgitation with evidence of damage to the valve by the infection *(1,10)*.

There are many occult cases of infective endocarditis in which the clinical circumstances should raise the possibility of this infection despite the presence of perhaps only one or two clinical manifestations. The most important consideration in infective endocarditis is to suspect the diagnosis. There is at times a need to diagnose this illness in the absence of appropriate clinical stigmata. In the 1990s, there has been further evolution of infective endocarditis criteria in a very vital direction.

In the early years of infective endocarditis, the criteria were based on the astute clinical observations of Sir William Osler *(2)*. In the 1980s, a set of criteria developed by von Reyn were of paramount importance and these are shown in Table 1 *(11)* as detailed by Bayer and co-workers *(1)*. However, the von Reyn criteria were hampered in the 1980s by the lack of inclusion of echocardiographic data *(11)*. This omission was corrected by the Duke criteria developed and pioneered by the Duke endocarditis team *(10)*. These important criteria, which have come into common use in the 1990s, are detailed in Tables 2 and 3 *(1)*. The improved diagnostic accuracy of the Duke criteria to the von Reyn criteria is dependent upon inclusion of echocardiography and the superiority of TEE to the earlier TTE. In the 1990s it was shown that the TTE is clearly inferior to the TEE in delineating the cardiac valves, and, in particular, prosthetic cardiac valves *(12,13)*. Further developments of TEE include multiplane studies and color studies, which also may be of great use in clarifying infective endocarditis. A recent study has shown that 80% of vegetations on prosthetic valves can be demonstrated by TEE *(12)*. Moreover, studies continue to show that the elderly greatly benefit from this superiority of TEE and that diagnosis in the elderly is greatly helped by the Duke criteria *(1,12)*.

Despite these developments in diagnosis, there is no substitute for great care in pursuing all aspects of infective endocarditis diagnosis, including the very careful examination of the patient for various stigmata, regular monitoring for fever, auscultation for new or changing murmurs, attention to new echocardiographic results, and monitoring blood culture results. Even with the current advances, there still is a delay in diagnosis

Table 1
Criteria for infective endocarditis

Definite	Direct evidence of infective endocarditis based on histology from surgery or autopsy, or on bacteriology (Gram's stain or culture) of valvular vegetation or peripheral embolus.
Probable	Persistently positive blood cultures[a] plus one of the following: 1. New regurgitant murmur 2. Predisposing heart disease[b] and vascular phenomena[c] Negative or intermittently positive blood cultures[d] plus all of the following: 1. Fever 2. New regurgitant murmur 3. Vascular phenomena
Possible	Persistently positive blood cultures plus one of the following: 1. Predisposing heart disease 2. Vascular phenomena Negative or intermittently positive blood cultures with all of the following: 1. Fever 2. Predisposing heart disease 3. Vascular phenomena For viridans streptococcal cases only: at least two positive blood cultures without an extracardiac source and fever.

[a] At least two blood cultures obtained, with two of two positive, three of three positive, or at least 70% of cultures positive if four or more cultures are obtained.
[b] Definite valvular or congenital heart disease, or a cardiac prosthesis (excluding permanent pacemakers).
[c] Petechiae, splinter hemorrhages, conjunctival hemorrhages, Roth's spots, Osler's nodes, Janeway lesions, aseptic meningitis, glomerulonephritis, and pulmonary, central nervous system, coronary or peripheral emboli.
[d] Any rate of blood culture positivity that does not meet the definition of persistently positive.
Adapted from ref. *(11)* with permission.

of infective endocarditis in the hospital, which ranges between 14 d and 30 d in various studies *(4,12)*.

4. TREATMENT

4.1. General Recommendations

Therapy of infective endocarditis has been evolving over all the years of its recognition and should be guided by the organism involved. The streptococci are the easiest organisms to eradicate in bacterial endocarditis, but there still is a 100% mortality in patients who are not treated for this organism. In the case of streptococci, there are

Table 2
Proposed New Criteria for Diagnosis of Infective Endocarditis

Definite infective endocarditis	Pathologic criteria: Microorganisms: demonstrated by culture or histology in a vegetation, or in a vegetation that has embolized, or in an intracardiac abscess, or Pathologic lesions: vegetation or intracardiac abscess present, confirmed by histology showing active endocarditis Clinical criteria, using specific definitions listed in Table 3: 2 major criteria, or 1 major and 3 minor criteria, or 5 minor criteria
Possible infective endocarditis	Findings consistent with infective endocarditis that fall short of "Definite," but not "rejected"
Rejected	Firm alternate diagnosis for manifestations of endocarditis, or Resolution of manifestations of endocarditis, with antibiotic therapy for 4 days or less, or No pathologic evidence of infective endocarditis at surgery or autopsy, after antibiotic therapy for 4 d or less

unique therapeutic regimens because they are more easily killed than other organisms and on most occasions can be treated simply with penicillin intravenously for 2 wk. Another situation where there may be a special regimen in many cases is the HACEK organisms *(14)*. These pathogens are more difficult to eradicate and thus a 4–6 wk antibiotic regimen of intravenous therapy is usually recommended.

Staphylococcal endocarditis (*S. aureus* and *S. epidermidis*) can present the clinician with some special problems, especially the risk of embolization and resistance to β lactam drugs. Many intravenous antibiotics may be chosen to treat staphylococcal endocarditis, including nafcillin, oxacillin, cefazolin, and vancomycin (β-lactam-resistant strains). Often, two or more antibiotics are used for a synergistic effect; generally an aminoglycoside and/or rifampin are added to a β-lactam or vancomycin. In many cases, the 6-wk duration of treatment is considered to be much safer than a 4-week duration especially if the aortic valve is involved, a prosthetic valve is infected, the organism is relatively resistant to antibiotics (e.g., Gram-negative bacilli, fungi), or the patient suffered complications of infective endocarditis (e.g., emboli, heart failure) *(15)*.

Each bacterial species in infective endocarditis therapy can be expected to respond best according to its specific antibiotic sensitivities. Ample references and reviews are available to guide the clinician in selecting appropriate drugs (3–7,14). It should be noted that the antibiotic sensitivity data for *Enterococcus* spp. may not correlate with clinical outcome; thus, high-dose ampicillin plus an aminoglycoside has been recom-

Table 3
Definitions of terminology used in the proposed new criteria

Major Criteria

Positive blood culture for infective endocarditis

Typical microorganism for infective endocarditis from two separate blood cultures

Viridans streptococci,* *Streptococcus bovis*, HACEK group, or Community-acquired *Staphylococcus aureus* or enterococci, in the absence of a primary focus.

OR

Persistently positive blood culture, defined as recovery of a microorganism consistent with infective endocarditis from:

1. Blood cultures drawn more than 12 hours apart, or
2. All of three or a majority of four or more separate blood cultures, with first and last drawn at least 1 hour apart

Evidence of endocardial involvement

Positive echocardiogram for infective endocarditis

1. Oscillating intracardiac mass, on valve or supporting structures, or in the path of regurgitant jets, or on implanted material, in the absence of an alternative anatomic explanation, or
2. Abscess, or
3. New partial dehiscence of prosthetic valve.

OR

New valvular regurgitation (increase or change in pre-existing murmur not sufficient)

Minor Criteria

Predisposition: predisposing heart condition or intravenous drug use

Fever: $\geq$ 38.0°C (100.4°F)

Vascular phenomena: major arterial emboli, septic pulmonary infarcts, mycotic aneurysm, intracranial hemorrhage, conjunctival hemorrhages, Janeway lesions

Immunologic phenomena: glomenulonephritis, Osler's nodes, Roth spots, rheumatoid factor

Microbiologic evidence: positive blood culture but not meeting major criterion as noted previously† or serologic evidence of active infection with organism consistent with infective endocarditis

Echocardiogram: consistent with infective endocarditis but not meeting major criterion as noted previously

HACEK = *Haemophilus* spp., *Actinobacillus actinomycetemcomitans, Cardiobacterium hominis, Eikenella* spp., and *Kingella kingae*

*Including nutritional variant strains

†Excluding single positive cultures for coagulase-negative staphylococci and organisms that do not cause endocarditis

85

mended. In some instances vancomycin is preferred over ampicillin (plus an aminoglycoside) *(15)*. Care should be taken to use bactericidal antibiotic therapy when available. Antibiotic levels in the patient's serum should exceed the minimum bactericidal concentration for the particular causative agent.

4.2. Empiric Therapy

In older patients with suspected infective endocarditis and who are clinically stable with no complications, antimicrobial therapy can be withheld until a specific pathogen is identified (48 h). Antibiotics should be initiated empirically in suspected cases of infective endocarditis with the following conditions: (1) hypotension or sepsis, (2) new regurgitant murmur, (3) congestive heart failure, (4) embolic events, or (5) aortic valve involvement *(15)*. However, if the index of suspicion for infective endocarditis is high, empiric treatment may be started and then therapy adjusted after culture and sensitivity data return. Appropriate empiric regimens include ampicillin (or penicillin G), nafcillin (or oxacillin) and an aminoglycoside. Vancomycin may be substituted for patients with penicillin allergy. For prosthetic valve endocarditis, treatment can be empirically begun with vancomycin and an aminoglycoside with or without rifampin. The latter regimen may also be useful for "culture-negative" endocarditis (negative blood cultures off antibiotics). Careful monitoring for drug toxicity, especially with aminoglycosides and vancomycin, is essential in the elderly.

4.3. Indications for Surgery

It is important during the therapy of infective endocarditis to always be alert for the possible indications for surgery. Cardiac surgery to remove and replace a diseased valve is often absolutely necessary. A higher mortality will result if surgery is delayed, and especially if cardiac complications (e.g., heart failure) are present. The findings that would usually indicate that surgery is necessary include, the development of new-onset or worsening heart failure; the development of an audible new murmur on therapy, especially a regurgitant lesion, and onset of large numbers of emboli, and, in particular, emboli to crucial organs *(12)*. Another possible indication for surgery would be a mobile large vegetation seen on TEE or TTE. This is an area of continued debate, but with the availability of TEE, it seems that this may become a more common indication for surgery, in particularly in the elderly because of the severe sequelae that result from embolization in elderly patients *(4,12)*.

4.4. Embolic Complications

When assessing an ongoing infective endocarditis case, one of the most important things to consider is the risk of embolization *(16)*. In native valves, some of the risks associated with embolization include double valve endocarditis, mitral valve endocarditis, and certain organisms (e.g., fungi, staphylococci). It is also worth noting that about 50% of all embolic events still occur before the admission of the patient or before the patient's diagnosis is reached. One of the features that appears to decrease the risk of embolization is aspirin therapy *(17)*. Whether other forms of anticoagulation also decrease the risk of embolization is not yet established. Emboli may create a need for further surgery, for instance, splenectomy or drainage of a paraspinous abscess, or resection of a mycotic aneurysm *(4)*. Because of the risk of embolization in the elderly,

Table 4
Infective Endocarditis Chemoprophylaxis
for Oral and Respiratory Tract Procedures

Standard regimen[a]
  Amoxicillin, 3 g orally, given 1 h before procedure.
  For penicillin-allergic patients, give erythromycin ethylsuccinate 800 mg or
    erythromycin stearate 1 g orally 2 h before procedure.

Alternative regimens
  Ampicillin 2 g intravenously or intramuscularly 30 min before procedure.
  Clindamycin 300 mg intravenously 30 min before procedure.
  Vancomycin 1 g intravenously infused over 60 min, beginning 1 h before procedure.
    No repeat dose necessary.

---

[a]Includes prosthetic heart valves and high-risk patients. Notice that postprocedure doses are eliminated.

Table 5
Infective Endocarditis Chemoprophylaxis
for Gastrointestinal and Genitourinary Procedures

Ampicillin 2 g intravenously or intramuscularly and gentamicin[a] 1.5 mg/kg (not to
  exceed 80 mg) intravenously or intramuscularly 30 min before the procedure (adjust
  dose and interval for gentamicin in patients with renal dysfunction). (Amoxicillin 1.5 g
  orally 6 h after initial dose may replace parenteral ampicillin.)[b]

In penicillin-allergic patients, ampicillin is replaced by vancomycin 1 g intravenously
  (infused over 60 min) before procedure (or adjusted for renal dysfunction).
  Gentamicin[a] is administered as previously described.[b]

---

[a]Equivalent aminoglycoside may be substituted.
[b]Notice that post-procedure doses are eliminated.
Data from ref. *(24)*.

which produces many adverse later effects, all measures that could decrease the risk of embolization should be considered.

5. PREVENTION OF ENDOCARDITIS

In the area of prevention, there is a very extensive literature and a continuing evaluation of the necessity of prophylaxis against infective endocarditis in patients with various valvular or endocardial lesions. Tables 4 and 5 show the latest American Heart Association guidelines for prophylaxis of infective endocarditis *(18)*. Note that postprocedure antibiotics are no longer recommended. These prophylaxis guidelines are not meant to apply to all oral-dental procedures but to procedures that are likely to lead to bleeding and bacteremia, such as extraction or scaling and root planing. In the area of urological and gastrointestinal procedures, high risk for bacteremia is also the concern.

Prophylaxis is complex and much debated because of the concerns of the larger dental and medical community about the possible adverse effects of the use of antibiotics in their outpatients and the use of antibiotics before various procedures. The research underpinnings of the need for prophylaxis are not complete. It appears that prophylaxis is very clearly indicated in the prosthetic valve patient *(19)*. However, the effectiveness of the prophylaxis given (antibiotics) may not entirely be related to killing of the microorganisms by the antibiotic. There may be effects on organism adherence. Microorganisms that are causing bacteremia must adhere to the native or prosthetic valve and form a colony there in order to cause infective endocarditis. There are very complex mechanisms by which organisms adhere to native or prosthetic valves *(20)*.

Because it would be unethical to return to a situation of zero prophylaxis, it may be impossible to complete our knowledge about the necessity of prophylaxis once and for all. It would not be ethical to have the no-therapy arms of the study, which would be necessary for such a determination.

It is possible, due to the changes in oral flora that are present in the elderly, that prophylaxis needs may change in the future. For instance, the overwhelming presence of streptococci in the mouths of many people may change to other organisms as they age *(21)*. The new predominant oral organism after antibiotics, dentures, or implantations may be *S. aureus*, lactobacilli, yeast, or still other organisms *(21)*.

There also may be increased prophylaxis required for the elderly for a variety of in-hospital procedures. As much as possible, we should base prophylaxis on the true rates of bacteremia in the elderly who undergo various in-hospital procedures. However, the study of such rates of bacteremia is difficult. Bacteremia with some oral procedures has been carefully studied *(22)*. Often it is necessary to proceed with prophylaxis in the absence of full knowledge about risks. The risk of reaction to the antibiotic given in prophylaxis is usually low compared with the risk of bacteremia and infective endocarditis resulting from the procedure. Ongoing studies and evaluation of the various needs for prophylaxis need to continue.

The overall prevention of infective endocarditis still depends not only on prophylactic antibiotics or other measures but on care to avoid unnecessary bacteremia in the elderly. Bacteremia from dental procedures and oral diseases can ultimately be prevented only by good dental and oral care, usually initiated by the patients themselves. Good dental care and self-care are probably associated with a lower risk of bacteremia due to dental sources *(22)*. In addition, ignored skin problems are a frequent source of bacteremia in the elderly, which can only be avoided by the person's own careful care of their skin and attention to periodic skin infections such as boils, which will arise throughout the person's life. In a recent review, Kjerulf and colleagues have pointed out the need not only for earlier detection of infective endocarditis and earlier antibiotic therapy, but the need for educating patients who already have cardiac disease or cardiac valve prostheses *(23)*. The patient's own vigilance for reducing the risk of infective endocarditis or for being aware of the early symptoms and signs of this infection may become one of the patient's best protective mechanisms. In addition, there is need to develop further early diagnostic tests that are able to detect the presence of infective endocarditis *(23)*. Overall, it is to be expected that infective endocarditis will become an ever more important infection in the elderly. The older patient will continue to benefit from the astute clinician's attention to the clinical manifestations, to the latest diagnostic tests and criteria, to ongoing improvements in therapy, and to the prevention of infective endocarditis.

REFERENCES

1. Bayer, A. S., Ward, J. I., Ginzton, L.E., et al. (1994) Evaluation of new criteria for the diagnosis of infective endocarditis. *Am. J. Med.* **96,** 211–219.
2. Osler, W. (1885) Gulstonian lectures on malignant endocarditis. *Lancet* **1,** 415.
3. Korzeniowski, O. M. and Kaye, D. (1992) Endocarditis, in *Infectious Diseases* (Gorbach, S.L., Bartlett, J.G., and Blacklow, N.R., eds.), W.B. Saunders Co., Philadelphia, PA, pp. 548–555.
4. Terpenning, M. S., Buggy, B. P., and Kauffman, C. A. (1987) Infective endocarditis: clinical features in young and elderly patients. *Am. J. Med.* **83,** 626–634.
5. Fisher, E. A., Fisher, L. L., Fuster, V., et al (1998) Infective endocarditis: New perspectives on an old disease. *Infect. Dis. Clin. Pract.* **7,** 12–24.
6. Cantrell, M. and Yoshikawa, T. T. (1984) Infective endocarditis in the aging patient. *Gerontology* **30,** 316–326.
7. Yoshikawa, T. T. (1987) Antimicrobial therapy: special considerations, in *Aging and Clinical Practice: Infectious Diseases. Diagnosis and Treatment* (Yoshikawa, T. T., Norman, D., eds.), Igaku–Shoin, New York, pp. 32–54.
8. Terpenning, M. S. and Dominguez, B. L. (1994) Endocarditis of oral origin (abstr.), in *Proceedings of the International Association for Dental Research*, March 9–13, Seattle, WA.
9. Hamada, S. and Slade, H. D. (1980) Biology, immunology and cariogenicity of *Streptococcus mutans. Microbiol. Rev.* **44,** 331–336.
10. Durack, D. T., Lakes, A. S., Bright, D. K., et al, and the Duke Endocarditis Service (1994) New criteria for diagnosis of infective endocarditis: Utilization of specific echocardiographic findings. *Am. J. Med.* **96,** 200–209.
11. von Reyn, C. F., Levy, B. S., Arbeit, R. D., et al. (1981) Infective endocarditis: an analysis based on strict case definitions. *Ann. Intern. Med.* **94,** 505–518.
12. Schulz, R., Werner, G. S., Fuchs, J. B., et al. (1996) Clinical outcome and echocardiographic findings of native and prosthetic valve endocarditis in the 1990s. *Eur. Heart J.* **17,** 281–288.
13. Daniel, W. G., Mugge, A., Grote, J., et al. (1993) Comparison of transthoracic and transesophageal echocardiography for detection of abnormalities of prosthetic and bioprosthetic valves in the mitral and aortic positions. *Am. J. Cardiol.* **71,** 210–215.
14. Wilson, W. R., Karchmer, A. W., Dajani, A. S., et al. (1995) Antibiotic treatment of adults with infective endocarditis due to streptococci, enterococci, staphylococci, and HACEK microorganisms. *JAMA* **274,** 1706–1713.
15. Terpenning, M. S. (1992) Infective endocarditis, in *Clinics in Geriatric Medicine* (Yoshikawa, T. T., ed.), vol. 8, W. B. Saunders Co., Philadelphia, PA, pp. 903–912.
16. Heinle, S., Wilderman, N., Harrison, J. K., et al and the Duke Endocarditis Service (1994) Value of transthoracic echocardiography in predicting embolic events in active infective endocarditis. *Am. J. Cardiol.* **74,** 799–801.
17. Schünemann, S., Werner, G. S., Schulz, R., et al. (1997) Embolische komplikationem bei bakterieller endokarditis. *Z. Kardiol.* **86,** 1017–1025.
18. American Heart Association Guidelines for the Treatment of Infective Endocarditis (1990) *JAMA* **264,** 2929, adapted to 1999.
19. Santinga, J. T., Kirsh, M., and Fekety, F. R. (1984) Factors affecting survival in prosthetic valve endocarditis. Review of the effectiveness of prophylaxis. *Chest* **85,** 471–481.
20. Jones, G. (1977) The attachment of bacteria to the surfaces of animal cells, in *Microbial Interactions: Receptors and Recognition* (Reissig, J. L., ed.), Chapman and Hall, New York, pp. 139–176.
21. Loesche, W. J., Schork, A., Terpenning, M. S., et al. (1995) Factors which influence levels of selected organisms in saliva of older individuals. *J. Clin. Microbiol.* **33,** 2550–2557.

22. Hockett, R. N., Loesche, W. J., and Sodeman, T. M. (1977) Bacteraemia in asymptomatic human subjects. *Arch. Oral Biol.* **22,** 91–98.
23. Kjerulf, A., Trede, M., and Aldershvile, J. (1998) Bacterial endocarditis at a tertiary hospital–How do we improve diagnosis and delay of treatment? *Cardiology* **89,** 79–86.
24. Dajani, A. S., Bisno, A. L., Chung, K. J. et al. (1990) Prevention of bacterial endocarditis. Recommendations by the American Heart Association. *JAMA* **264,** 2919.

9

Intraabdominal Infections

Brian Scott Campbell and Samuel E. Wilson

Intraabdominal infections are becoming more common in the geriatric patient, which is the fastest-growing segment of the population in North America. Due to varied and sometimes masked manifestations of illnesses in this population, the diagnosis of an intraabdominal infection may be challenging. The causes and incidence of intraabdominal infections are different in older patients when compared with younger patients. In older adults cholecystitis, diverticulitis, and intestinal obstruction, perforation, and ischemia are more common (*see* Table 1). Different or atypical presentations of these disorders may lead to delays in the diagnosis of abdominal complaints in elderly patients. Lack of fevers and leukocytosis are common in older patients with intraabdominal infections *(1)*. Furthermore, mental confusion or dementia, as well as coexisting illnesses, may confound and complicate the history and physical examination. Despite these difficulties the diagnosis of intraabdominal infections in the elderly should not be delayed because this leads to higher morbidity and mortality.

1. DIVERTICULITIS AND DIVERTICULOSIS

1.1. Epidemiology and Clinical Relevance

In 20th century Western civilization, diverticula of the colon is becoming increasingly prevalent in older patients. This disorder is associated with increasing age and low-fiber diets favored in North America. Colonic diverticula are herniations of mucosa and submucosa through the circular muscle of the bowel wall. These are "false" diverticula because only two of the three layers of the intestine are represented in the wall; the lack of a muscularis portion makes these more susceptible to perforation. The prevalence of diverticular disease in Western countries ranges between 35 and 50% *(2)*. In the elderly the prevalence increases dramatically—from 5% at age 40 to as high as 65% at age 65 *(3)*. Only about 10–25% of persons with colonic diverticulosis will develop symptomatic diverticulitis *(4)*. Although colon carcinoma is the most common source of gastrointestinal blood loss, diverticulosis, especially right-sided lesions, may cause massive lower gastrointestinal bleeding in the elderly.

The inflammation of one or more diverticula of the colon is termed diverticulitis. The severity of this process ranges from a localized inflammation to free perforation and peritonitis. The sigmoid colon is involved in 90% of diverticulitis *(5)*. Right-sided diverticulitis represents only 5% of cases; however, it can have presenting symptoms and signs indistinguishable from appendicitis, and this should be included in the differential diagnosis when evaluating patients with right lower-quadrant pain.

From: *Infectious Disease in the Aging*
Edited by: Thomas T. Yoshikawa and Dean C. Norman
© Humana Press Inc., Totowa, NJ

Table 1
Rates of Disease in 2406 Patients >50 Yr Old and 6317 Patients ≤50 Yr Old
Presenting with Acute Abdominal Pain from the OMGE Series

Disease	Patients ≤50 yr old (%)	Patients >50 yr old (%)
Nonspecific abdominal pain	39.5	15.7
Appendicitis	32.0	15.2
Cholecystitis	6.3	20.9
Obstruction	2.5	12.3
Pancreatitis	1.6	7.3
Diverticular disease	<0.1	5.5
Cancer	<0.1	4.1
Hernia	<0.1	3.1
Vascular	<0.1	2.3

OMGE = Organisation Mondiale de Gastroenterologie. From ref. *(26)*.

1.2. Clinical Manifestations

Acute diverticulitis has a similar presentation to acute appendicitis; however, it usually presents in the left lower quadrant. Gradual onset of pain, described as a dull ache, which is steady or colicky in nature, can be variable in location due to redundancy in the sigmoid colon. This may lead to suprapubic, generalized lower-quadrant pain and/or right lower-quadrant pain. Defecation may exacerbate the pain, but constipation is the rule. Anorexia and nausea are common, but vomiting is a rare complaint. In the elderly suprapubic pain and dysuria may be a sign of diverticulitis and should not necessarily be assumed to be cystitis. Physical findings consist of a low-grade fever, mild abdominal distention, left lower-quadrant tenderness, palpable mass, and/or leukocytosis. Rectal examination may elicit tenderness, and in 25% of patients guaiac (blood)-positive stools may be found. Bowel sounds are usually present.

1.3. Diagnostic Tests

Acute abdominal radiographic series may show nonspecific findings of ileus or obstruction, free air in the bladder indicating colovesicular fistulae, soft-tissue mass in left lower quadrant, and/or pneumoperitoneum from free perforation. The initial radiographic study of choice is abdominal computed tomographic (CT) scan with water-soluble contrast. This imaging study is 93% sensitive and 100% specific for diverticulitis. In identification of complications of diverticulosis, a CT scan is superior to barium enema, which was formerly the study of choice. Findings on CT scan include inflammation of pericolonic fat, single or multiple diverticula, thickened bowel wall to 4 mm, and/or peridiverticular abscess. Barium enema and lower endoscopy should be avoided during the acute attack due to possible leakage of barium into the peritoneal cavity, and the risk of perforation from high pressure.

1.4. Treatment

The initial treatment of uncomplicated acute diverticulitis is conservative medical therapy. This consists of bowel rest, intravenous fluid hydration, and antibiotics that are active against normal gut flora (aerobic and anaerobic bacteria). Once resolution of the inflammatory process is appreciated, oral feeding may slowly be advanced. The patient should also be started on a high-fiber diet. The patient will need to be evaluated with colonoscopy and/or barium enema several weeks after the resolution of the attack. Patients who fail to respond within 24–48 h may need urgent surgical intervention. A diverticular abscess can be temporarily drained by CT guidance for stabilization prior to definitive surgical treatment.

Surgical treatment of complicated diverticulitis, such as peritonitis, abscess, obstruction, or fistula is mandatory. Patients with recurrent diverticulitis or a first episode of acute diverticulitis before the age of 50 yr are at high risk and should undergo elective resection after resolution the disease.

2. CHOLECYSTITIS

2.1. Epidemiology and Clinical Relevance

The most common cause for surgical intraabdominal infections in the elderly is acute cholecystitis, and the number of cholecystectomies in the elderly is increasing *(6)*. The incidence of this disease is higher in the female. However, the female-to-male ratio lowers from 3:1 in younger adults to 1.5:1 in patients older than 50. Cholelithiasis accounts for 95% of acute cholecystitis, with the other 5% termed acalculous cholecystitis. The incidence of cholelithiasis increases with age, ranging from 25–40% for those in their sixties to over 50% in those 70 yr and older *(7)*. Acute cholecystitis appears to be caused by obstruction of the cystic duct by an impacted stone. The sequelae of this may be simple acute cholecystitis, gangrenous cholecystitis, perforation of the gallbladder with possible bile peritonitis, or cholecystoenteric fistula. If a cholecystoenteric fistula is found in the presence of small bowel obstruction, the possibility of a gallstone lodged in the distal ileum should be considered.

2.2. Clinical Manifestations

In the elderly, biliary disease should be considered foremost in the differential diagnosis of the physician when eliciting the history of upper abdominal pain. The pain may be steady and persistent in the right subcostal, epigastric region or both. Often the pain may develop after ingestion of a meal. Radiation of this pain may be to the back or to the tip of the right scapula. Also, irritation of the diaphragm may cause right shoulder pain. Nausea and vomiting are common in about 65% of patients. Fever, which is found in 80% of all acute cholecystitis patients, may be absent in the elderly, especially if they are taking nonsteroidal anti-inflammatory drugs. The physical examination should elicit tenderness in the right upper quadrant, epigastrium, or both. A common physical finding is inspiratory arrest during deep palpation of the right upper quadrant, which is called Murphy's sign. Rigidity, rebound tenderness, and/or a palpable mass may be found as well. In 10% of patients with acute cholecystitis, jaundice can occur due to bile pigments entering into the circulation from the damaged mucosa of the gallbladder *(8)*. Choledocholithiasis should always be suspected in the presence of jaundice. This is because the incidence of common bile duct stones increases with age to about 20% in the elderly patient with acute cholecystitis.

2.3. Diagnostic Tests

Laboratory studies may show increased leukocytosis, increase in serum bilirubin, and/or an increase in serum amylase. Ultrasound examination of the right upper quadrant is highly sensitive, approximately 95%, in showing gallstones. Other findings of acute cholecystitis with ultrasonography are dilated and thickened gallbladder wall, pericholecystic fluid, and or ultrasonographic Murphy's sign. When the diagnosis is still in question, a cholescintigraphic study using 99m-labeled derivative of iminodiacetic acid (HIDA) may be used. In the presence of acute cholecystitis, the gallbladder will not be seen. This indicates cystic duct obstruction. The HIDA scan is 100% sensitive and 95% specific for the diagnosis of acute cholecystitis *(9)*.

2.4. Treatment

In the presence of symptomatic cholelithiasis, elective laparoscopic cholecystectomy is associated with reduced morbidity and mortality when compared with emergent surgery. Acute cholecystitis in the elderly is associated with a higher morbidity when compared with the general population with the same disease. Emergent cholecystectomy is associated with a mortality rate of 10% in the elderly. Furthermore, the conversion rate of laparoscopic cholecystectomy to open cholecystectomy can be as high as 50% *(10)*. In the majority of elderly patients, medical therapies for acute cholecystitis will fail *(11)*. Early cholecystectomy has a lower morbidity and mortality than medical management with elective cholecystectomy *(12)*. Intraoperative cholangiography is encouraged in the elderly due to the increased risk of concomitant common bile duct stones. In the unstable patient, cholecystostomy may be an immediate alternative to emergent cholecystectomy. This may be performed through a limited incision under local or general anesthesia, or by image-guided percutaneous catheter placement.

3. APPENDICITIS IN THE ELDERLY

3.1. Epidemiology and Clinical Relevance

Appendicitis in the elderly is associated with a higher mortality rate, approximately 10% in patients 70 and older, when compared with the general population *(13,14)*. Although the incidence is more common in the second and third decade of life, appendicitis still accounts for 15% of all surgical emergencies in the elderly *(15)*. Prompt diagnosis, followed by definitive surgical treatment, reduces morbidity and mortality in this age group.

The diagnosis of appendicitis may not be as simple as in the young adult and this may delay treatment. The classic findings of nausea, vomiting, anorexia, fever, right lower-quadrant pain, and leukocytosis may not all be found in the elderly patient. Furthermore, the symptoms and signs of acute appendicitis are similar to other disease processes common in the older patient, resulting in the delayed diagnosis of appendicitis *(see* Table 2). Physical examination will indicate tenderness to palpation, involuntary guarding, and/or rebound tenderness in the right lower quadrant, which are similar in the younger patient. Typical physical findings in younger patients, which may not be present in the elderly patient, are fever, leukocytosis, abdominal distention, psoas sign, decreased bowel sounds, and/or rectal tenderness.

3.2. Diagnostic Tests

Radiographic studies can be used to help confirm the diagnosis of appendicitis or exclude other causes of the patient's symptoms. Plain radiographs are not sensitive or specific; however, plain abdominal radiographs may show appendiceal fecaliths, gas in the appendix, localized paralytic ileus, loss of right psoas shadow, and/or free air. It

Table 2
Difference in Presentation of Acute Appendicitis in 366 Patients >50 Yr Old and 1970 patients ≤50 Yr Old From the OMGE Series

Clinical feature	Patients ≤ 50 yr old (%)	Patients > 50 yr old (%)
Generalized pain	2.2	13.1
Pain duration >24 h	57.2	75.4
Previous surgery	3.2	21.0
Distention	6.2	23.8
Generalized tenderness	2.1	14.2
Rigidity	18.9	40.1
Decreased bowel sounds	19.0	38.0
Mass	4.0	12.1

OMGE = Organisation Mondiale de Gastroenterologie. From ref. *(26)*

is more useful in excluding other illness common to the elderly. Ultrasonography can be used in the evaluation of acute appendicitis and is associated with 85% sensitivity and 92% specificity *(16)*. The two primary criteria used for ultrasonic diagnosis of appendicitis are noncompressible appendix with a diameter of 7 mm or greater or appendicolithiasis. Findings of gas bubbles in the appendicial lumen, localized fluid collection, and/or periappendiceal abscess are also suggestive of the diagnosis. CT scan may also be used in the diagnosis of acute appendicitis. This study has a higher sensitivity and similar specificity as ultrasonography. Presence of pericecal inflammation or fluid collections are suggestive of appendicitis on CT scans.

3.3. Treatment

The treatment of acute appendicitis in the elderly is emergent appendectomy. This should be undertaken within 24 h of symptoms because of the increased risk of perforation past this time frame. If the diagnosis is unclear, diagnostic laparoscopy may be used in the elderly patient to avoid untimely delays in diagnosis *(17,18)*. This procedure can include laparoscopic appendectomy when the diagnosis is made intraoperatively.

4. BOWEL OBSTRUCTION IN THE ELDERLY

Causes of bowel obstruction usually specific to the elderly include sigmoid volvulus, Ogilvie's Syndrome, colon carcinoma, and gallstone ileus. These conditions in the elderly patient can lead to gangrene with resulting perforation.

4.1. Sigmoid Volvulus

Sigmoid volvulus is 20 times more likely in the patient age 60 yr and greater *(19)*. This age association may be due to acquired redundancy of the sigmoid colon. High-residue diets are believed to be the causative factor in developing a redundant sigmoid *(20)*. Other factors associated with volvulus are Parkinson's disease, dementia including Alzheimer's disease, bedridden state, and prior abdominal operations, all of which increase in frequency in the elderly patient. Sigmoid volvulus usually presents as acute onset of colicky abdominal pain, distention, and obstipation. When strangulation has occurred, the patient can present with generalized abdominal pain, tenderness to palpation, fevers, leukocytosis, and hypotension. Plain abdominal radiographs characteristically show a dilated sigmoid loop with a "bird's beak" pointing to the site of obstruction. If the plain abdominal radiographs are equivocal, a barium enema may be used. However, this test is contraindicated if strangulation is suspected. Decompression with endoscopy and rectal tube placement should be performed in the absence of peritoneal signs. This is successful in 70–80% of patients. The risk of recurrence of sigmoid volvulus is high (approximately 55–90%), therefore the patient should be evaluated for elective sigmoid resection. If the sigmoid volvulus has progressed to gangrene, mortality approaches 50–70%. When peritoneal signs are present emergent laparotomy is indicated.

4.2. Ogilvie's Syndrome

Ogilvie's syndrome, also called colonic pseudo-obstruction, usually occurs in the elderly bedridden patient. When cecal distension approaches 12 cm, the risk of gangrene, infarction, and perforation increases. When perforation and gangrene occur, mortality is 50%. As in sigmoid volvulus, colonoscopic decompression is the treatment of choice. However, if endoscopy fails or the patient is unstable, cecostomy or laporatomy with resection may be indicated.

4.3. Gallstone Ileus

An interesting, yet rare, cause for small bowel obstruction in the elderly is gallstone ileus. This is caused by the passage of a large biliary calculus from the gallbladder to the distal iliem through a cholecystenteric fistula. This disorder carries an overall mortality rate of 15%. Rigler's triad, which includes small bowel obstruction, ectopic gallstones, and pneumobilia, characterizes this disorder. Enterolithotomy, which carries an operative mortality of 12%, is the procedure of choice *(21)*. A one-stage procedure of enterolithotomy, cholecystectomy, and fistula repair carries a mortality of 17% *(22)*.

4.4. Carcinoma of the Colon

Cancer of the colon and rectum is the second most common cancer in western countries with an incidence of 150,000 new cases per year. The incidence increases with age, with up to three-quarters of the cases occurring in patients 65 yr and older. Colorectal cancers may present with obstruction and/or peritonitis. The mortality from complicated obstruction from colorectal cancer is as high as 50%, and long-term survival after resection is greatly reduced. This is partially due to more advanced disease and metastasis in patients with this complication *(23)*. In the critically ill elderly patient with perforation or obstruction, a bypass or diversionary procedure should be considered. Definitive treatment may then be performed on an elective basis.

5. ACUTE MESENTERIC INFARCTION

5.1. Epidemiology and Clinical Relevance

Acute mesenteric infarction can lead to a catastrophic intraabdominal infection in the elderly with mortality rates as high as 90%. Arterial emboli to the mesenteric vessels occur in 30% of patients with this disorder. These emboli originate most commonly from a mural thrombus in an infarcted left ventricle or a fibrillating left atrium. Thrombosis of a mesenteric vessel occurs in 25% of patients and is due to atherosclerotic stenosis. This is usually preceded by intestinal angina. Other less common causes of acute mesenteric infarction are thrombosis of mesenteric veins, dissecting aneurysms, fusiform aneurysms, and connective tissue disorders. Mesenteric vascular occlusion leads to necrosis of villi, mucosal sloughing, ulceration, and bleeding. Even without full-thickness necrosis, perforation, sepsis, multiorgan failure, and death may occur.

5.2. Clinical Manifestation

Pain out of proportion to the physical examination is one of the hallmarks of acute mesenteric ischemia. This pain is severe, poorly localized, and can be associated with nausea, vomiting, diarrhea, and/or constipation. When late in the presentation or when perforation occurs the patient may develop abdominal distention, tenderness to palpation, hypotension, and/or generalized peritonitis. Guaiac-positive stools are present in 75–95% of patients. Leukocytosis, hyperamylasemia, increased alkaline phosphatase, elevated serum lactate, hyperphosphatemia, and acidosis may be observed.

5.3. Diagnostic Tests

Acute abdominal radiographic series are commonly unremarkable early in ischemia. However, as the disease progresses the radiographs can show dilated loops of small intestine containing air–fluid levels, "thumbprinting" of the bowel wall, intramural gas, and/or free air *(24)*. CT scans of the abdomen can be useful, especially to exclude other abdominal pathology. Findings on CT scan may show bowel wall thickening, intramural gas, dilatation of bowel loops, fluid-filled loops, increase attenuation of mesenteric fat, and/or mesenteric or portal venous gas. In evaluation of mesenteric venous thrombosis CT scan is the study of choice and may detect superior mesenteric artery thrombosis. Despite large numbers of negative studies angiography can be a precise method for diagnosing occlusive intestinal ischemia *(25)*.

5.4. Treatment

If peritoneal signs are present, exploratory laparotomy is warranted. Treatment will be focused on resection of nonviable bowel and restoration of intestinal blood flow. Transarterial embolectomy may be attempted in the stable patient. Thrombolytic therapy has yet to be proven an effective treatment, however, anticoagulant therapy may be used for prophylaxis against further emboli.

REFERENCES

1. Potts, F. E. and Vukov L. F. (1999) Utility of fever and leukocytosis in acute surgical abdomens in octogenarians and beyond. *J. Gerontol.* **54A (No2),** 54–58.
2. Hughes, L. E. (1969) Postmortem survey of diverticular disease of the colon: I. Diverticulosis and diverticulitis. *Gut* **10,** 344–351.
3. Painter, N. S. and Burkitt, D. P. (1975) Diverticular disease of the colon, a 20th century problem. *Clin. Gastroenterol.* **4,** 3–21.
4. Parks, T. G. (1975) Natural history of diverticular disease of the colon. *Clin. Gastroenterol.* **4,** 53–69.
5. Rodkey, G. V. and Welch, C. E. (1984) Changing patterns in the surgical treatment of diverticular disease. *Ann. Surg.* **200,** 466–478.

6. Dietrick, N. A., Cacioppo, J. C., and Davis, R. P. (1988) The vanishing elective cholecystectomy. *Arch. Surg.* **123,** 810–814.

7. Crump, C. (1932) The incidence of gallstones and gallbladder disease. *Surg. Gynecol. Obstet.* **55,** 666–667.

8. Ostrow, J. D. (1967) Absorption of bile pigments by the gallbladder. *J. Clin. Invest.* **46,** 2035–2052.

9. Weissmann, H. S., Badia, J., Sugarman, G. A., et al. (1981) Spectrum of 99m-Tc-IDA cholescintigraphic patterns in acute cholecystitits. *Radiology* **138,** 167–175.

10. Magnuson, T. H., Ratner, L. E., Zenilman, M. E., et al. (1997) Laparoscopic cholecystectomy: applicability in the geriatric population. *Am. Surg.* **63,** 91–96.

11. Morrow, D. J., Thompson, J., Wilson, S. E., et al. (1978) Acute cholecystitis in the elderly. *Arch. Surg.* **113,** 1149–1152.

12. Edlund, G. and Ljungdahl, M. (1990) Acute cholecystitis in the elderly. *Am. J. Surg.* **159(3),** 414–416.

13. Owens, B. J. and Hamit, H. F. (1978) Appendicitis in the elderly. *Ann. Surg.* **187,** 392–396.

14. Addis, D. G., Shaffer, N., and Fowler, B. S. (1990) The epidemiology of appendicitis and appendectomy in the United States. *Am. J. Epidemiol.* **132,** 910–925.

15. Telfer, S., Fenyo, G., Holt, P. R., et al. (1988) Acute abdominal pain in patients over 50 yr of age. *Scand. J. Gastroenterol.* **23(Suppl) 144,** 47–55.

16. Orr, R. K., Porter, D., Hartman, D., et al. (1995) Ultrasonography to evaluate adults for appendicitis: decision-making based on meta-analysis and probabilistic reasoning. *Acad. Emerg. Med.* **2,** 644–650.

17. Geis, W. P. and Kim, H. C. (1995) Use of laparoscopy in the diagnosis and treatment of patients with surgical abdominal sepsis. *Surg. Endoscopy* **9,** 178–182.

18. Hubbel, D. S., Barton, W. K., and Solomon, O. D. (1960) Appendicitis in older people. *Surg. Gynecol. Obstet.* **110,** 289–292.

19. Ballantyne, G. H., Brender, M. D., and Beard, R. W (1985) Volvulus of the colon. *Ann. Surg.* **205,** 83–92.

20. Ballantyne, G. H., (1982) Review of sigmoid volvulus: clinical patterns and pathogenesis. *Dis. Colon Rectum* **25,** 823–830.

21. Reisner, R. M. and Cohen, J. R. (1994) Gallstone ileus: a review of 1001 reported cases. *Am. Surg.* **60,** 441–446.

22. Berliner, S. D. and Burson, L. C. (1965) One stage repair for cholecystoduodenal fistula and gallstone ileus. *Arch. Surg.* **90,** 313–316.

23. Kyllonen, L. (1987) Obstruction and perforation complicating colorectal carcinoma: an epidemiologic and clinical study with special references to incidence and survival. *Acta. Chir. Scand.* **153,** 607–614.

24. Klein, H. M., Lensing, R., Klosterhalfen, B., et al. (1995) Diagnostic imaging of mesenteric infarction. *Radiology* **197,** 79–82.

25. Boley, S. J., Sprayregan, S, Siegelman, S. S., et al. (1977) Initial results from an aggressive roentgenological and surgical approach to acute mesenteric ischemia. *Surgery* **82,** 848–855.

26. Telfer, S., Fenyo, G., Holt, P. R., et al. (1988) Acute abdominal pain in patients over 50 yr of age. *Scand. J. Gastroenterol.* **23(Suppl 144),** 47–50.

10

Urinary Tract Infection

Lindsay E. Nicolle

1. CLINICAL RELEVANCE

Urinary infection is an important problem in elderly populations. As with any clinical problem in this group, the significance and manifestations vary depending on the characteristics of the population. Thus, urinary infection needs to be considered within a continuum from the ambulant, well elderly in the community to the highly functionally disabled long-term care facility resident. There are also special considerations for elderly subjects with long-term indwelling catheters.

The kidney, ureters, bladder, and proximal urethra are normally sterile. Urinary tract infection is the presence of significant numbers of bacteria within the genitourinary tract, and may be asymptomatic or symptomatic. Bacteriuria simply means bacteria in the urine. It is usually used in the context of "significant bacteriuria" and is interchangeable with the term urinary tract infection. While the term "bladder colonization" is sometimes used in the context of asymptomatic urinary infection, it has no identified clinical relevance for urinary infection in the elderly. An elderly individual with bacteriuria usually has evidence for a host response within the genitourinary tract. Thus, the term "colonization" is not used here, and the term "bacteriuria" is used interchangeably with asymptomatic urinary tract infection.

1.1. Prevalence and Incidence

Urinary tract infection is the most common bacterial infection in elderly populations. Young, sexually active women have a prevalence of positive urine cultures of 2–5%, but this increases to 5–10% for women aged 65 yr and older (1). A positive urine culture is uncommon in younger men, but the prevalence for those aged 65 yr and older is 5% or higher. Residents of long-term care facilities have an extraordinary prevalence of bacteriuria, 25–50% for women and 15–40% for men. The prevalence increases in frequency with increasing levels of functional disability in the institutionalized populations.

The incidence of urinary infection is also high. There are no population-based studies of urinary infection for the well, ambulant elderly living in the community, so for this group the incidence of infection is not well described. In one cohort of elderly male outpatients at a veteran's hospital, 10% of 209 men initially not bacteriuric developed bacteriuria during a mean follow-up of 2.8 yr (2). However, 76% of these elderly ambulatory men cleared their asymptomatic bacteriuria spontaneously.

From: *Infectious Disease in the Aging*
Edited by: Thomas T. Yoshikawa and Dean C. Norman
© Humana Press Inc., Totowa, NJ

There are high rates of acquisition of bacteriuria in any institutionalized elderly population. For male residents of one nursing home, an incidence of urinary infection of 45/100 patient yr was observed, and 10% of nonbacteriuric residents become bacteriuric every 3 mo *(3)*. Women in a nursing home initially identified as bacteriuric and not treated with antibiotics had 87 new infections/100 patient yr *(4)*. The high frequency of urinary infection in institutionalized populations is also described by the "turnover" of bacteriuria *(1)*. From 10–20% of initially nonbacteriuric institutionalized men or women will have become bacteriuric at 6–12 mo, whereas 25–30% of those with bacteriuria will become nonbacteriuric in the same time period. Thus, urinary infection is extremely common and dynamic in elderly populations.

The burden of symptomatic infection in elderly community populations is not well described. One clinical parameter, hospitalization rates for pyelonephritis, was reported to be 10–15/10,000 population over age 70 yr, with similar rates for men and women *(5)*. Mims and colleagues *(2)* reported a frequency of symptomatic urinary infection of 0.17/1000 d in elderly ambulatory men. Elderly ambulant women resident in a geriatric apartment had an incidence of symptomatic infection of 0.9/ 1000 d *(6)*. The incidence of symptomatic urinary infection for the institutionalized population has been reported to be 1.0–2.4 per 1000 resident days *(7)*, but as low as 0.11–0.15 symptomatic infections per bacteriuric year (number of symptomatic infections divided by total number of symptomatic and asymptomatic infections for entire year) when more restrictive definitions are used *(3,4)*. The incidence of urinary infection with fever was reported to be 0.49–1.04/10,000 resident days in two large nursing homes *(8)*.

1.2. Pathogenesis

The reasons for the very high frequency of urinary infection in elderly ambulatory populations, although not fully described, are multiple *(1)*. Changes in the immune system with aging have not been shown to be associated with increased urinary infection. For men, prostatic hypertrophy resulting in urinary retention and turbulent urethral urine flow is the most important contributing factor *(9)*. When bacterial prostatitis occurs, recurrent urinary infection from a prostatic source is common because of limited diffusion of antimicrobials into the prostate or the presence of infected stones. Other genitourinary abnormalities that promote infection and occur with increased frequency in elderly men include urethral or ureteric strictures due to fibrosis or tumors, and renal or bladder stones.

Older women with a history of recurrent urinary infection in the premenopausal period have an increased occurrence of urinary infection. Postmenopausal women with an increased residual urine volume after bladder emptying or a history of genitourinary surgery are more likely to have bacteriuria. An aging-associated decline in the estrogen effect on the genitourinary mucosa may contribute to an increased frequency of urinary infection, but further study to clarify this observation is needed. Sexual intercourse is the most important precipitating factor for urinary infection in premenopausal women, but its contribution to infection in postmenopausal women has not been studied.

For institutionalized men and women, the prevalence of bacteriuria is greatest in the most functionally impaired. These individuals usually have incontinence of bladder or

Table 1
Bacteriology of Urinary Infection in Asymptomatic Elderly Populations

Organisms	Percent of infections with organisms isolated			
	Community		Institution	
	Men	Women	Men	Women
E. coli	19	68	11	47
P. mirabilis	5	1	30	27
K. pneumoniae	5	10	6	7
P. stuartii			16	7
P. aeruginosa	5		19	5
Other Gram-negative bacteria	2		7	6
Enterococcus spp	25	5	5	6
S. agalactiae	39	10	—	1
Coagulase-negative staphylococci		6	2	—
Other Gram-positive bacteria			3	—

bowel, are confused or demented, and have impaired mobility *(6,10)*. Comorbid diseases that necessitate institutional care, such as Alzheimer's disease, Parkinson's disease, or cerebrovascular accidents, are usually accompanied by a neurogenic bladder. The resultant impaired bladder function leads to incomplete bladder emptying and ureteric reflux, promoting the very high frequency of infection in these residents. For men, external condom catheters are frequently used to manage incontinence. A condom catheter is associated with a twofold increase in frequency of infection, and is more likely when twisting and obstruction of the drainage tube occurs.

1.3. Microbiology

For elderly women resident in the community *Escherichia coli* is the most common infecting organism, as it is in younger populations (*see* Table 1). The proportion of infections from which this organism is isolated, however, is lower than in younger populations. Other organisms isolated include *Klebsiella* spp., *Proteus* spp., and group B streptococcus (*Streptococcus agalactiae*). Coagulase-negative staphylococci are frequently isolated from ambulatory elderly men but are seldom associated with symptomatic infection *(2)*. When symptomatic infection is present, *E. coli* and *Proteus mirabilis* are the most frequent infecting organisms. *Enterococcus* spp. is also a common infecting organism.

E. coli remains the most frequent infecting organism isolated in institutionalized women but occurs in only 50–60% of episodes *(4)*. *P. mirabilis* and other Enterobacteriaceae bacteria are isolated with increased frequency in elderly women relative to other female populations. For men, *P. mirabilis* is isolated more frequently than *E. coli* *(3)*. The intensity of antimicrobial use in long-term care facilities, and transfer of organisms between patients in the institutional setting, promotes infection with organisms characterized by a higher likelihood of antimicrobial resistance. Organisms frequently isolated, including *Providencia stuartii*, *Pseudomonas aeruginosa*, and Enterobacteriaceae, such as *Klebsiella* spp., *Enterobacter* spp., *Serratia* spp., and *Citrobacter* spp., are frequently resistant to multiple antimicrobials.

Polymicrobial bacteriuria is common in the bacteriuric institutionalized elderly. From 15–25% of women and 10–15% of men with bacteriuria may have more than one organism isolated *(3,4)*. Men with incontinence managed by external condom catheter drainage have an increased frequency of polymicrobial bacteriuria. Thus, although in younger populations isolation of more than one organism is generally interpreted as contamination of the urine specimen, this is not the case for many elderly residents of long-term care facilities.

1.4. Morbidity and Mortality

Urinary infection is an important cause of morbidity in elderly populations, but the burden is surprisingly limited given the extraordinary frequency of infection. Short-term morbidity is associated with symptomatic urinary infection presenting along a spectrum of lower tract irritative symptoms (acute cystitis), through acute pyelonephritis, bacteremia, and, rarely, death. Local infectious complications may include epididymitis and prostatitis in men, or bladder and renal stone formation associated with urease-producing organisms such as *P. mirabilis* or *P. stuartii*. An additional problem in institutionalized populations is the emergence of organisms of increased antimicrobial resistance following repeated antimicrobial exposure, as asymptomatic bacteriuria in residents is a substantial reservoir for such resistant organisms *(7)*.

Urinary infection is the most frequent cause of community-acquired bacteremia in elderly populations. The majority of elderly patients with bacteremia from a urinary source, however, will have abnormalities of the genitourinary system such as retention, tumor, or an indwelling catheter. Urinary infection is also the most frequent source of bacteremia in long-term care populations and a common precipitating cause for acute care hospitalization of long-term care residents in some facilities *(7)*. Urinary infection may lead to sepsis and death due to Gram-negative septicemia. This is a relatively infrequent occurrence, however, given the very high frequency of urinary infection and usually occurs in individuals with significant structural genitourinary abnormalities, including long-term indwelling catheters. Death of residents in long-term care facilities is only rarely attributed to urinary infection *(7)*.

Bacteriuria is commonly persistent, sometimes for years. There is no evidence that this prolonged bacteriuria is associated with poorer long-term outcomes for institutionalized elderly populations. Asymptomatic bacteriuria is not associated with an increased frequency of hypertension or renal failure. In addition, despite the very high occurrence of infection with urease-producing organisms in many long-term care facilities, complications secondary to urolithiasis are infrequent.

Early studies reported an association between decreased survival and asymptomatic bacteriuria in elderly populations in both Greece and Finland *(1)*. These studies did not adjust for different functional or medical status between bacteriuric and nonbacteriuric subjects. Subsequent studies from community populations in Finland and Sweden *(11)*, and in an institutionalized population in the United States *(12)*, did not document an association between asymptomatic bacteriuria and survival. In fact, a survival difference between bacteriuric and nonbacteriuric elderly might be anticipated, as the group with bacteriuria clearly differ in functional status. Currently, however, there is no evidence to support a negative impact of asymptomatic bacteriuria on survival in elderly men or women.

1.5. Long-Term Indwelling Urethral Catheters

A subset of elderly individuals, most of whom are institutionalized, have voiding of urine managed through use of a long-term indwelling urethral catheter *(13)*. From 5–10% of residents in long-term care facilities have chronic indwelling catheters. The most frequent indications for catheter use are urinary retention in men and urinary incontinence in women. Individuals with chronic indwelling catheters are always bacteriuric, usually with 2–5 organisms isolated at any time. Urease-producing organisms such as *P. mirabilis* and *P. stuartii* occur with high frequency. These organisms may also cause catheter obstruction through development of a bacterial biofilm on the interior surface of the catheter.

Residents with long-term urethral catheters have a higher incidence of invasive urinary infection, manifested by fever or bacteremia, than bacteriuric residents without indwelling catheters *(8,13)*. Local complications of urinary infection are also more common in the presence of a chronic urethral catheter. These include urethritis, urethral fistula, epididymitis, prostatitis and prostatic abscess, and scrotal abscesses. Bladder stones may occur where urease-producing organisms are present. At autopsy, histologic evidence for acute pyelonephritis occurs more frequently in nursing home residents with chronic indwelling catheters compared to those with asymptomatic bacteriuria without chronic indwelling catheters *(14)*. Thus, bacteriuria with a chronic indwelling catheter *in situ* is associated with greater morbidity than asymptomatic bacteriuria in noncatheterized elderly subjects. Residents of long-term care facilities with chronic indwelling catheters have also been reported to have decreased survival *(15)*. The extent to which this is attributable to the catheter or catheter-acquired bacteriuria is not clear, as the catheterized and noncatheterized populations differ in clinical and functional characteristics.

2. CLINICAL MANIFESTATIONS

Urinary infection in elderly populations is usually asymptomatic *(1)*. That is, the urine culture is positive but there are no acute local genitourinary or systemic symptoms attributable to the infection. When symptomatic infection does occur, different clinical presentations may be seen. There may be acute lower tract irritative symptoms such frequency, dysuria, urgency, or suprapubic discomfort and, particularly in elderly women, acute deterioration of continence status. Infection may also present with systemic manifestations including pyelonephritis with fever and costrovertebral angle pain and tenderness, or as fever with hematuria without other localizing findings. Fever with obstruction of a chronic indwelling catheter is also consistent with urinary infection. Bacteremic infection is most likely to occur in the setting of ureteral or urethral obstruction or mucosal trauma.

A clinical diagnosis of acute symptomatic urinary infection in elderly populations is often not straightforward *(8)* (*see* Table 2). It is most problematic in the institutionalized population where chronic symptoms from comorbid diseases and difficulties in communication interfere with clinical assessment. Chronic genitourinary symptoms such as chronic incontinence and nocturia are not due to urinary infection, although many elderly individuals with these symptoms have a positive urine culture *(1,16)*. Where a patient has fever and findings localizing to the genitourinary tract such as acute retention, catheter obstruction, hematuria, or symptoms of pyelonephritis, clini-

Table 2
Clinical Presentations of Urinary Tract Infection in Elderly Bacteriuric Subjects

Probable urinary infection
    Acute onset or deterioration in lower tract symptoms: frequency, dysuria,
        suprapubic pain, urgency
    Fever with:
        Costovertebral pain/tenderness
        Hematuria
        Retention
        Catheter obstruction

Possible urinary infection
    Acute deterioration in continence status
    Fever without localizing findings:
        Indwelling catheter (30% probability)
        No indwelling catheter (10% probability)

Unlikely symptomatic urinary infection
    Chronic incontinence, or other chronic genitourinary symptoms
    Clinical deterioration without fever or localizing genitourinary findings

cal diagnosis of urinary infection may be made with a degree of certainty. For the elderly subject with fever and without localizing findings to the genitourinary tract a diagnosis of urinary tract infection is frequently incorrect *(8)*. A positive urine culture is present in 25–50% of the institutionalized population at any time, and residents with symptoms for any cause have a high probability of a positive urine culture. As many as one third of episodes of fever without localizing genitourinary symptoms may be due to urinary infection in residents with a chronic indwelling urethral catheter *(8)*. However, only 10% of such episodes of fever in residents without indwelling catheters have a urinary source. In this setting, then, a definitive diagnosis of urinary infection cannot be made, and the limitations in diagnostic accuracy must be appreciated.

There are several other diagnostic dilemmas in identifying symptomatic urinary infection in institutionalized populations. "Foul-smelling urine" in residents of long-term care facilities is frequently attributed to urinary infection and sometimes considered an indication for antimicrobial therapy. Urinary infection may be associated with an unpleasant odor, likely secondary to polyamine production by bacteria in the urine. Not all subjects with bacteriuria, however, will have an unpleasant odor to the urine, and not all individuals with an unpleasant odor have a positive urine culture *(17)*. When the odor is associated with urinary infection it may be ameliorated by antimicrobial therapy. However, alternate approaches, such as improved continence management, are more appropriate and effective in the longer term than repeated antimicrobial courses.

Another confusing clinical scenario is the elderly subject who has deteriorated clinically without fever or localizing findings. Again, many of these individuals will have positive urine cultures because of the high frequency of asymptomatic bacteriuria in this population, but there is currently no evidence that this clinical scenario is frequently, if ever, due to urinary infection. In this situation the appropriate management is likely observation and reassessment rather than antimicrobial therapy.

3. DIAGNOSTIC TESTS

3.1. Urine Culture

A positive urine culture is necessary for a microbiologic diagnosis of urinary infection. A urine specimen for culture should be obtained whenever a diagnosis of symptomatic urinary infection is considered. This specimen will not only confirm the presence of bacteriuria, but also identify the infecting organism and antimicrobial susceptibilities so antimicrobial therapy may be optimized. In every case, the urine specimen should be collected prior to the institution of antimicrobial therapy to ensure that causative organisms are isolated.

An appropriate method for specimen collection that minimizes bacterial contamination must be used. For symptomatic men, a single clean-catch urine specimen is usually adequate. For men with external condom catheters used to manage incontinence, a urine specimen may be obtained immediately postvoiding from a freshly applied leg bag *(1)*. A clean-catch specimen is preferred for women. For highly functionally impaired institutionalized women, it may not be possible to obtain a voided urine specimen. Where a woman is not able to cooperate in voiding, specimen collection through methods such as a bedpan or pedibag lead to contamination with periurethral or vaginal flora. These collection methods have not been validated for diagnostic criteria for urinary infection and should be discouraged. When a urine specimen is indicated to assist with clinical management in these patients, the specimen should be obtained by in-and-out urethral catheterization.

A urine specimen obtained from the urinary catheter in residents with long-term indwelling catheters reflects the bacterial flora of the biofilm on the interior surface of the catheter and may not be representative of bladder bacteriuria *(18)*. For urine specimen collection from subjects with chronic indwelling catheters, the catheter should be changed and a urine specimen obtained from the freshly inserted catheter. For short-term indwelling catheters (<30 d), catheter replacement prior to specimen collection is not recommended as biofilm formation is not as frequent in this situation.

A urine culture growing $\geq 10^5$ colony-forming units (CFU/mL) of one or more organisms on two consecutive specimens is required to diagnose asymptomatic urinary infection. A single urine culture with $\geq 10^5$ CFU/mL is adequate for bacteriologic diagnosis in subjects with acute symptoms referable to the genitourinary tract. With a clinical presentation consistent with acute pyelonephritis $\geq 10^4$ CFU/mL is sufficient. In younger women, quantitative counts of Enterobacteriaceae of $\geq 10^2$ CFU/mL are isolated from 30% of episodes in women with acute cystitis. Whether this is also the case for postmenopausal women presenting with a similar clinical syndrome has not been studied. However, for older women with symptoms consistent with acute cystitis, the lower quantitative count of organisms may be relevant.

Lower quantitative counts of organisms also occur with certain less common infecting organisms, such as *Candida albicans*. Patients with renal failure or receiving diuretics may also have dilute urine and lower quantitative bacterial counts. Some uncommon infecting organisms, such as *Ureaplasma urealyticum* or *Haemophilus influenzae* are not identified through routine culture methods, and urine cultures may be negative unless special cultures are requested. In the presence of complete obstruction to urinary drainage with infection proximal to the obstruction, as in ureteric obstruction due to a stone, stricture, or tumor, the voided urine culture may be negative, and a percutaneous aspirate from the proximal infected site is necessary to identify infecting organisms.

3.2. Pyuria

Pyuria, the presence of excess leukocytes in the urine, is virtually universal with acute symptomatic urinary infection. The presence of pyuria, however, cannot differentiate asymptomatic from symptomatic infection, as asymptomatic infection is also usually accompanied by pyuria *(1)*. About 90% of elderly subjects with asymptomatic bacteriuria have pyuria, whether assessed by routine urinalysis or leukocyte esterase. Where urease-producing organisms such as *P. mirabilis* or *P. stuartii* are present, leading to an alkaline urine, pyuria may not be identified due to rapid disintegration of leukocytes in the alkaline urine. Conversely, about 30% of residents of nursing homes with negative urine cultures also have pyuria. Thus, pyuria by itself is not a diagnostic test for urinary infection and cannot replace urine culture. In addition, as pyuria cannot differentiate symptomatic from asymptomatic infection, the presence or absence of pyuria in an individual with a positive urine culture does not determine whether or not antimicrobial therapy is indicated.

3.3. Other Tests

Bacteremia occurs in some subjects with symptomatic urinary infection. These are often patients with obstruction or trauma to the genitourinary tract. Blood cultures should be obtained in patients presenting with a high fever, hypothermia, acute systemic clinical deterioration, or hemodynamic instability.

The site of infection within the genitourinary tract may be the bladder, kidney, and, for men, the prostate. At least 50% of infections in elderly institutionalized women with asymptomatic bacteriuria are present in the kidney *(1)*. No available reliable tests can identify the site of infection. In most cases, in fact, determination of the site of infection has not been shown to be clinically relevant. Although presence of infection in the kidney is manifested by increased pyuria, there is no evidence that it is associated with poorer short- or long-term outcomes than infection localized only to the bladder.

A number of other markers of inflammation are present in urinary infection but have not been shown to have diagnostic or prognostic utility *(1)*. Patients with significant systemic manifestations such as fever have an increase in C-reactive protein, and urine antibodies and interleukin (IL)1α, IL6, or IL8 are present. These parameters decline or disappear following treatment of the infection. However, these cytokines are also present in a substantial proportion of subjects with asymptomatic bacteriuria, some of whom also have elevated urinary and systemic antibodies to the infecting organisms. Virtually all of these mediators are nonspecific indicators of infection, and infection at other sites may lead to similar alterations.

4. THERAPY

4.1. Asymptomatic Infection

Asymptomatic urinary infection in elderly populations should not be treated. Prospective, randomized, comparative trials of therapy compared with no therapy for the treatment of asymptomatic infection in institutionalized men or women have not documented improvements in morbidity or mortality with treatment *(4,5,12)*. For long-term care residents with chronic incontinence and bacteriuria, antimicrobial treatment of urinary infection does not improve continence *(16)*. Attempts to treat asymptomatic infection with antimicrobial therapy are, in fact, harmful due to increased adverse effects from medication, emergence of resistant organisms, and increased cost *(4)*. Thus, the evidence is consistent that there are no benefits and some adverse effects with treatment of asymptomatic bacteriuria. The presence of pyuria with bacteriuria is not an indication for antimicrobial therapy, as pyuria does not differentiate symptomatic from asymptomatic infection. It follows, then, that elderly asymptomatic subjects should not be screened for the presence of pyuria or bacteriuria, as there is no indication for treatment even if infection is identified.

Treatment of asymptomatic bacteriuria is recommended for individuals who are to undergo invasive genitourinary procedures with a risk of mucosal trauma, such as transurethral resection of prostate or cystoscopy *(19)*. There is a high frequency of bacteremia and sepsis in this situation. Urine cultures to identify bacteriuria should be obtained and, if infection is present, antimicrobial therapy selected based on the organisms isolated. The antimicrobial should be started immediately prior to the surgical procedure. Antimicrobial therapy is given for prophylaxis to prevent urosepsis, rather than for treatment of asymptomatic bacteriuria.

4.2. Symptomatic Infection

Symptomatic infection should, of course, be treated. The goal of therapy is to ameliorate symptoms, not to sterilize the urine. Antimicrobial treatment is selected on the basis of the organisms isolated from the urine and the antimicrobial susceptibilities. Where the patient is sufficiently ill that empiric antimicrobial therapy must be given before urine culture results are available, a broad-spectrum antimicrobial agent effective against Gram-negative organisms and enterococci is most appropriate. Oral therapy is usually adequate, but where there are concerns about patient tolerance, drug absorption, or antimicrobial resistance, parenteral therapy is more appropriate. Parenteral therapy is changed to oral therapy once the patient is stabilized and results of pretherapy urine cultures are available, usually after 2–4 d of therapy.

4.3. Antimicrobial Selection

Many antimicrobials are effective for the treatment of urinary infection in the elderly. Few studies, however, have specifically addressed the comparative efficacy of different antimicrobial regimens to allow an informed assessment of the balance of efficacy against adverse effects. Recommendations for antimicrobial selection in elderly populations are primarily based on studies from younger populations, frequently done in clinical settings that may not be relevant for the elderly.

With the foregoing provisos, a list of antimicrobials that may be used for oral or parenteral therapy are provided in Table 3. Initial empiric oral therapy with trimethoprim/sulfamethoxazole (TMP/SMX) is usually recommended. If there is a possibility of TMP/SMX-resistant organisms, a quinolone may be the best alternate, although nitrofurantoin should also be considered. Other agents would be selected based on tolerance of the patient or anticipated susceptibility of the organism. An aminoglycoside with or without ampicillin remains excellent empiric parenteral

Table 3
Antimicrobials for Treatment of Urinary Tract Infection in Elderly Populations

Agent	Dose	
	Oral	Parenteral
Penicillins		
Amoxicillin	500 mg tid	1–2 g q6h
Amoxicillin/clavulanic acid	500 mg tid	
Piperacillin		3 g q4h
Piperacillin/tazobactam		4 g/500 mg q8h
Cephalosporins		
Cephalexin	500 mg qid	
Cefazolin		1–2g q8h
Cefadroxil	1 g qd or bid	
Cefixime	400 mg qd	
Cefuroxime axetil	250 mg bid	
Cefotaxime		1–2 g q8h
Ceftriaxone		1–2 g q12h
Ceftazidime		500 mg – 2 g q8h
Quinolones		
Norfloxacin	400 mg bid	
Ciprofloxacin	250–500 mg bid	400 mg q12h
Ofloxacin	200–400 mg bid	400 mg q12h
Lomefloxacin	400 mg q24h	
Levofloxacin	250 mg q24h	250 mg q24h
Aminoglycosides		
Gentamicin		1–1.5 mg/kg q8h or 4–5 mg/kg q24h
Tobramycin		1–1.5 mg/kg q8h or 4–5 mg/kg q24h
Amikacin		5 mg/kg q8h or 15 mg/kg/q24h
Other		
Aztreonam		1–2 g q6h
Imipenem/cilastatin		500 mg q6h
Nitrofurantoin	50–100 mg qid	
Trimethoprim	100 mg bid	
Trimethoprim/sulfamethoxazole	160/800 mg bid	

qd, once a day; bid, two times a day; tid, three times a day; qid, four times a day; q, every; h, hour.

therapy. Although there are concerns about aminoglycoside nephrotoxicity, the expectation is that therapy will be altered at 48–72 h when culture results are available. Thus, the duration of empiric therapy with the aminoglycoside is minimized, and there is little risk of toxicity. In patients with renal failure, an aminoglycoside is not appropriate for initial empiric therapy, and an extended-spectrum cephalosporin or quinolone is preferred.

4.4. Duration of Therapy

A treatment course of 7 d is recommended for women with acute lower tract irritative symptoms. Shorter courses of therapy of three days are effective for many well elderly women, but are generally less effective than 7 d therapy *(20,21)*. One optional approach, however, is a 3-d course of therapy with retreatment with a longer course if early symptomatic relapse occurs. When women present with more severe systemic symptoms, such as fever or pyelonephritis, 14 days of therapy is recommended. Men with any presentation of symptomatic infection should be treated with an initial course of 10–14 d. Symptomatic relapse from a prostatic source requires a more prolonged course of therapy of 6–12 wk. A prostatic source is usually only suspected, however, when recurrent relapse with the same organism is identified *(22,23)*.

More prolonged courses of antimicrobial therapy for treatment of urinary infection are generally discouraged in elderly patients. Such courses may occasionally be indicated for suppressive therapy in highly selected and infrequent circumstances. In this situation, an individual with an underlying abnormality of the genitourinary tract that predisposes them to symptomatic recurrent urinary infection or progressive renal impairment is given antimicrobial therapy to suppress infection where it cannot be eradicated. For instance, in patients with struvite stones that may not be removable, prolonged antimicrobial therapy will prevent further enlargement of stones and will preserve renal function. Where suppressive therapy is used, a full dose of the antimicrobial is initially given, and this may be decreased by half if it is effective and the patient remains stable. It must be emphasized, however, that the use of long-term antimicrobial therapy should be infrequent, and initiated only where there are compelling indications.

Treatment courses should be as short as possible in individuals with chronic indwelling catheters. Antimicrobial therapy in this setting will not prevent bacteriuria but will lead to emergence of more resistant organisms. Hence, therapy is limited in duration to 7 d, if possible, to limit antimicrobial pressure that may lead to the emergence of more resistant organisms.

5. PREVENTION

The extent to which prevention of urinary infection in elderly populations is feasible is unclear. The very high frequency of urinary infection is primarily due to associated comorbidity, and usually this cannot be modified. Adequate nutrition, optimal management of comorbidities, and maintenance of maximal function certainly seem reasonable recommendations, but the impact of these interventions in decreasing urinary infection is not known. For a small subset of elderly well women who are experiencing repeated episodes of acute cystitis, the use of prophylactic antibiotics, a strategy similar to younger female populations, may be effective. An alternate approach in selected postmenopausal women may be the use of topical estrogen therapy *(24)*, although the relative efficacy of estrogen compared to antimicrobial prophylaxis remains to be determined. Studies of the impact of oral estrogen in reducing urinary infection have given conflicting results. Long-term antimicrobial prophylaxis should only be used in selected women and likely should be avoided for institutionalized subjects.

Avoidance of devices such as chronic indwelling catheters or condom catheters will also decrease the frequency of infection. This is not always possible for the individual patient. Intermittent catheterization is an option for subjects with incontinence and a flaccid bladder. One prospective randomized study in institutionalized men has shown that frequency of infection was similar with clean or sterile intermittent catheterization *(25)*. Thus, clean catheterization, which is less costly, is recommended.

There has been substantial interest, including in the popular press, in the use of "natural antiseptics" such as cranberry juice for the management of urinary infection in elderly populations. Cranberry juice was associated with a decrease in the presence of pyuria in association with bacteriuria but not a change in bacteriuria itself in one study *(26)*. There was no evidence that there was a decrease in the frequency of symptomatic infections. There is no reason to discourage the use of cranberry juice in elderly populations. Current evidence, however, does not support a significant benefit on the presence of or complications from urinary infection with cranberry juice.

Although asymptomatic bacteriuria may not be preventable, some symptomatic episodes may be avoided. Strategies that are effective include prophylactic antimicrobials prior to invasive procedures and optimal catheter care. Preventing obstruction to catheter drainage and avoiding catheter trauma will prevent episodes of systemic infection.

REFERENCES

1. Nicolle, L. E. (1997) Asymptomatic bacteriuria in the elderly. *Infect. Dis. Clin. North Am.* **11,** 647–662.
2. Mims, A. D., Norman, D. C., Yamamura, R. H., et al. (1990) Clinically inapparent (asymptomatic) bacteriuria in ambulatory elderly men: epidemiological, clinical, and microbiological findings. *J. Am. Geriatr. Soc.* **38,** 1209–1214.
3. Nicolle, L. E., Bjornson, J., Harding, G. K. M., et al. (1983) Bacteriuria in elderly institutionalized men. *N. Engl. J. Med.* **309,** 1420–1426.
4. Nicolle, L. E., Mayhew, J. W., and Bryan, L. (1987) Prospective randomized comparison of therapy and no therapy for asymptomatic bacteriuria in institutionalized women. *Am. J. Med.* **83,** 27–33.
5. Nicolle, L. E., Friesen, D., Harding, G. K. M., et al. (1996) Hospitalization from acute pyelonephritis in Manitoba, Canada during the period 1989–1992. Impact of diabetes, pregnancy, and aboriginal origin. *Clin. Infect. Dis.* **22,** 1051–1056.
6. Boscia, J. A., Kobasa, W. D., Knight, R. A., et al. (1986) Epidemiology of bacteriuria in an elderly ambulatory population. *Am. J. Med.* **80,** 208–214.
7. Nicolle, L. E., Strausbaugh, L. J., and Garibaldi, R. A. (1996) Infections and antibiotic resistance in nursing homes. *Clin. Microbol. Rev.* **9,** 1–17.
8. Orr, P., Nicolle, L. E., Duckworth, H., et al. (1996) Febrile urinary infection in the institutionalized elderly. *Am. J. Med.* **100,** 71–77.
9. Nickel, J. C. (1996) Prostate, in *Antibiotic Therapy in Urology* (Mulholland, S. G., ed.) Lippincott-Raven, Philadelphia, pp. 57–69.
10. Nicolle, L. E., Henderson, E., and Bjornson, J. (1987) The association of bacteriuria with resident characteristics and survival in elderly institutionalized males. *Ann. Intern. Med.* **106,** 682–686.
11. Nordenstam, G. R., Brandberg, C. A., Oden, A. S., et al. (1986) Bacteriuria and mortality in an elderly population. *N. Engl. J. Med.* **314,** 1152–1156.
12. Abrutyn, E., Mossey, J., Berlin, J. A., et al. (1994) Does asymptomatic bacteriuria predict mortality and does antimicrobial treatment reduce mortality in elderly, ambulatory women. *Ann. Intern. Med.* **120,** 827–833.

13. Warren, J. W. (1997) Catheter-associated urinary tract infections. *Infect. Dis. Clin. North Am.* **11,** 609–622.
14. Warren, J. W., Muncie, H. L. Jr., and Hall-Craggs, M. (1988) Acute pyelonephritis associated with the bacteriuria of long-term catheterization. A prospective, clinico-pathological study. *J. Infect. Dis.* **158,** 1341–1346.
15. Kunin, C. M., Douthitt, S., Dancing, J., et al. (1992) The association between the use of urinary catheters and morbidity and mortality among elderly patients in nursing homes. *Am. J. Epidemiol.* **135,** 291–301.
16. Ouslander, J. G., Shaperia, M., and Schnelle, J. F. (1995) Does eradicating bacteriuria affect the severity of chronic urinary incontinence in nursing home residents. *Ann. Intern. Med.* **122,** 749–754.
17. Nicolle, L. E. (1994) Consequences of asymptomatic bacteriuria in the elderly. *Internat. J. Antimicrob. Agents* **4,** 107–111.
18. Grahn, D., Norman, D. C., White, M. L., et al. (1985) Validity of urinary catheter specimen for diagnosis of urinary tract infection in the elderly. *Arch. Intern. Med.* **145,** 1858–1860.
19. Cafferkey, M. T., Falkiner, F. R., Gillespie, W. A., et al. (1982) Antibiotics for the prevention of septicemia in urology. *J. Antimicrob. Chemother.* **9,** 471–477.
20. Saginur, R., Nicolle, L. E., and the Canadian Infectious Diseases Society Clinical Trials Study Group (1992) Single dose compared with three days norfloxacin for treatment of uncomplicated urinary infection in women. *Arch. Intern. Med.* **152,** 1233–1237.
21. Harding, G. K. M., Nicolle, L. E., Ronald, A. R., et al. (1991) Management of catheter-acquired urinary tract infection: therapy following catheter removal. *Ann. Intern. Med.* **114,** 713–719.
22. Gleckman, R., Crowley, M., and Natsios, G. A. (1991) Therapy for recurrent invasive urinary tract infections in men. *N. Engl. J. Med.* **301,** 878–880.
23. Smith, J. W., Jones, S. R., and Reed, W. P. (1979) Recurrent urinary tract infections in men: characteristics and response to therapy. *Ann. Intern. Med.* **91,** 544–548.
24. Raz, R. and Stamm, W. (1993) A controlled trial of intravaginal estriol in post-menopausal women with recurrent urinary tract infections. *N. Engl. J. Med.* **329,** 753–757.
25. Duffy, L. M., Cleary, J., and Ahern, S. (1995) Clean intermittent catheterization: safe, cost-effective bladder management for male residents of VA nursing homes. *J. Am. Geriatr. Soc.* **43,** 865–870.
26. Avorn, J., Monane, M., and Gurwitz, J. A. (1994) Reduction of bacteriuria and pyuria after ingestion of cranberry juice. *JAMA* **271,** 751–754.

11

Bacterial Meningitis

Chester Choi

1. EPIDEMIOLOGY AND CLINICAL RELEVANCE

Bacterial meningitis in the older adult continues to be associated with high case fatality rates and significant morbidity. Improved modes of diagnosis may be on the horizon; however, atypical presentations in the older adult make early diagnosis more difficult in this population. Effective, early treatment is important in decreasing the morbidity and mortality but has become more complicated due to antimicrobial resistance. The prevention of some forms of bacterial meningitis may be feasible, but even currently available vaccines are markedly underutilized in at-risk populations.

1.1. Case Fatality and Attack Rates

In epidemiologic studies, an increased incidence of bacterial meningitis was noted in older adults, particularly with etiologic organisms such as *Streptococcus pneumoniae, Listeria monocytogenes*, group B streptococci (*Streptococcus agalactiae*), and Gram-negative organisms such as *Escherichia coli, Klebsiella pneumoniae, Proteus* spp., *Enterobacter* spp., and *Pseudomonas aeruginosa (1–4)*. Viral meningitis, on the other hand, appears to be a rare infection in the older adult. The most recent, comprehensive examination of the epidemiology of bacterial meningitis, based on 1995 data from surveillance studies in Georgia, Tennessee, Maryland and California, showed that *S. pneumoniae* caused almost 70% of the cases of meningitis in those over the age of 60, and that the case fatality rate (CFR) for this organism was 21%. *Listeria monocytogenes* accounted for almost 25% of the cases with an overall CFR of 15%. In the older adult population, *Haemophilus influenzae*, group B streptococci, and *Neisseria meningitidis* together accounted for approximately 6% of the cases. In summarizing these data, the authors noted that the attack rate for bacterial meningitis in older adults due to these five pathogens remained about the same in comparison to 1986 data, a marked difference from the situation in the pediatric population (those from 1–23 mo of age) where the annual number of cases fell from 7270 to 948, an 87% decrease felt to be largely due to the widespread use of *H. influenzae* vaccine *(5)*.

Other estimates of the overall attack rate in individuals over 60 yr of age range from 2–9 per 100,000 per year, accounting for 1000–3000 cases per year in the U.S. It is estimated that the costs of treatment alone for these infections would be in excess of $11–33 million per year. A summary of these data and the case fatality rates for the responsible etiologic organisms is shown in Table 1.

From: *Infectious Disease in the Aging*
Edited by: Thomas T. Yoshikawa and Dean C. Norman
© Humana Press Inc., Totowa, NJ

Table 1
Surveillance Studies of Bacterial Meningitis in Older Adults

Organisms	Studies					
	Wenger et al.[a]		Schlech et al.[b]		Schuchat et al.[c]	
	AR	CFR	AR	CFR	AR	CFR
S. pneumoniae	1.5	31	0.5	54	1.9	20
L. monocytogenes	0.5	—	0.1	41	0.6	—
H. influenzae	0.2	—	0.09	24	0.07	—
N. meningitidis	0.1	—	0.2	29	0.1	—
Group B streptococcus	0.2	51	0.02	23	0.1	18

AR, attack rate per 100,000; CFR, case fatality rate (percent).
[a]Data from ref. *(1)*.
[b]Data from ref. *(2)*.
[c]Data from ref. *(4)*.

1.2. Pathogenesis

Bacterial meningitis usually results from the hematogenous spread of organisms or from local invasion from areas of colonization or local infection. Once the organisms reach the meninges, however, they encounter limited host defenses and can proliferate to large numbers, stimulating the production of inflammatory mediators. This results in increased intracranial pressure and altered intracerebral vascular autoregulation, phenomena that can lead to complications such as cerebral ischemia or infarction, hydrocephalus, subdural effusion or empyema, and sagittal sinus or cortical vein thrombosis. Patients may manifest these complications in the form of seizures, stroke syndromes, cranial nerve deficits, coma, or death (3).

1.3. Etiologic Organisms

S. pneumoniae is recognized on Gram-stained smears in the form of Gram-positive diplococci or short chains of cocci with an elongation along their axis of division. Exposure to antibiotics or anaerobic conditions may cause the organism to appear Gram negative. Its growth may be inhibited by allowing specimens to dry at room temperature or by placing them in sterile solutions. In cultures, the organism is alpha hemolytic and optochin-disk susceptible, features that facilitate identification. Serotyping based on antigenic differences in the capsular polysaccharides allows for differentiation into 84 types, but most disease is caused by a relatively small number of serotypes *(1,3,4,7–9,12,14)* that tend to have larger capsules *(6)*.

L. monocytogenes is an aerobic, Gram-positive bacillus that is often associated with foodborne illness. Outbreaks have been associated with a variety of foods including cheeses (Mexican and Brie), hot dogs, prepared meats, and ice cream or other dairy products *(7)*. *L. monocytogenes* must be differentiated from diphtheroids, as misidentification or the assumption that the diphtheroid-like organisms represent contaminants has resulted in clinical catastrophes. *L. monocytogenes* causes beta hemolysis and has a characteristic "end-over-end" or tumbling motility. Infections with this organism are often associated with alterations in cell-mediated host immunity but may occur in the absence of recognized immunodeficiencies *(8)*.

N. meningitidis is an occasional cause of meningitis in the older adult. The organism is nonmotile and Gram-negative and often appears as kidney-shaped diplococci on Gram stain. Most disease is caused by serogroups A, B, C, Y, and W135 with serogroup B accounting for more than 50% of cases in many developed countries. Prompt inoculation of specimens of cerebrospinal fluid (CSF) onto blood or chocolate agar plates and use of optimal growth conditions including 10% CO_2 increase diagnostic yields. Group B streptococci (*S. agalactiae*) may be recognized in smears as Gram-positive cocci forming longer chains. The organism is generally beta hemolytic, although 1–2% of strains are nonhemolytic. They can be differentiated from other beta hemolytic streptococci by serologic tests for the group B specific cell wall antigen (staphylococcal coagglutination and latex agglutination tests are used most commonly) or by nonserologic methods (bacitracin or trimethoprim sulfamethoxazole resistance, hippurate hydrolysis, and the like). Infection with this organism is often associated with diabetes mellitus, malignancy, liver or renal failure, or genital tract infection *(6,9,10)*.

H. influenzae is a pleomorphic Gram-negative organism that often appears coccobacillary on Gram stain. Meningitis and most other forms of invasive disease are caused by serotype B, and many strains of this organism contain plasmids, which enable them to produce beta lactamase, leading to penicillin and ampicillin resistance. Aerobic Gram-negative bacilli such as *K. pneumoniae* or *E. coli* have increasingly been found as the cause of meningitis, primarily in the hospitalized patient, but also occasionally in those with community-acquired disease. Infection with these organisms may result from postsurgical or traumatic conditions that allow them to gain access to the meninges, or it may be a consequence of infection at a distant site with subsequent hematogenous seeding of the meninges *(11)*.

2. CLINICAL MANIFESTATIONS

The usual symptoms and signs of meningitis include fever, headache, alteration of sensorium, photophobia, and neck stiffness. In major reviews of these findings in the older adult, however, fever was noted in less than 60% in one study and nuchal rigidity was found in less than 60% in another (*see* Table 2) *(4,6,12)*. Similarly, the classical, discriminating signs of meningitis may not be entirely specific since a significant percentage of older adults may have nuchal rigidity or other signs usually attributed to meningeal irritation. Puxty and colleagues noted that nuchal rigidity was found in 35% of older patients without meningitis on acute-care and rehabilitation wards *(13)*. This physical finding and the associated ones of Kernig's and Brudzinski's signs were often found in those patients with a history of cerebrovascular disease, confusion, abnormal plantar responses, and primitive reflexes. However, the presence of meningeal signs in patients without the underlying history of cerebrovascular disease, neurologic deficit, cognitive disorder, or primitive reflexes should greatly increase the suspicion for meningitis *(13)*.

The evaluation of nuchal rigidity should assess for limitation of range of motion of the neck in all directions. Limitations to rotation or lateral flexion are seen more frequently with cervical arthritis, and flexion with this condition often results in limitation at the extremes of range of motion. Meningitis, on the other hand, usually causes immediate resistance to flexion due to the meningeal irritation and muscle spasm. Kernig's sign is determined by passive flexion of the hip and then extension

Table 2
Frequency of Symptoms and Signs of Meningitis
in the Older Adult

Symptom or sign	Frequency (%)
Fever	59–100
Confusion	57–96
Headache	21–81
Nuchal rigidity	57–92

Source: Adapted from refs. *(3,6,12)*.

of the knee with resultant extensor spasm at the knee at 135° in the presence of meningeal irritation, whereas Brudzinski's sign is elicited by neck flexion with resultant hip and knee flexion.

Patients suspected of having bacterial meningitis should be investigated for accompanying or inciting infections such as pneumonia. Other predisposing conditions in the study by Gorse and colleagues included neurosurgical procedures, trauma, sinusitis, diabetes mellitus, alcohol abuse, and neoplastic disease or corticosteroid therapy *(12)*.

2.1. Fever and Altered Mental Status

Older adults frequently present with fever and altered or changed mental function. It is well-recognized, however, that nonmeningeal or non-central nervous system infection, such as urinary tract infection or pneumonia, can result in either a state of delirium or of depressed mental function and even coma *(14)*. Ruling out meningitis may be important in that the antibiotic choices and doses may be significantly different for bacterial meningitis. Given the lack of sensitivity or specificity of the physical findings and history, the clinician often must perform a lumbar puncture to assess for meningitis. However, the interpretation of these CSF results may be complicated by prior antibiotic therapy for the urinary tract infection or pneumonia *(3,6)*.

2.2. Evaluation of Dementia

Lumbar punctures are often performed to evaluate older patients for the cause of their dementia. Rarely, however, are syphilis or bacterial meningitis found in these evaluations without a prior history or suspicion of these diseases. Thus, CSF analysis should be performed only with a heightened index of suspicion based on history or physical findings in patients with dementia of uncertain cause *(15)*.

2.3. Effect of Corticosteroids or Immunosuppression

Many older adults may be receiving corticosteroids or immunosuppressants for underlying conditions such as asthma, polymyalgia rheumatica, and others. In such patients, clinical evaluation for the possibility of bacterial meningitis can be difficult, as they would be at increased risk of serious infections including meningitis, but corticosteroids or immunosuppression may alter the expression of such invasive infections. Nuchal rigidity would be a less reliable sign in these individuals, and fever may also be seen less often. A high index of suspicion should result from any combination of findings of fever, headache, altered mental state, neck stiffness, or photophobia *(3,16)*.

2.4. Parameningeal Infection

Bacterial meningitis may result from or be mimicked by parameningeal infections such as sinusitis, mastoiditis, vertebral osteomyelitis, or epidural abscess. A careful physical examination and appropriate diagnostic tests for these conditions should be carried out in patients with suspected bacterial meningitis. Examination for sinus, mastoid, and vertebral tenderness can be quickly performed, and appropriate computed tomographic (CT) or magnetic resonance imaging (MRI) scans (when patients are sufficiently stable and initial therapy has begun) may be indicated *(3,16)*.

3. DIAGNOSTIC TESTS

The diagnosis of bacterial meningitis rests largely on examination of the CSF, but the rapidity of the patient's course may dictate the appropriate timing of the lumbar puncture. Patients with a rapid clinical course (< 24 h) and/or focal neurological signs, seizures, altered consciousness, or evidence of intracranial hypertension (e.g., papilledema) require initial empiric antibiotic therapy prior to a lumbar puncture; the antibiotic choice may be based upon available history including age, underlying medical conditions, prior antibiotic therapy, and the status of immunity *(17,18)*.

In patients without papilledema or focal neurologic signs on physical examination, the risk of herniation due to lumbar puncture is felt to be low; however, older adults are more commonly afflicted with space-occupying lesions such as brain abscess, tumors, or other masses that might predispose to herniation. Additionally, some epidemiologic studies have documented the frequent occurrence (39–43%) of focal neurologic findings in older adults with bacterial meningitis *(3, 12)*. Thus, CT scan of the brain may be deemed necessary in the majority of older adults suspected of bacterial meningitis. Talan and colleagues reviewed the issue of administration of antibiotic therapy prior to performance of the lumbar puncture and concluded that empiric therapy probably did not adversely affect the diagnostic properties of examination of the CSF, particularly if the delay before the lumbar puncture was not prolonged. Similar conclusions were reached by others utilizing rabbit models of bacterial meningitis *(18)*.

With bacterial meningitis, the CSF generally has the characteristics shown in Table 3 and, in surveys of this disease in older adults, no differences were noted in the diagnostic criteria including pleocytosis, hypoglycorrhachia, or positive cultures. Additionally, the rate at which blood cultures were positive also seemed similar to that in younger patients. The determination of hypoglycorrhachia may be more difficult in patients with peripheral blood hyperglycemia or hypoglycemia. A serum glucose drawn at approximately the same time as the lumbar puncture is mandatory; ratios of CSF glucose to serum glucose of less than 0.31 are consistent with hypoglycorrhachia and bacterial meningitis *(20)*. A minority of patients with bacterial meningitis may demonstrate atypical CSF parameters, particularly a lymphocytic response or lower percentage of neutrophils or a Gram stain without organisms *(19)*. This scenario is especially seen with *L. monocytogenes* meningitis in which the Gram stain is positive in fewer than one third of cases, and with Gram-negative bacillary meningitis where the pleocytosis may be less and the percentage of neutrophils may be somewhat lower than with typical bacterial meningitis. Usually, however, the glucose, Gram stain and other tests strongly suggest a bacterial etiology *(8)*.

Table 3
Cerebrospinal Fluid Findings in Meningitis

CSF findings	Normal CSF	Acute bacterial	Viral	Tuberculous
Opening pressure (cm H$_2$O)	6–20	Usually elevated	Normal to moderately elevated	Usually elevated
WBC's (per mm^3)	0–5, (about 85% lymphocytes)	Usually several hundred to >60,000, PMNs predominate	5 to a few hundred but may be more than 1000. Lymphocytes predominate but may be >80% PMNs in the first few days	Usually 25–100, rarely >500. Lymphocytes predominate except early stages where PMNs may account for >80% of cells
Protein (mg/dL)	18–45	Usually 100–500, occasionally >1000	Frequently normal or slightly elevated <100; may show greater elevation in severe cases	Nearly always elevated, usually 100–200 but may be much higher if dynamic block
Glucose (mg/dL)	45–80 or 0.6 X serum glucose	Usually 5–40 or <0.3X serum glucose	Usually normal, but can be low with mumps, HSV 2	Usually reduced; <45 in 3/4 of cases
Miscellaneous	For traumatic taps add 1 WBC and 1 mg/dL protein for each 1000 RBCs	Gram-stain + in about 60–80%; Sp = Gram + diplococci; Nm = Gram neg diplococci; Lm = Gram + bacillus	Usually do not need to find specific causal virus	AFB + stain in 25%, culture + in >2/3 of cases (but may take 4–8 wk for growth)

Source: Adapted from refs. *(5,6,19).*

Sp, *S. pneumoniae*; Nm, *N. meningitidis*; Lm, *L. monocytogenes*; AFB, acid-fast bacilli; HSV 2, Herpes simplex type II; CSF, cerebrospinal fluid; PMNs, polymorphonuclear neutrophils; RBCs, red blood cells; WBCs, white blood cells; +, positive; cmH$_2$O, centimeter of water; neg, negative.

The frequent use of antibiotics in the community generates many cases of meningitis where this prior antibiotic administration clouds the etiologic diagnosis. Several studies have concluded that prior antibiotics can alter the Gram-stain results, delay the growth of organisms on culture, and occasionally change the CSF parameters. In general, however, the CSF results are sufficiently unaltered to allow appropriate suspicion of a bacterial rather than a viral or aseptic etiology and to permit the growth of the etiologic agent *(3,6,19,22).* The delay in specific diagnosis, particularly due to the effect of prior antibiotics on the Gram-stain results, is of concern and may prevent the use of specific antibiotic therapy. To address this issue, bacterial antigen testing of the CSF is indicated, with tests available for *S. pneumoniae*, *N. meningitidis*, *H. influenzae*, group B streptococci, and *E. coli*. The overall sensitivities of these tests is approximately 50–75% and the specificities approach 100%; thus, a positive test is quite helpful as it is likely to be a true positive, whereas a negative test is not helpful as it may be either a true negative or a false negative *(3,6,23)*. Improved diagnostic testing is currently being sought and polymerase chain reaction (PCR) or DNA probe technology to identify specific bacteria in the CSF may be clinically useful in the near future.

The differential diagnosis of bacterial meningitis includes conditions that can cause altered mental status and fever, with or without meningeal signs. Thus, conditions that should also be considered include encephalitis, brain abscess, subdural empyema, epidural abscess, cancers (either primary or metastatic malignancies of the CNS), cerebrovascular disease, or vasculitis. A clinical prediction rule has been proposed to help in the diagnosis of acute bacterial meningitis *(24,25)*.

Encephalitis in the older adult may be secondary to viral etiologies such as herpes simplex, equine encephalitis viruses, or others. The presentation of this syndrome is usually one of more profound alteration of level of consciousness or mental function with less prominent meningeal signs; seizures occur more commonly than with bacterial meningitis. The differentiation of these entities on clinical grounds, however, may be difficult, and the clinician may need to rely on the CSF examination to exclude bacterial meningitis. The diagnosis of encephalitis is more highly suspected with demonstration of areas of inflammation of the brain on CT or MRI (especially with herpes encephalitis) scan and by serologic tests for etiologic viruses or, in the case of herpes simplex, with a PCR of the CSF.

Patients with brain abscess may present in varying fashions. Fever is found in less than 75% of cases, and even headache or alteration of mental function are not universal symptoms. The diagnosis of brain abscess is best determined by imaging studies such as CT or MRI scan of the brain.

Individuals with subdural empyema may have clinical courses indistinguishable from bacterial meningitis, and indeed, this syndrome may be a complication of bacterial meningitis. The diagnosis is suspected in individuals whose response to antibiotic therapy is incomplete or delayed, and the presence of subdural fluid may be confirmed with CT or MRI scan. The precise diagnosis and treatment is best obtained with drainage of the subdural collection and appropriate antibiotic therapy based on culture results.

Epidural abscesses are generally of hematogenous origin, and are generally best treated with aspiration or debridement and appropriate antibiotics *(26)*.

4. TREATMENT

The management of bacterial meningitis requires consideration of several factors. First, the clinician should be cognizant of the clinical progression of disease and be prepared to institute empiric antibiotics in those with more severe manifestations or more rapid downhill course, since delays in those with seizures, hypotension, or severely altered mental status are associated with worsened outcomes *(27)*. Second, because the disease is occurring in an area of poor host resistance, administering

Table 4
Antibiotic Penetration of CSF

Excellent	Good (with inflammation)	Poor or negligible
Rifampin	Penicillins	Most 1st and 2nd generation cephalosporins
TMP-SMZ	3rd-generation cephalosporins	Aminoglycosides
Chloramphenicol	Cefuroxime	Clindamycin
Metronidazole	Vancomycin (variable) Erythromycin (variable) Tetracyclines (variable)	

TMP-SMZ, Trimethoprim-sulfamethoxazole.
Source: Adapted from refs. *(6,17,21,29)*.

bactericidal antibiotics with rapid killing is essential. Third, the degree of penetration of antibiotics into the CSF must be considered. Many antibiotics that act by inhibition of cell wall synthesis (penicillins, cephalosporins, carbapenems, vancomycin) cross the blood–brain barrier relatively poorly unless inflammation of the meninges is present. Other antibiotics such as trimethoprim-sulfamethoxazole, rifampin, chloramphenicol, and many quinolones cross this barrier with or without the presence of inflammation, whereas agents such as aminoglycosides, clindamycin, and first-generation cephalosporins do not cross in quantities sufficient to inhibit most bacteria in the CSF (*see* Table 4) *(6,28,29)*. Fourth, the clinician should be aware of the antibiotic susceptibilities of meningopathogens in the community. In many areas of the U.S. and other areas of the world, *S. pneumoniae* is frequently relatively resistant to penicillin (minimum inhibitory concentration [MICs] ≥ 0.1 µg/mL) and sometimes highly resistant to this agent (MICs ≥ 2.0 µg/mL). In the former situation, (MICs ≥ 0.1–<2.0 µg/mL) third-generation cephalosporins such as ceftriaxone or cefotaxime may be used for treatment of *S. pneumoniae* since these agents have sufficient affinity for the altered penicillin-binding proteins of the relatively resistant *S. pneumoniae*; however, in the latter situation (MICs ≥ 2.0 µg/mL), vancomycin should be selected, as cephalosporins would not be adequate therapy for the highly resistant *S. pneumoniae*, and vancomycin does not rely on attachment to penicillin-binding proteins for its antibacterial activity *(21)*.

Thus, the empiric treatment of bacterial meningitis in the older adult should provide antibiotic activity against the most likely pathogens. In areas where *S. pneumoniae* resistance to penicillin is seen, a combination of antibiotics may be necessary. Recommendations have included vancomycin for penicillin-resistant *S. pneumoniae;* ceftriaxone or cefotaxime for *S. pneumoniae*, Gram-negative bacilli, *N. meningitidis, H. influenza* and group B streptococci; and ampicillin for *L. monocytogenes*. Vancomycin has demonstrated activity against *L. monocytogenes* in vitro; however there have been treatment failures utilizing this drug in patients with *Listeria* meningitis, and there is a relative lack of clinical data documenting vancomycin's efficacy in this condition *(18)*.

Table 5
Recommended Antibiotic Therapy for Bacterial Meningitis

Organism	Antibiotic	Total Daily Dose
Empirical treatment for bacterial meningitis[a]	Cefotaxime or ceftriaxone plus ampicillin	8–12 g 4–6 g 12 g
S. pneumoniae (penicillin sensitive)	Penicillin G	20–24 million units
S. pneumoniae (moderately penicillin resistant)	Cefotaxime or ceftriaxone	8–12 g 4–6 g
S. pneumoniae (highly penicillin resistant)	Vancomycin	2 g
L. monocytogenes	Ampicillin plus an aminoglycoside: gentamicin, tobramycin, amikacin	12 g 5 mg/kg 15 mg/kg
N. meningitidis	Penicillin G or ampicillin	20–24 million units 12 g
H. influenzae	Cefotaxime or ceftriaxone	8–12 g 4–6 g
Enterobacteriaceae (Gram-negative bacilli)	Cefotaxime or ceftriaxone[b]	8–12 g 4–6 g
S. aureus (methicillin sensitive)	Nafcillin or oxacillin	8–12 g
S. aureus (methicillin resistant)	Vancomycin	2 g

[a]Add vancomycin if highly penicillin resistant *Streptococcus pneumoniae* is suspected
[b]Ceftazidime if *P. aeruginosa* is suspected or proven.
Source: Adapted from refs. *(6,17,21)*.

Penicillins and cephalosporins demonstrate the phenomenon of time-dependent kill-ing; thus, these drugs should be administered in a manner that ensures high levels in the CSF for prolonged durations. For example, ceftriaxone should be administered on a twice-daily schedule and cefotaxime should probably be given no less frequently than every 6 h. Penicillin G should be given either as a continuous infusion or dosed every 4 h, and ampicillin should be given no less frequently than every 6 h. Similarly, vanco-mycin should be dosed every 12 hours to ensure adequate CSF levels throughout the day *(28)*. Because of limitations of the penetration of most of these agents across the blood–brain barrier and the presence of the infection in an area of limited host resis-tance, high doses of bactericidal antibiotics are required. Table 5 lists current antibiotic dosing recommendations for adults with bacterial meningitis.

Adjunctive therapy with dexamethasone to decrease the inflammatory affects of meningitis and prevent some of its complications has been recommended for pediatric patients with *H. influenzae* meningitis. No similar recommendations exist for adults or older adults, and no controlled studies exist to support the use of corticosteroids in this population; however, if evidence of significant cerebral edema, particularly with findings of brain "shift" is present, corticosteroid therapy may be warranted to decrease cerebral edema *(3,30)*. Other measures to decrease intracranial pressure may be needed in the treatment of bacterial meningitis. Elevation of the head of the bed to 30°, administration of mannitol, and the use of hyperventilation may be required for patients with significant cerebral edema *(3,6)*.

No well-controlled, prospective clinical trials have been performed to establish with certainty the duration of treatment for bacterial meningitis in the older adult. Most authorities recommend a duration of at least 10–14 d for patients with *S. pneumoniae*. Studies done in younger patients suggest that the duration of therapy for those with *N. meningitidis* can be significantly more brief, and recommendations for 5–7 d have been promulgated. The treatment of *L. monocytogenes* meningitis, particularly in the older adult, should extend over at least 14–21 d, and similar durations of therapy have been recommended for those patients with aerobic Gram-negative bacillary (21 d) and group B streptococcal (14–21 d) meningitis *(17)*.

The performance of an end-of-treatment lumbar puncture to gauge the duration of therapy has largely been abandoned, as cell counts and differentials, glucose levels, and protein amounts can remain signifantly abnormal even after weeks of effective therapy. In the study by Durack and others, these parameters were not useful to guide the discontinuation of therapy, and symptomatic improvement was a more useful indicator *(31)*.

5. PREVENTION

Given that a significant number of cases of bacterial meningitis in the older adult are caused by *S. pneumoniae*, its prevention should be a high priority for clinicians. Surveys from 1993 showed that fewer than one-third of patients for whom *S. pneumoniae* vaccine was indicated had, in fact, received it. Whether this vaccine can adequately prevent invasive forms of S. *pneumoniae* has been controversial, but the vaccine does appear to be at least partially effective (56–81% for invasive disease including meningitis) and to be both safe and well tolerated. Thus, increased utilization of pneumococcal vaccine is a major health care goal of the Centers for Disease Control and Prevention and a number of other agencies with an aim to achieve 60% vaccination rates of eligible persons (80% for institutionalized older adults) by the year 2000 *(33)*.

The currently available vaccine contains 23 serotypes of *S. pneumoniae* and would afford putative protection against the 6 serotypes that have been associated with invasive disease and drug resistance. The development of an improved pneumococcal vaccine is also a major goal, and the testing of a protein conjugate vaccine utilizing elements of the capsule of *S. pneumoniae* is underway. Early results suggest improved protection in tests carried out in the pediatric population, and it is hoped that similar results may be obtained in older adults and immunocompromised individuals.

Widespread use of the *H. influenzae* b vaccine has resulted in a dramatic decrease in the number of pediatric *Haemophilus* meningitis cases. Because *H. influenzae* is an uncommon cause of meningitis in the older adult, the use of this vaccine in the geriatric population would not be expected to have a significant impact. Similarly, *N. meningitidis* vaccine is available and utilized for outbreaks of invasive disease or to protect some travelers and longer-term visitors and residents in areas of high endemnicity for this disease; however, there are no recommendations for its routine use in the older adult population. Additional factors that would limit the use of *N. meningitidis* vaccine in the older adult are the difficulty of immunizing individuals to serotype B, which causes more than 50% of cases in the U.S. overall, and the short duration of immunity engendered by the vaccine. The vaccine is recommended, however, for those individuals who have had prior serious infections with this organism and in those with complement deficiencies. Current preventive efforts for *L. monocytogenes* focus on decreasing exposure to this pathogen by improving food safety and awareness. Research efforts toward the development of a group B streptococcal vaccine are underway, largely directed toward its use to prevent perinatal transmission of this organism and the subsequent invasive disease in the neonate. No trials in the older adult, including those with risk factors such as diabetes mellitus or renal failure, have been published.

REFERENCES

1. Wenger, J. D., Hightower, A. W., Facklam, R. R., et al. (1990) Bacterial meningitis in the United States, 1986: report of a multistate surveillance study. *J. Infect. Dis.* **162,** 1316–1323.
2. Schlech, W. F. III, Ward, J. I., Band, J. D., et al. (1985) Bacterial meningitis in the United States, 1978 through 1981: the national bacterial meningitis surveillance study. *JAMA* **253,** 1749–1754.
3. Behrman, R. E., Meyers, B. R., Mendelson, M. H., et al. (1989) Central nervous system infections in the elderly. *Arch. Intern. Med.* **149,** 1596–1599.
4. Schuchat, A., Robinson, K., Wenger, J. D., et al. (1997) Bacterial meningitis in the United States in 1995. *N. Engl. J. Med.* 337, 970–976
5. Roos, K. L., Tunkel, A. R., and Scheld, W. M. (1997) Acute bacterial meningitis in children and adults, in *Infections of the Central Nervous System*, 2nd ed. (Scheld, W. M., Whitley, R. J., and Durack, D. T., eds.), Lippincott-Raven, Philadelphia, pp. 335–402.
6. Choi, C. (1992) Bacterial meningitis. *Clin. Geriatr. Med.* **8,** 889–902.
7. Tappero, J. W., Schuchat, A., Deaver, K. A., et al. (1995) Reduction in the incidence of human listeriosis in the United States: effectiveness of prevention efforts? *JAMA* **273,** 1118–1122.
8. Nieman, R. E. and Lorber, B. (1980) Listeriosis in adults: a changing pattern. Report of eight cases and review of the literature, 1968–1978. *Rev. Infect. Dis.* **2,** 207–227.
9. Cabellos, C., Viladrich, P. F., Corredoira, J., et al. (1999) Streptococcal meningitis in adult patients: current epidemiology and clinical spectrum. *Clin. Infect. Dis.* **28,** 1104–1108.
10 Domingo, P., Barquet, N., Alvarez, M., et al. (1997) Group B streptococcal meningitis in adults: report of twelve cases and review. *Clin. Infect. Dis.* **25,** 1180–1187.
11. Berk, S. L. and McCabe, W. R. (1980) Meningitis caused by gram-negative bacilli. *Ann. Intern. Med.* **93,** 253–260.
12. Gorse, G. J., Thrupp, L. D., Nudelman, K. L., et al. (1984) Bacterial meningitis in the elderly. *Arch. Intern. Med.* **144,** 1603–1607.
13. Puxty, J. A. H., Fox, R. A., and Horan, M. A. (1983) The frequency of physical signs usually attributed to meningeal irritation in elderly patients. *J. Am. Geriatr. Soc.* **31,** 590–592.
14. Roos, K. L. (1990) Meningitis as it presents in the elderly: diagnosis and care. *Geriatrics* **45,** 63–75.
15. Becker, P. M., Feussner, J. R., Mulrow, C. D., et al. (1985) The role of lumbar puncture in the evaluation of dementia: the Durham Veterans Administration/Duke University study. *J. Am. Geriatr. Soc.* **33,** 392–396.

16. Lambert, H. P. (1991) Meningitis: diagnostic problems, in *Infections of the Central Nervous System* (Lambert, H. P., ed.), B. C. Decker, Philadelphia, pp. 32–39.
17. Quagliarello, V. J. and Scheld, W. M. (1997) Treatment of bacterial meningitis. *N. Engl. J. Med.* **336,** 708–716.
18. Talan, D. A., Hoffman, J. R., and Yoshikawa, T. T. (1988) Role of empiric parenteral antibiotics prior to lumbar puncture in suspected bacterial meningitis: state of the art. *Rev. Infect. Dis.* **10,** 365–372.
19. Fishman, R. A. (1992) CSF findings in diseases of the nervous system, in *Cerebrospinal Fluid in Diseases of the Nervous System*, 2nd ed. (Fishman, R. A., ed.), W. B. Saunders, Philadelphia, pp. 253–343.
20 Powers, W. J. (1981) Cerebrospinal fluid to serum glucose ratios in diabetes mellitus and bacterial meningitis. *Am. J. Med.* **71,** 217–220.
21. Quagliarello, V. J. and Scheld, W. M. (1993) New perspectives on bacterial meningitis. *Clin. Infect. Dis.* **17,** 603–610.
22. Mandal, B. K. (1976) The dilemma of partially treated bacterial meningitis. *Scand. J. Infect. Dis.* **8,** 185–188.
23. Gray, L. D. and Fedorko, D. P. (1992) Laboratory diagnosis of bacterial meningitis. *Clin. Microbiol. Rev.* **5,** 130–145.
24. Spanos, A., Harrell, F. E., and Durack, D. T. (1989) Differential diagnosis of acute meningitis, an analysis of the predictive value of initial observations. *JAMA* **26,** 2700–2707.
25. McKinney, W. P., Heudebert, G. R., Harper, S. A., et al. (1994) Validation of a clinical prediction rule for the differential diagnosis of acute meningitis. *J. Gen. Intern. Med.* **9,** 8–12.
26. Yoshikawa, T. T. and Quinn, W. (1988) The aching head. Intracranial suppuration due to head and neck infections. *Infect. Dis. Clin. North Am.* **2,** 265–277.
27. Aronin, S. I., Peduzzi, P., and Quagliarello, V. J. (1998) Community-acquired bacterial meningitis: risk stratification for adverse clinical outcome and effect of antibiotic timing. *Ann. Intern. Med.* **129,** 862–869.
28. Lutsar, I., McCracken, G. H. Jr., and Friedland, I. R. (1998) Antibiotic pharmacodynamics in cerebrospinal fluid. *Clin. Infect. Dis.* **27,** 1117–1129.
29. Scheld W. M. (1989) Drug delivery to the central nervous system: general principles and relevance to therapy for infections of the central nervous system. *Rev. Infect. Dis.* **11 (Suppl 7),** S1669–S1690.
30 McGowan, J. E. Jr, Chesney, J. P., Crossley, K. B., et al. (1992) Guidelines for the use of systemic glucocorticosteroids in the management of selected infections. *J. Infect. Dis.* **165,** 1–13.
31. Durack, D. T. and Spanos, A. (1982) End-of-treatment spinal tap in bacterial meningitis: is it worthwhile? *JAMA* **248,** 75–80.
32. Centers for Disease Control and Prevention (1995) Influenza and pneumococcal vaccination coverage levels among persons aged > 65 yr. *M. M. W. R.* 44, 506–507; 513–515.
33. Centers for Disease Control and Prevention (1997) Prevention of pneumococcal disease. Recommendations of the advisory committee on immunization practices (ACIP). *M. M. W. R.* 46RR-8, 1–19.

12

Osteomyelitis and Septic Arthritis

Jack D. McCue

In comparison with lower respiratory tract, urinary tract, and skin and soft tissue infections, infections of bones and joints are relatively uncommon in the elderly, accounting for no more than a few percent of the infectious diseases treated by geriatricians. However, some bone and joint infections disproportionately afflict the elderly, such as osteomyelitis contiguous to pressure ulcers, septic arthritis of joints damaged by rheumatoid arthritis, or periprosthetic hip joint septic arthritis. As is true of many infectious illnesses in the elderly, diagnosis of bone and joint infections may be complicated by subtle, masked, or atypical clinical presentations. The consequences of delay in diagnosis and treatment of these infections, moreover, are no less serious in the elderly than in younger patients, and in the frail elderly inadequate diagnosis and treatment may increase mortality and cause great morbidity. Although definitive antibiotic treatment is similar to that of bone and joint infections in younger patients, empiric therapy in most cases must be broader.

1. OSTEOMYELITIS

1.1. Clinical Relevance

At any age, infections of the periosteum, medullary cavity, and cortex of bones are usually caused by pyogenic bacteria, and less commonly by mycobacteria or fungi; infections by other types of organisms are extremely rare. Osteomyelitis is classified primarily according to route and duration of infection, and secondarily by anatomic location and etiologic agent. Such a classification is useful in ensuring a careful evaluation of the patient, as well as determining antibiotic and surgical treatment choices. The terms *acute* and *chronic*, while clinically useful, are not sharply demarcated temporally, and are often used loosely as descriptors (1). In general, acute osteomyelitis evolves over weeks, and chronic osteomyelitis evolves over many months or years, and may be associated with dead bone (sequestra), fistulous tracts, or foreign bodies.

1.1.1. Pathogenesis

Three types of osteomyelitis are usually distinguished: contiguous focus infection, hematogenous osteomyelitis, and that which is secondary to vascular insufficiency. Whereas most cases of osteomyelitis in elderly patients treated by geriatricians are the result of contiguous spread from an infected wound or cellulitis, hematogenous seeding from a distant infection, postoperative complications resulting from orthopaedic surgery, or penetrating wounds may also be the underlying causes. In all circumstances,

From: *Infectious Disease in the Aging*
Edited by: Thomas T. Yoshikawa and Dean C. Norman
© Humana Press Inc., Totowa, NJ

however, healthy bone is highly resistant to infection, so trauma, ischemia, or foreign bodies are usually necessary preconditions.

Once bacteria are introduced into or near injured or ischemic bone, the phagocytic reaction that is mobilized to contain the infection releases enzymes that may lyse bone. The inflammatory response also impairs blood flow and may cause bone necrosis, which may eventually lead to the development of a devascularized sequestra of bone. Once bone infection is well established, the bacteria protect themselves from host defenses with the production of a polysaccharide-rich biofilm—especially when a foreign body is involved—making it more difficult to eradicate infection. As a result, most treatment regimens for osteomyelitis are longer than those for acute infections such as pneumonia or urinary tract infection.

1.1.1.1. CONTIGUOUS FOCUS OSTEOMYELITIS

Osteomyelitis in elderly patients most often develops by direct, contiguous extension of infection from infected adjacent soft tissues. Clinically, contiguous focus osteomyelitis may be indolent and its presence obscured by the skin and soft-tissue infection. The usual underlying infection in elderly patients is infected pressure ulcers (decubitus ulcers). Whereas penetrating injuries, compound comminuted fractures, and postoperative complications of surgical procedures are more typical of the type of contiguous focus osteomyelitis encountered in younger patients, they may also be responsible for contiguous focus osteomyelitis in elderly patients. When pressure ulcers or smoldering cellulitis fail to respond to wound care and antibiotic therapy, underlying contiguous focus osteomyelitis must be suspected *(2)*.

In the usual case of contiguous focus osteomyelitis in an elderly patient, poor tissue perfusion and repeated trauma to soft tissue produce conditions that are conducive to polymicrobial and anaerobic infection. Thus, it should be assumed that contiguous focus bone infection in elderly patients is polymicrobial in etiology, although *Staphylococcus aureus* (the most prevalent cause of bone infection in younger patients) is still incriminated as a pathogen or copathogen in the majority of cases. Consequently, a mixture of staphylococci, streptococci, enteric gram-negative organisms, and anaerobic bacteria may be found in bone biopsy cultures when contiguous focus osteomyelitis is due to a diabetic foot infection or underlying pressure ulcer. Similarly, osteomyelitis from soft tissue infection of the oropharynx, paranasal sinuses, gastrointestinal tract, or female genital tract is usually due to an unpredictable mixture of anaerobic and Gram-positive and Gram-negative bacteria. When osteomyelitis results from a postoperative wound infection, the cause is most often *S. aureus*, although coagulase-negative staphylococci are common when osteomyelitis follows implantation of orthopedic appliances. *Pseudomonas aeruginosa* osteomyelitis may be the result of puncture-wound infections of the foot, especially when the foot wound is soaked in water, which may introduce pseudomonas organisms. Antibiotic-resistant organisms, such as *Enterobacter aerogenes*, *Acinetobacter calcoaceticus*, or *P. aeruginosa,* may be selected out when polymicrobially infected pressure ulcers are treated with narrow-spectrum antibiotics.

1.1.1.2. HEMATOGENOUS (VERTEBRAL) OSTEOMYELITIS

Acute hematogenous osteomyelitis primarily occurs as an infection of intravenous drug abusers and young children. The only type of hematogenous infection ordinarily encountered in older adults is the relatively indolent vertebral osteomyelitis. In vertebral osteomyelitis, bacteria reach the vertebral end plate and disk space via the spinal arteries and spread to the adjacent vertebral body. The urinary tract is often the source of the infection, and in older men bacteria are believed to reach the spine via the prostatic venous (Batson's) plexus. The source of bacteremia in cases that are unrelated to urinary tract infection is usually obvious—less-obvious primary sources of vertebral body infection include subacute bacterial endocarditis, remote soft tissue infections, or an infected intravenous line or other medical device.

Spine pain with no apparent cause or a fever of unknown origin are typical presentations for vertebral osteomyelitis; atypical presentations, such as referred pain to chest or abdomen, may result from nerve root irritation. The lumbar spine is involved most often, followed by the thoracic and cervical spine. In the case of now-rare Pott's disease, tuberculous spondylitis most often affects the thoracic vertebrae. The majority of cases of vertebral osteomyelitis have a subacute course with vague pain that gradually intensifies over several months and low-grade fever. Fever may be absent, however, and the white blood cell count is usually not elevated. There may be spasm of the paraspinal muscles and limitation of spine motion. In patients suspected of having an occult vertebral osteomyelitis, diagnosis may be reliably suggested by the simple physical examination finding of localized percussion tenderness over the involved vertebrae. Posterior extension may cause epidural and subdural abscesses or meningitis, and anterior or lateral extension may lead to paravertebral, retropharyngeal, mediastinal, subphrenic, or retroperitoneal abscesses.

Because of the protracted course typical of vertebral osteomyelitis, before it is clinically recognized the erythrocyte sedimentation rate (ESR) is elevated and plain X-rays show irregular erosions in the end plates of adjacent vertebral bodies and narrowing of the disk space—a radiographic pattern that is virtually diagnostic of bacterial infection because tumors and other diseases of the spine rarely cross the disk space. Computed tomographic (CT) or magnetic resonance imaging (MRI) scans are still prudent for confirmation of diagnosis because they may demonstrate paraspinal or epidural abscesses. When the cause of vertebral pain, radicular pain, and muscle weakness is unrecognized as coming from an epidural abscess, the clinical course may be one of rapid progression over several weeks to irreversible paralysis.

When nonvertebral hematogenous osteomyelitis is diagnosed in older adults, it is often a relapse of an infection that occurred many years or even decades after the initial episode of infection. In these cases of nonvertebral hematogenous chronic osteomyelitis, recurrent exacerbations typically punctuate long periods of quiescence. Patients are usually afebrile, and a relapse may be manifest only by increased purulence of drainage from sinus tracts between bone and skin, or an increase in the ESR. Rare late complications of chronic hematogenous osteomyelitis include pathologic fractures, squamous cell carcinoma of the sinus tract, and amyloidosis.

The microbiology of vertebral osteomyelitis is different from contiguous focus osteomyelitis in that more than 95% are caused by a single organism. The majority of all cases of hematogenous osteomyelitis are caused by *S. aureus*, although in vertebral osteomyelitis *Escherichia coli* or other enteric bacilli are often the cause. The literature is replete with cases that have unusual causes of hematogenous osteomyelitis, including fungi—such as those resulting from disseminated histoplasmosis, coccidioidomycosis, blastomycosis, cryptococcosis, and *Candida* or aspergillus tissue infections. Atypical mycobacteria, syphilis, yaws, or even viruses such as varicella and vaccinia may also infect bone. The great variety of causes makes culture verification of etiology, either by bone biopsy (always preferred) or blood culture, imperative. Sinus or urine cultures alone are never sufficient to determine antibiotic therapy.

1.1.1.3. OSTEOMYELITIS SECONDARY TO VASCULAR INSUFFICIENCY

When osteomyelitis occurs in the setting of peripheral vascular disease or diabetic neuropathy, it nearly always involves the small bones of the feet. Poor vascular supply to the infected bone and soft tissue impairs normal healing and defenses against infection; in the case of diabetic or other types of peripheral neuropathy, there may be delayed recognition of osteomyelitis because of lack of normal sensation. Microbiologically there is little difference in etiologies between contiguous focus osteomyelitis and that caused by vascular insufficiency: a wide range of Gram-positive cocci, Gram-negative bacilli, and anaerobic pathogens must be considered. Cultures of skin ulcers are unreliable for identification of pathogens, and cultures of bone biopsies are mandatory if precise bacteriologic data are needed *(3,4)*.

1.2. Clinical Manifestations

As with other infections in the elderly, the clinical manifestations of osteomyelitis may be blunted by muted fever or reduced inflammatory response, and the diagnosis can be unrecognized or delayed by difficulties in communication with patients who frequently have neurological diseases. Moreover, because the debilitated elderly may be less mobile, the physical movements or weight bearing that elicit musculoskeletal pain in younger patients may not be present or pain may occur only when they are passively moved by caregivers. As a result, an indolent bone infection may become well-established, and the diagnosis of osteomyelitis only becomes apparent weeks or months later. The initial indication that osteomyelitis is present may thus be the occurrence of complications such as sinus tract formation or disseminated infection. The diagnosis of vertebral osteomyelitis may be the surprising conclusion of a search for the cause of a low-grade fever that had been incorrectly attributed to cellulitis, urinary tract infection, or aspiration and has failed to resolve with treatment. Although the diagnosis of osteomyelitis may be suspected clinically, the definitive diagnosis must be made on the basis of radiological studies or examination of pathological specimens.

1.3. Diagnostic Tests

Prompt diagnosis and institution of antibiotic therapy of osteomyelitis may prevent bone necrosis or serious septic complications. An elevated ESR or C-reactive protein (CRP) level is present in most cases of active osteomyelitis, including in patients who do not have constitutional symptoms or an elevated white blood cell count. Although these are nonspecific laboratory tests, and especially in early infections the ESR may occasionally be normal, the diagnosis of osteomyelitis should be called into doubt when the ESR and CRP are normal.

The targeted evaluation of suspected osteomyelitis usually begins with plain radiographs, although they frequently show no abnormalities during early infection because, on average, 1–2 wk are required for infection to cause necrosis of bone. Plain radiographs may initially show nonspecific soft-tissue swelling; radiographic findings of periosteal reaction, if they occur, are not visible for at least 10 d after the onset of infection. Definitive indications of possible infection, such as lytic changes that do not appear until more than half of bone has been lost, sequestra, or sclerotic new bone formation, may require many weeks to appear on plain radiographs. A CT scan is more sensitive than plain films for the detection of sequestra, sinus tracts, and soft-tissue abscesses. Both CT and ultrasonography are useful for guiding percutaneous aspiration of subperiosteal and soft-tissue fluid collections.

Bone scans are very sensitive indicators of osteomyelitis. In nearly all cases, the technetium radionuclide scan (99mTc diphosphonate) is positive within 24 h of symptomatic infection. Consequently, a negative radioisotope bone scan virtually excludes osteomyelitis. Bone scans are, however, not at all specific for infection. Uptake of technetium merely indicates osteoblastic activity and increased vascularity, so technetium bone scanning cannot differentiate osteomyelitis from fracture, tumor, adjacent soft-tissue infection, or infarction. Although less convenient and more expensive than technetium scans, an abnormal gallium or indium scan (with 67Ga citrate, or 111In-labeled leukocyte or immunoglobulin isotopes) are evolving diagnostic techniques that may be helpful in distinguishing infectious from noninfectious processes found by plain radiographs and technetium scanning, and may prove especially useful in patients with diabetic ulcers *(5)*.

At present, however, the definitive radiographic study for delineating the presence and extent of infection is the MRI scan, which is as sensitive as radioisotope bone scans for the diagnosis of osteomyelitis but is far more specific for infection. It yields better anatomic resolution of epidural abscesses and other soft-tissue processes, and it is preferable to CT scan for delineation of anatomical changes. An MRI scan gives detailed information about the activity and the anatomic extent of infection but cannot always distinguish osteomyelitis from healing fractures and tumors. The MRI scan is particularly useful in distinguishing cellulitis from osteomyelitis in the diabetic foot.

"Probing to bone" is a relatively specific procedure for verifying the presence of osteomyelitis, and may be very useful in the evaluation of nursing facility patients with pressure ulcers. If bone is palpable during examination of the base of an ulcer with a blunt surgical probe, osteomyelitis is highly likely, and further diagnostic testing may be avoidable.

Blood cultures are positive in more than 25% of cases of vertebral osteomyelitis. Cultures of sinus tract drainage or the base of an ulcer correlate poorly with the organisms infecting the bone *(4,6)*. The gold standard is aerobic and anaerobic culture of a biopsy specimen obtained under direct vision during surgery. Multiple aerobic and anaerobic cultures by percutaneous needle biopsy under ultrasound or radiographic guidance or biopsy at the time of debridement are mandatory before antibiotic therapy for chronic osteomyelitis is initiated. Cultures positive for multiple organisms and organisms of low virulence, such as coagulase-negative staphylococci, should not be assumed to be contaminants, especially if foreign bodies are present. Special culture media for less common pathogens, such as mycobacteria or fungi, may be required in some cases, and ultimately histopathologic examination of biopsy specimens may be the only way to make a diagnosis.

1.4. Treatment

1.4.1. Antibiotic Therapy

Antibiotic treatment should not be initiated until appropriate cultures have been obtained. The antibiotics selected should be bactericidal and in most cases, at least initially, should be given intravenously. When possible, empiric therapy may be initiated by Gram staining of a specimen from the bone or abscess. If Gram stains are unavailable, after cultures are obtained, prompt broad-coverage empiric therapy against the most likely pathogens is prudent. Empiric therapy should always include high doses of an antistaphylococcal antibiotic, such as nafcillin, a cephalosporin, or vancomycin; if Gram-negative organisms are likely to be involved, as is usually the case for vertebral osteomyelitis, a third-generation cephalosporin such as ceftazidime or a newer fluoroquinolone such as levofloxacin, may be used. If, methicillin-resistant staphylococci and *P. aeruginosa* are possible infecting organisms, a combination of vancomycin and an antipseudomonal antibiotic, such as a parenteral fluoroquinolone or an antipseudomonal third-generation cephalosporin, may be needed *(7,8)*. Success in animal models of staphylococcal osteomyelitis using rifampin have led some to use the drug in combination with usual antistaphylococcal therapy *(9)*. Typical initial antibiotic regimens for elderly patients based on the presumed infecting organism are listed in Table 1.

Doses must be modified for the reduced lean-body weight and reduced renal function of elderly patients, especially those residing in long-term care facilities. Aminoglycosides should be avoided in the elderly because of their unpredictable ototoxicity and nephrotoxicity, both of which are more frequent and, when they occur, more debilitating in the elderly. If they must be used, serum levels of aminoglycosides should be monitored closely and renal function checked frequently to minimize toxicity.

Duration of intravenous and oral therapy for osteomyelitis is 4–6 wk. When well-absorbed antibiotics such as fluoroquinolones are employed, the switch to oral therapy may be made after defervescence to reduce the complications and expense of immobilization and parenteral therapy. When more than a week of parenteral antibiotic therapy is required, use of agents that require infrequent dosing, such as ceftriaxone, vancomycin, or once-daily newer fluoroquinolones, is preferred *(10,11)*.

When oral therapy is prescribed, the bioavailability and gastrointestinal tolerance of antibiotics must be considered carefully. For example, most oral penicillins or cephalosporins are incompletely absorbed, absorption may be reduced by food (or, paradoxically, by fasting) and the doses required for the treatment of osteomyelitis are several times higher than the doses of these drugs prescribed for other common infections, which may not be tolerated by older adults. Except for the fluoroquinolones, such as ciprofloxacin (500–750 mg twice daily) or levofloxacin (500 mg once daily) there are limited clinical data to support the use of oral antibiotics by adults for the treatment of chronic osteomyelitis. Caution should be exercised in the use of fluoroquinolones as the sole agents for treatment of infection caused by *S. aureus* or *P. aeruginosa* because resistance may develop during therapy. Clindamycin (300–450 mg every 6 h) or metronidazole (500 mg every 6–8 h) are also highly bioavailable and may be useful for oral regimens.

Table 1
**Intravenous Antibiotic Regimens for the Initial Treatment of Bone
and Joint Infections in Elderly Patients, Based on Presumed or Known Pathogens**[a]

- Penicillin-sensitive staphylococci and streptococci:
    Penicillin G (3–4 million units every 4–6 h)
- Penicillin-resistant, methicillin-sensitive staphylococci
    Nafcillin or oxacillin (2 g every 4–6 h), or cefazolin (1–2 g every 8–12 h)
- Methicillin-resistant staphylococci
    Vancomycin (15 mg/kg (up to 1 g) every 12 h)
- Gram-negative bacilli (based on in vitro susceptibility)
    Ampicillin (2 g every 4–6 h), cefazolin, cefuroxime (1.5 g every 8–12 h), or a
      fluoroquinolone such as levofloxacin (500 mg every 24 h)
- Resistant Gram-negative bacilli, such as *P. aeruginosa*:
    Two antibiotics known to be active against the organism, such as piperacillin (3 g every
      6–8 h), or ceftazidime (1 to 2 g every 8–12 h), plus gentamicin or tobramycin
      (1.7 mg/kg every 8 h, or 5–7 mg/kg every 24 h) or a fluoroquinolone, such as
      ciprofloxacin (750 mg every 12 h) or levofloxacin (500 mg every 24 h), or
      aztreonam (1–2 g every 8–12 h) have been recommended by some clinicians

[a]Usually continued for 4–6 wk, although shorter courses may be appropriate for some infections. If response to therapy is rapid, a shorter course of parenteral therapy followed by high doses of oral antibiotics known to be active against the infecting bacteria for the remainder of the course of therapy may be effective.

The ESR may be useful to monitor treatment of chronic osteomyelitis, and in particular, vertebral osteomyelitis. Failure of the ESR to drop to about half of pretreatment levels after a 4–6 wk course of treatment with an appropriate antibiotic is an indication for longer treatment.

1.4.2. Nonantibiotic Therapy

Surgery is seldom necessary for noncontiguous-focus osteomyelitis, even in cases of many months' duration, except in instances of spinal instability, new or progressive neurologic deficits, large soft-tissue abscesses that cannot be drained percutaneously, or a failure of medical treatment. Immobilization, which is always hazardous for elderly patients, should be prescribed only for relief of symptoms—when back pain has declined to the point at which ambulation is possible, bed rest should be terminated. Spontaneous fusion of involved vertebrae occurs in the majority of cases after successful treatment.

Even when diagnosed early, however, cure of contiguous-focus osteomyelitis usually requires at least surgical debridement in addition to 4–6 wk of antibiotic therapy *(12)*. Risks and benefits of aggressive therapy for chronic osteomyelitis in the elderly, however, should be considered carefully. For nursing home patients, for example, intermittent courses of suppressive therapy with oral antibiotics are an attractive option when compared with enduring multiple surgical procedures, prolonged courses of parenteral antimicrobial therapy, and in some cases the risk of loss of an extremity. If surgical intervention is chosen, biopsy and culture performed preoperatively permits the administration of targeted antibiotic therapy before surgery to reduce active infection and inflammation. If the specific etiology is not known, antibiotics should be given intraoperatively—after debridement with culture obtained for definitive therapy. Management of "dead space" created by debridement surgery is mandatory—the goal of dead-space management is to replace dead bone and scar tissue with durable vascularized tissue, as scar tissue that fills the defect may later become avascular. Complete wound closure should be attempted.

The effectiveness of treatment of osteomyelitis of the small bones of the feet related to vascular insufficiency is obviously is limited by the poor blood supply and impaired ability to heal. When appropriate, revascularization should be considered. In the case of decreased perfusion due to diabetic small-vessel disease, the only likely options are suppressive antibiotic therapy or amputation. If infected bone is entirely surgically removed, routine preoperative surgical prophylaxis is sufficient. Although employed at some medical centers, the routine use of hyperbaric oxygen to enhance the killing of microorganisms by phagocytes remains controversial.

1.5. Prevention

Prevention of osteomyelitis depends primarily on controlling the predisposing conditions—bacteremia from acute infection elsewhere, pressure ulcers, and the complications of diabetic neuropathy and vascular disease. Prevention of the latter conditions rests mostly with good skin care, rather than the use of antibiotic therapy once ulcers have developed. The role of antibiotics in the treatment on pressure or trophic ulcers has, moreover, always been controversial, and is, at best, only marginally beneficial unless acute cellulitis is present.

2. SEPTIC ARTHRITIS

2.1. Clinical Relevance

In the elderly, acute joint pain and swelling is much more likely to be caused by crystal-induced arthritis than septic arthritis; the consequences of joint infection, however, are so serious that the possibility of infection requires a targeted diagnostic evaluation to exclude septic arthritis in most patients with acute joint pain. Immediate antibiotic treatment is necessary—loss of cartilage and erosion of subchondral bone from invasion of the cartilage by bacteria and inflammatory cells, increased intra-articular pressure, and release of proteases and cytokines from chondrocytes, begins within days of infection (13). The vast majority of cases of septic arthritis is caused by bacteria and is nearly always hematogenous in origin; nongonococcal arthritis most often involves previously damaged or arthritic joints. The type of infecting organism, to a large degree, also determines the extent of damage: Neisseria gonorrhoeae, for example, causes limited infiltration by leukocytes and results in minimal joint destruction.

2.2. Clinical Manifestations

Sudden onset of articular or periarticular pain, or a change in the pattern of chronic joint pain suggests the possibility of septic arthritis. The presence of pain (100%) and limitation of motion of a joint (90–100%) in a previously normal joint are the most consistent findings in elderly patients with septic arthritis caused by bacteria (13). Most often a single joint is affected, but polyarticular septic arthritis is seen in approximately 10% of cases—patients with rheumatoid arthritis are particularly susceptible (13). In elderly patients with septic (bacterial) arthritis, the knee joint is most frequently involved (35–65%), followed by the hip joint (5–15%) (14). Fever may or may not be present. A complete examination of all joints should be performed even when monoarticular arthritis appears to be present; special attention should be devoted to examining the eyes, skin, mucous membrane, and heart as part of the differential diagnosis. Infection of the hip, shoulder, or sacroiliac joint may not be clinically detectable.

2.3. Diagnostic Tests

Diagnosis of septic arthritis ultimately depends on the results of examination of synovial fluid for leukocytes, crystals, and the presence of bacteria by Gram stain and culture. Although synovial fluid leukocytosis, (white blood cell count exceeding $10,000/mm^3$) with more than 85% neutrophils, is almost always present, it does not distinguish between septic and crystal-induced arthritis. Normal synovial fluid has <180 white blood cells/mm^3 and they are predominantly lymphocytes. In acute bacterial synovitis, white blood cell counts exceed 25,000–50,000 cells/mm^3, and typically reach 100,000 cells/mm^3, with more than 75–90% neutrophils. Noninfectious inflammatory arthritides and mycobacterial and fungal infections usually have fewer than 50,000 cells/mm^3, and more of a lymphocytic response.

When positive, a Gram stain can guide empiric therapy, but it is often negative for bacteria (15,16). Synovial fluid cultures should always be obtained, even when crystals are seen by polarized light examination of a wet mount. If available, polymerase chain reaction (PCR) techniques can detect minute quantities of bacterial DNA within synovial fluid and tissue, but the assay is susceptible to false positives from contamination and cannot distinguish between live and dead organisms. Blood cultures may be positive, especially in *S. aureus* septic arthritis. As in osteomyelitis, the ESR and CRP are usually positive, and may be helpful in monitoring response to treatment. In fact, a normal ESR and/or CRP should make the diagnosis of bacterial arthritis highly suspect (14,17).

Radiographs are of limited utility. MRI scans and, to a lesser extent, CT cans, may be useful for evaluating periarticular soft tissues for abscesses or cellulitis. As with osteomyelitis, radionuclide bone scans are very sensitive early indicators of septic arthritis. Scans with technetium (99mTc), gallium (67Ga), or indium (111In) localizes inflammation and increased bone metabolism, but cannot reliably distinguish between infection-induced and crystal-induced arthritis. For most patients from whom synovial fluid can be obtained, however, MRI scan or radionuclide imaging adds little to the diagnostic process.

Traditionally, bacterial arthritis is divided into nongonococcal and gonococcal etiologies, the latter of which has a better prognosis. Although a bacterial pathogen can be identified in most cases of nongonococcal septic arthritis, the source of infection is less commonly identified. When a source is found, most are cutaneous, respiratory, and genitourinary infections (18).

2.4. Specific Types of Septic Arthritis

2.4.1. Gonococcal Septic Arthritis

Although less common than in younger patients, disseminated gonococcal infection (DGI) must be considered in all sexually active older patients with septic arthritis (13,19). In a review of gonococcal arthritis in young women, the knee was most often affected, followed by hand and wrist synovitis *(20)*. Skin manifestations—small numbers of papules that progress to hemorrhagic pustules on the trunk and the extensor surfaces of the distal extremities—and/or migratory polyarthralgias were present in about half of patients. Joint fluid may be difficult to obtain, and cultures are consistently negative in DGI. Blood cultures were positive in only 13% of cases *(20)*. Although antibiotic resistance of gonococci is an international problem, resistance to ceftriaxone or ciprofloxacin have not been a problem in DGI in the U.S. An appropriate initial regimen is ceftriaxone (1 g parenterally once daily); alternate regimens include ceftizoxime (1 g intravenously (I.V.) every 8 h) or cefotaxime (1 g I.V. every 8 h) until 24–48 h after resolution of symptoms) *(21)*. Persons allergic to β-lactam drugs may be prescribed ciprofloxacin (500 mg I.V. every 12 h), ofloxacin (400 mg I.V. every 12 h), or spectinomycin (2 g intramuscularly (I.M.) every 12 h). Subsequent oral therapy should be with a ciprofloxacin (500 mg twice daily) or ofloxacin (400 mg twice daily), or cefixime (400 mg twice daily), plus empiric treatment for *Chlamydia trachomatis* infection with oral doxycycline (unless a week of ofloxacin is used for followup therapy) *(21)*.

2.4.2. Staphylococcal and Streptococcal Septic Arthritis

S. aureus accounts for the great majority of cases of septic arthritis in older adults *(14)*, and for more than 80% of cases in rheumatoid arthritis or hemodialysis patients *(22,23)*. As a result, all empiric regimens for patients with nongonococcal septic arthritis should include coverage for *S. aureus*, and the probability of bacteremia with possible endovascular infection considered. There is now an increasing prevalence of methicillin-resistant *S. aureus* (MRSA) and *S. epidermidis*, especially in patients with prosthetic joint septic arthritis. Suspected staphylococcal joint infection should be treated initially with vancomycin (1 g I.V. every 12 h), until methicillin resistance can be excluded, with follow-up therapy with a cephalosporin for the remainder of the 4–6 wk course.

The streptococci (nongroup A β-hemolytic streptococci—groups B, C, and G, and pneumococci) and enterococci are the second most common causes of nongonococcal septic arthritis. Group B streptococcal infection may be particularly virulent in diabetic patients. Enterococci can infect native or prosthetic joints. If the Gram stain shows Gram-positive cocci, empiric therapy with vancomycin provides sufficient coverage, including activity against penicillin-resistant *S. pneumoniae*.

2.4.3. Gram-Negative Bacilli

Up to 20% of cases of septic arthritis cases at teaching hospitals are caused by a variety of Gram-negative bacilli, especially among immunosuppressed patients *(18,24)*. In addition, predispositions typical of elderly nursing facility patients—prior antibiotic use, urinary tract infections, and pressure ulcers—are associated with Gram-negative bacilli as causes of septic arthritis. If Gram-negative bacilli are seen on Gram's stain, empiric therapy should include a fluoroquinolone such as ciprofloxacin (500 mg twice daily) or levofloxacin (500 mg daily), or a third-generation cephalosporin such as ceftazidime (2 g twice daily), or imipenem (500 mg every 6 h).

2.4.4. Unusual Causes

Anaerobic joint infections are rare, but should be considered if abdominal abscess or anaerobic soft-tissue infection, such as that associated with pressure ulcers, is present.

Pasteurella multocida, a Gram-negative coccobacillus that is sensitive to penicillin, may cause septic arthritis following an animal bite. Quite rarely, *Mycobacterium marinum*, from exposure to freshwater, saltwater, swimming pools, or fish tanks, may cause mildly painful septic arthritis, without systemic symptoms. Other rare causes that are included in a broad differential diagnosis are *M. tuberculosis* and other mycobacterial species (chronic monoarticular arthritis), *Ureaplasma urealyticum*, *Brucella* spp. (ingestion of unpasteurized dairy products), oral flora such as *Eikenella corrodens* (human bites), and *Treponema pallidum*. Other pathogens to consider in relevant circumstances include *Borrelia burgdorferi* (Lyme disease), *Coccidiodes immitis* (endemic areas), *Sporothrix schenkii* (thorns or splinters), and *Streptobacillus moniliformis* (rat bites). Several viruses, such as mumps, rubella, and parvovirus, may cause infectious arthritis, but are not likely to be encountered in the elderly.

3. ISSUES OF SPECIAL RELEVANCE TO THE ELDERLY

3.1. Prosthetic Joint Infection

Most joint replacement surgery is performed for elderly patients. (*See also* Chapter 17) In a few percent of cases their postoperative course is complicated by infection, and the outcome is poorer with higher mortality and morbidity than in younger patients *(25,26)*. Patients with rheumatoid arthritis have both a higher incidence of joint infection following surgery, and have a poorer outcome when infection occurs. Other groups of patients said to be at greater risk include those with previous surgery on that joint, diabetes mellitus, poor nutritional status, and very old patients. In general, the range of infecting organisms is much broader in the latter susceptible patients, and the fluid should be cultured for less common pathogens such as anaerobic bacteria, fungi, and mycobacteria.

A classic acute presentation of prosthetic joint infection with fever, pain, and inflammation, suggests infection with *S. aureus*, streptococci, or enteric bacilli. On the other hand, many months or even years after surgery less virulent organisms, such as coagulase-negative staphylococci, viridans streptococci, or diphtheroids, or rarely anaerobic bacteria, may be cultured during an evaluation for chronic joint pain or for radiographically noted loosening of the prosthesis. When joint infection follows wound infection, multiple pathogens may be present. Some advocate preoperative treatment of asymptomatic bacteriuria, with the hope of reducing infection risk *(25)*. Radiography, including various types of scans, is of uncertain usefulness—the gold standard for diagnostic testing remains joint aspiration and examination of synovial fluid. In contrast to routine aspiration of nonprosthetic joints, the presence of a foreign body in a joint means that accidental inoculation of organisms during needle aspiration is a special hazard.

The best hope of cure requires a two-stage surgical procedure—removal of the prosthesis and cement is accompanied by a 6-wk course of bactericidal antibiotic therapy chosen on the basis of in vitro susceptibility studies *(26)*. Reimplantation is performed at the conclusion of the 6-wk antibiotic course. A new prosthesis may not be feasible at all, however, and the realistic options for some elderly patients may be limited to joint fusion or amputation. Simple surgical drainage with retention of the prosthesis plus a defined course of antibiotic therapy is generally not successful, and should be reserved only for acute cases (symptoms no longer than 5 d) that are promptly diagnosed, drained, and treated vigorously *(27)*—even then, success with this approach is achieved in only about a third of patients *(25)*. Antibiotic therapy should be continued longer than 6 wk if the prosthesis is left in place *(28,29)*. There are no studies of suppressive or follow-up oral therapy, although the availability of excellent new oral antibiotics makes this a reasonable choice for some patients.

3.2. Rheumatoid Arthritis and Septic Arthritis

Patients with rheumatoid arthritis have the highest incidence of septic arthritis, most often due to *S. aureus*. As many as half of elderly patients with septic arthritis have underlying rheumatoid arthritis, and about 20% of patients with rheumatoid arthritis develop joint infections at some time during the illness *(22)*. Polyarticular infection that can resemble an excerbation of their underlying disease is peculiar to patients with rheumatoid arthritis. Their predispositions to infection include chronically inflamed joints, corticosteroid and other antiinflammatory therapy, breakdown of rheumatoid nodules, and ulcers in the skin overlying deformed joints. Symptoms of infection tend to be insidious and the diagnosis of infection is delayed or ascribed to the underlying disease; perhaps as a result, outcomes tend to be worse than septic arthritis in patients without rheumatoid arthritis *(22)*. In most circumstances, an acutely inflamed joint in a patient with rheumatoid arthritis should be considered to be septic arthritis until infection has been excluded.

4. NONANTIBIOTIC THERAPY

The decision to employ surgical drainage and the type of drainage procedure chosen is more often based on individual clinical decision-making and custom than data. If the joint, e.g., hip septic arthritis, is difficult to aspirate or monitor, a scarred rheumatoid joint is infected, or there has been inadequate response to antibiotics, open drainage may be chosen. Patients with a rapid response to antibiotics and those with gonococcal septic arthritis rarely require open drainage and lavage. An initial attempt at percutaneous drainage or multiple aspirations is preferable in most cases, although arthroscopic lavage is preferred by some orthopedic surgeons. The impulse to lavage joints with antibiotics, which may cause chemical irritation, should be resisted.

Joint immobilization for a few days may improve pain control, but range-of-motion exercises and mobilization should be instituted as soon as possible to reduce deconditioning and maintain joint function *(14)*. Immobilization and deconditioning are especially detrimental for elderly patients.

5. ANTIBIOTIC TREATMENT

Once cultures of blood and synovial fluid have been obtained, empiric antibiotics should be started promptly. There are no standard regimens that are subscribed to universally, but most regimens include a second- or third-generation cephalosporin and specific antistaphylococcal therapy, such as ceftazidime (1–2 g every 8 h) or ceftriaxone (1–2 g every 24 h), and nafcillin (2 g every 6 h), respectively, until culture data are available. Intravenous vancomycin (1 g every 12 h) should be given if methicillin-resistant *S. aureus* is a possible pathogen—particularly in hospitalized or long-term care patients. If *P. aeruginosa* is a possible pathogen, an antipseudomonal antibiotic, such as ceftazidime, piperacillin, imipenem, or ciprofloxacin, should be prescribed. Some clinicians recommend prescribing two antipseudomonal antibiotics.

Definitive therapy with vancomycin, nafcillin, or a first-generation cephalosporin should be continued for at least 4 wk for infections due to staphylococci. Nonstaphylococcal bacterial arthritis, such as that due to *Haemophilus influenzae* or streptococci, may respond to 2–3 wk of therapy, or an abbreviated course of intravenous therapy followed by several weeks of an oral antibiotic with excellent bioavailability. DGI should be treated with standard regimens employed in younger patients. Therapy for unusual organisms must be individualized, with the assistance of infectious disease consultation.

6. PREVENTION

The most preventable form of septic arthritis in the elderly is periprosthetic joint infection. Joint replacement candidates with higher rates of infection—patients with rheumatoid arthritis or other medical conditions requiring immunosuppressive therapy, and those who have undergone previous surgery on the joint—should be evaluated and treated with care. Preoperative antibiotic prophylaxis with cefazolin and laminar air flow in the operating room can lower infection rates. Postoperative care to prevent hematogenous spread of bacteria to the prosthesis requires special attention to intravenous catheters, avoidance of indwelling bladder catheters, and prompt treatment of respiratory, urinary, and cutaneous infections during the perioperative period. The role of prophylactic antibiotics for the prevention of periprosthetic infection following dental procedures or gastrointestinal and genitourinary tract instrumentation is unclear, and they are probably of little or no benefit.

REFERENCES

1. Waldvogel, F. A., Medoff, G., and Swartz, M. N. (1970) Osteomyelitis: a review of clinical features, therapeutic considerations, and unusual aspects. *N. Engl. J. Med.* **282,** 198–316.
2. Darouiche, R. O. (1994) Osteomyelitis associated with pressure sores. *Arch. Intern. Med.* **154,** 753–758.
3. Waldvogel, F. A. and Vasey, H. (1980) Osteomyelitis: the past decade. *N. Engl. J. Med.* **303,** 360–370.
4. Mackowiak, P. A., Jones, S. R., and Smith, J. W. (1978) Diagnostic value of sinus-tract cultures in chronic osteomyelitis. *JAMA.* **239,** 2772–2775.
5. Harvey, J. and Cohen, M. M. (1997) Technetium99–labeled leukocytes in diagnosing diabetic osteomyelitis in the foot. *J. Foot Ankle Surg.* **36,** 209–214.
6. Patzakis, M. J., Wilkins, J., Kumar, J., et al. (1994) Comparison of the results of bacterial cultures from multiple sites in chronic osteomyelitis of long bones: a prospective study. *J. Bone Joint Surg. Am.* **76,** 664–666.
7. Lew, D. P. and Waldvogel, F. A. (1995) Quinolones and osteomyelitis: state of the art. *Drugs,* **49(Suppl 2),** 100–111.
8. Galanakis, N., Giamarellou, H., Moussas, T., et al. (1997) Chronic osteomyelitis caused by multiresistant gram negative bacteria: evaluation of treatment with newer quinolones after prolonged followup. *J. Antimicrob. Chemother.* **39,** 241–246.
9. Norden, C. W. and Keleti, E. (1980) Treatment of experimental staphylococcal osteomyelitis with rifampin and trimethoprim, alone and in combination. *Antimicrob. Agents Chemother.* **17,** 591–194.
10. Rissing, J. P. (1997) Antimicrobial therapy for chronic osteomyelitis in adults: role of the quinolones. *Clin. Infect. Dis.* **25,** 1327–1333.

11. Mauceri, A. A. (1995) Treatment of bone and joint infections utilizing a third generation cephalosporin with an outpatient drug delivery device. *Am. J. Med.* **97(2a),** 14–22.
12. Tetsworth, K. and Cierny, G. 3rd (1999) Osteomyelitis debridement techniques. *Clin. Orthop.* **360,** 87–96.
13. Smith, J. W. and Piercy, E. A. (1995) Infectious arthritis. *Clin. Infect. Dis.* **20,** 225–231.
14. Yoshikawa TT. (1996) Aging and bacterial arthritis. *Infect. Dis. Clin. Pract.* **5,** 548–550.
15. Goldenberg, D. L. and Cohen, A. S. (1976) Acute infectious arthritis: a review of patients with nongonococcal joint infections (with emphasis on therapy and prognosis) *Am. J. Med.* **60,** 369–377.
16. Krey, P. R. and Bailen, D. A. (1979) Synovial fluid leukocytosis: a study of extremes. *Am. J. Med.* **67,** 436–42.
17. Kortekangas, P. (1999) Bacterial arthritis in the elderly. An overview. *Drugs Aging* **14,** 165–171.
18. Le Dantec, L., Maury, F., Flipo, R. M., et al. (1996) Peripheral pyogenic arthritis: a study of one hundred seventy-nine cases. *Rev. Rheum. Engl. Ed.* **63,** 103–110.
19. Geelhold, P. H. L. M., vander Meer, J. W. M., Lichtendahl-Bernards, A. T., et al. (1986) Disseminated gonococcal infection in elderly patients. *Arch. Intern. Med.* **146,** 1739,1740.
20. Wise CM, Morris CR, Wasilauskas BL, et al. (1994) Gonococcal arthritis in an era of increasing penicillin resistance: presentations and outcomes in 41 recent cases (1985–1991) *Arch. Intern. Med.* **154,** 2690–2695.
21. Centers for Disease Control and Prevention (1998) 1998 guidelines for treatment of sexually transmitted diseases. *M. M. W. R.* **47(No. RR-1),** 1–116.
22. Gardner, G. C. and Weisman, M. H. (1990) Pyarthrosis in patients with rheumatoid arthritis: a report of 13 cases and a review of the literature from the past 40 years. *Am. J. Med.* **88,** 503–511.
23. Slaughter, S., Dworkin, R. J., Gilbert, D. N., et al. (1995) Staphylococcus aureus septic arthritis in patients on hemodialysis treatment. *West. J. Med.* **163,** 128–132.
24. Dubost, J. J., Fis, I., Denis, P., et al. (1993) Polyarticular septic arthritis. *Medicine (Baltimore),* **72,** 296–310.
25. Saccente, M. (1998) Periprosthetic joint infections: a review for clinicians. *Infect. Dis. Clin. Pract.* **7,** 431–441.
26. Powers, K. A., Terpenning, M. S., Voice, R. A. et al. (1990) Prosthetic joint infections in the elderly. *Am. J. Med.* **88,** (5N), 9N–13N.
27. Tattevin, P., Cremieux, A. -C., Pottier, P., et al. (1999) Prosthetic joint infection: when can prosthesis salvage be considered? *Clin. Infect. Dis.* **29,** 292–295.
28. Bose, W. J., Gearen, P. F., Randall, J. C., et al. (1995) Longterm outcome of 42 knees with chronic infection after total knee arthroplasty. *Clin. Orthop. Rel. Res.* **319,** 285–296.
29. Ivey, F. M., Hicks, C. A., Calhoun, J. H., et al. (1990) Treatment options for infected knee arthroplasties. *Rev. Infect. Dis.* **12,** 468–478.

13

Skin and Soft-Tissue Infections

Natalie C. Klein and Burke A. Cunha

Skin and soft-tissue infections are common problems in the elderly. In one study of nursing home residents, skin infections accounted for 35% of infections acquired in nursing homes in Maryland *(1)*. The presence of a skin ulcer was the major risk factor for developing an infected ulcer or cellulitis. In addition to the normal changes of the aging skin such as decreased turgor, elasticity, and atrophy, elderly patients often have coexisting peripheral vascular disease or small-vessel disease of diabetes mellitus, which makes them increasingly vulnerable to skin and soft-tissue infections, and may result in delayed healing. The elderly are at risk for all the usual pathogens causing skin and soft-tissue infections but in addition, because of their impaired host defenses and frequent coexisting vascular disease and diabetes mellitus, the elderly are at greater risk of developing necrotizing soft-tissue infection, infected pressure ulcers, and diabetic foot infections (*see* also Chapter 22). Skin and soft-tissue infections in the elderly consist of the primary pyodermas, erysipelas or cellulitis, necrotizing fasciitis, and the infected ulcer (*see* Table 1).

1. PRIMARY PYODERMAS

Superficial skin infections, also called primary pyodermas, are the most common skin infections occurring in all age groups. These include impetigo, folliculitis, furuncles, carbuncles, and paronychia. Most of these infections are caused by group A streptococci or by *Staphylococcus aureus*. *Pseudomonas aeruginosa* is a cause of hot tub folliculitis, an infection associated with recreational use of contaminated whirlpools and hot tubs resulting in a self-limited pruritic papular eruption in a characteristic bathing suit distribution. Some cases of folliculitis and paronychia are caused by *Candida albicans*.

S. aureus colonizes the anterior nares in 20–40% of the normal population. The rate of nasal *S. aureus* colonization is increased in insulin-dependent diabetics, patients undergoing hemodialysis, individuals receiving allergy injections, and in intravenous drug users. Because the elderly often have coexisting diabetes mellitus or renal insufficiency, it is not surprising that asymptomatic nasal *S. aureus* carriage may be increased in the older patient.

From: *Infectious Disease in the Aging*
Edited by: *Thomas T. Yoshikawa and Dean C. Norman*
© *Humana Press Inc., Totowa, NJ*

Table 1
Skin and Soft-Tissue Infections in the Elderly

Type	Major pathogens	Other pathogens
Primary pyoderma	*Staphylococcus aureus*, Group A streptococci	*Pseudomonas aeruginosa*, *Candida* spp.
Erysipelas/ cellulitis	Group A streptococci, *S. aureus*	Group B, C, G streptococci, *Vibrio vulnificus*, *Aeromonas hydrophila*, *Erysipelothrix*, *Pasteurella multocida*,
Necrotizing cellulitis/ fasciitis	Group A streptococci, Enterobacteriaceae	*Bacteroides* spp. *Mycobacterium ulcerans*
Infected ulcer	Streptococci, *S. aureus*, *Escherichia coli*	*Klebsiella*, *Enterobacter*

Colonization and infection with methicillin-resistant *S. aureus* (MRSA) has also become a problem in acute care hospitals, chronic care facilities, and hemodialysis units *(2)*. It is not known why infection with staphylococci develops in some individuals and not in others, but it seems likely that the presence of chronic diseases, wounds, especially skin ulcers, debilitation, and nasal *S. aureus* carriage are all predisposing factors.

In the elderly, localized skin infections due to *S. aureus* include folliculitis, furuncles, carbuncles, hydradenitis suppurativa, and staphylococcal wound infections. Folliculitis, furunculosis, and the carbuncle all involve inflammation and infection around the hair follicle. Folliculitis is the most benign of these infections and presents as painful, erythematous, indurated pustules and crusts around a hair follicle. A furuncle or boil is a deeper infection involving the hair follicle and presents as a painful red nodule or induration that develops a fluctuant center containing purulent creamy material. Carbuncles are deep-seated infections of several hair follicles that often have multiple sinus tracts draining purulent material. Patients with carbuncles may have associated symptoms of fever and chills.

Hydradenitis suppurativa is a recurrent infection of apocrine sweat glands, usually due to *S. aureus*. Patients most often present with recurrent axillary furuncles. Most superficial localized *S. aureus* skin infections can be treated with warm compresses and topical antimicrobial therapy with bacitracin or mupirocin. Antistaphylococcal antibiotics such as penicillinase-resistant penicillins (cloxacillin), first-generation cephalosporins, clindamycin, or alternately minocycline or vancomycin (for MRSA) should be reserved for more serious staphylococcal soft-tissue infections. Large fluctuant lesions usually require incision and draining.

2. ERYSIPELAS/CELLULITIS

Erysipelas and cellulitis are acute spreading infections of the skin, usually involving large confluent areas and accompanied by systemic toxicity. Erysipelas is a superficial skin infection involving the cutaneous lymphatic vessels, caused most commonly by group A streptococci and occasionally by group C or G streptococci. Erysipelas most often involves the face, has a characteristic, well-demarcated appearance with raised margins, and is accompanied by systemic symptoms of fever and chills. Streptococcal cellulitis is an acute, rapidly spreading infection that extends deeper than erysipelas and involves the skin and subcutaneous tissues. Cellulitis is generally associated with diffuse erythema, pain, swelling, lymphangitis, fever, chills, and sometimes bacteremia. Recurrent cellulitis of the extremities occurs in persons with impaired lymphatic drainage such as in lymphedema after radical mastectomy, or phlebectomy associated with coronary artery bypass surgery (CABG). An association between the presence of tinea pedis and post-CABG cellulitis of a lower extremity has been noted *(3)*.

Although most cases of cellulitis are caused by streptococci or staphylococci, a number of unusual organisms can cause cellulitis *(see* Table 2). *Pasteurella multocida,* the major pathogen in dog and cat bites, causes a rapidly progressive cellulitis, often with accompanying lymphangitis occurring several hours after the bite. Cellulitis caused by human bites is polymicrobial similar to bacteriology of oral flora, and usually include streptococci, *S. aureus, Fusobacterium, Bacteroides* spp. and other anaerobes, and *Eikenella corrodens (4)*. *Aeromonas hydrophila* is a Gram-negative bacillus causing cellulitis, wound infections, and rarely myonecrosis after exposure to contaminated fresh water. Usually there is a history of preceding trauma *(5)*. *A. hydrophila* is a normal inhabitant of the foregut of leeches, and *Aeromonas* soft-tissue infections have occurred after application of leeches *(6)*.

Vibrio vulnificus causes two distinct clinical syndromes involving the skin *(7,8)*. Primary bacteremia occurs after ingestion of contaminated raw oysters or other shellfish. Infection usually occurs in the elderly with chronic underlying disease, especially cirrhosis. Onset of disease is rapid and characterized by high fever, chills, shock in about 30%, and characteristic bullous skin lesions in more than 50% of patients. Primary wound infection occurs after exposure to sea water, and also typically causes a bullous cellulitis that varies from a mild infection to severe necrosis mimicking gas gangrene.

Erysipelothrix rhusiopathiae, a Gram-positive bacilli, is the causative agent of erysipeloid, a localized subacute cellulitis and a rare diffuse cutaneous form of cellulitis. Erysipelothrix is acquired from infected animals or fish, usually via trauma to the skin. Erysipeloid usually occurs on the fingers as a slightly raised, well-demarcated violaceous, very painful cellulitis that may be accompanied by lymphangitis *(9)*.

Nodular lymphangitis is a distinct syndrome characterized by superficial nodules developing along the dermal or subcutaneous lymphatics *(10)*. It is caused most often by *Sporothrix schenckii* or *Mycobacterium marinum (11)*. *S. schenckii* is a dimorphic fungus found in the soil, and lymphocutaneous infection characteristically occurs in

Table 2
Unusual Causes of Skin Infection

Risk factor	Pathogens	Therapy
Dog/cat bites	Pasteurella multocida, *Staphylococcus aureus*, streptococci, *Capnocytophaga*	Piperacillin-tazobactam or amoxicillin clavulanic acid
Human bite	Anaerobes, *Eikenella corrodens*, *S. aureus*, streptococci	Piperacillin-tazobactam or amoxicillin-clavulanic acid
Fresh water exposure	*Aeromonas hydrophila*	Trimethoprim-sulfamethoxazole
Cirrhosis	*Vibrio vulnificus*	Doxycycline or 3rd-generation cephalosporin
Salt water exposure	*Vibrio vulnificus*	Doxycycline or 3rd-generation cephalosporin
Shellfish, meat	*Erysipelothrix*	Penicillin
Aquarium	*Mycobacterium marinum*	Doxycycline or trimethoprim-sulfamethoxazole
Gardener	*Sporothrix schenckii*	Itraconazole
Immunosuppression	*Aspergillus*	Amphotericin or itraconazole
	Candida	Fluconazole
	Cryptococcus	Fluconazole
	Pseudomonas aeruginosa	Piperacillin or cefepime or meropenem

gardeners. *M. marinum* is an atypical mycobacterium found in fresh water and sea water. Most cases of lymphocutaneous infection occur in individuals who have contact with aquariums, swimming pools, or fish.

Immunosuppressed individuals are at risk for developing fungal infections of the skin and soft tissue. Ecthyma gangrenosum, a rapidly developing necrotic ulcer, is most often due to bacteremic *P. aeruginosa* infection and occurs predominantly in neutropenic patients. Occasionally, *Aeromonas*, *Candida* spp, and other Gram-negative bacilli can produce similar lesions.

3. NECROTIZING SKIN AND SOFT-TISSUE INFECTIONS

Necrotizing soft-tissue infections are a group of severe, rapidly progressing, often life-threatening infections characterized by extensive tissue damage, sometimes with gas production and frequently progressing to gangrene *(12)* *(see* Table 3). Most of these

Table 3
Necrotizing Soft-Tissue Infections

Clinical entity	Microbiology	Risk factor
Clostridial myonecrosis	*Clostridium perfringens*	Local trauma, surgery
Non-clostridial crepitant cellulitis	Peptostreptococci, *Bacteroides* spp., Enterobacteriaceae	Diabetes mellitus
Necrotizing fasciitis	Group A streptococci, Mixed Enterobacteriaceae and anaerobes	Minor trauma, abdominal surgery, perirectal infection
Progressive bacterial synergistic gangrene	Streptococci, *Staphylococcus aureus*, Enterobacteriaceae	Prior abdominal or thoracic surgery, retention sutures
Synergistic necrotizing cellulitis	Enterobacteriaceae, anaerobes (*Bacteroides* or *Peptostreptococcus*)	Diabetes mellitus, cardiorenal disease, perirectal abscess
Phycomycotic gangrene cellulitis	*Rhizopus*, *Mucor*, *Absidia*	Diabetes mellitus, leukemia, lymphoma, severe burns, elasticized adhesive tape

infections occur in patients with predisposing conditions of trauma, surgery, malignancy, ischemia and diabetes mellitus. (*See* also Chapter 22).

Clostridial myonecrosis caused by *Clostrium perfringens* is a necrotizing infection of subcutaneous tissues that usually occurs after trauma or surgery. Often, there is a history of wound contamination by bowel flora. Minimal gas is present in the tissues, and there is often serous to purulent drainage, and pain is often severe. Nonclostridial crepitant cellulitis caused by anaerobic and facultative bacteria including *Bacteroides* spp., peptostreptococci and Enterobacteriaceae occur predominantly in diabetic patients and, like clostridial cellulitis, is characterized by extensive gas formation in the tissues accompanied by moderate toxicity (*see* also Chapter 22).

Necrotizing fasciitis involves the superficial fascia and subcutaneous tissue causing extensive undermining of tissue, which can be demonstrated by lack of resistance to passage of a probe along the fascial plane *(13)*. Necrotizing fasciitis caused by group A streptococci is also known as streptococcal gangrene, but many other organisms including anaerobes and Enterobacteriaceae can produce this clinical entity. There is often a history of preceding trauma, abdominal surgery, or perirectal infection prior to development of necrotizing fasciitis. Necrotizing fasciitis is a much more painful infection than clostridial or nonclostridial crepitant cellulitis, and there are frequent skin changes of erythema, edema, cyanosis, and gangrene.

Progressive bacterial synergistic gangrene is a distinctive ulcerating lesion that occurs at an abdominal or thoracic operative wound site, often near retention sutures. The infection begins with erythema and induration that evolves into a painful shaggy ulcer with gangrenous margins. Enterobacteriaceae or *S. aureus* are characteristically cultured from the center of the ulcer, whereas anaerobic streptococci grow from the gangrenous margins.

Synergistic necrotizing cellulitis caused by a combination of anaerobe (*B. fragilis* or anaerobic streptococci) and a Gram-negative bacilli occurs predominantly in diabetic patients, often with perirectal infections. This infection causes extensive muscle and fascial necroses with overlying skin gangrene. Patients appear markedly toxic, there is severe pain, and wounds have a characteristic foul-odor drainage, so-called "dishwater" pus.

Phycomycotic gangrenous cellulitis caused by the nonseptate branching fungi, *Rhizopus*, *Mucor*, and *Absidia*, is seen predominantly in diabetics, immunocompromised patients, after severe burns, and after use of elasticized adhesive tape for surgical wounds *(12)* (*see* also Chapter 18). Typically, a black necrotic ulcer develops with raised borders, there is cutaneous anesthesia, and biopsy of the lesion shows fungal invasion. The management of necrotizing skin and soft-tissue infections requires prompt surgical debridement and broad-spectrum antibiotic therapy. If crepitus is present or gas is visualized on radiograph, immediate surgical incision with inspection of soft-tissue and fascia is required. Specimens should be obtained for Gram stain and culture. An appropriate empiric antibiotic regimen should include coverage for streptococci, anaerobes, Enterobacteriaceae, and *S. aureus*.

4. INFECTED ULCERS

Infected ulcers are a common problem in the elderly, especially in the diabetic patient and in patients with impaired motility. Pressure ulcers occur in 10% of patients residing in nursing homes *(14)*. The presence of an ulcer increases the risk of not only to local infection but also to cellulitis, osteomyelitis, and bacteremia. The bacteriology of infected pressure ulcers is polymicrobial. Frequently isolated bacteria include *Proteus mirabilis*, *Escherichia coli*, *Pseudomonas* spp., staphylococci, enterococci, and anaerobes *(15)*. Empiric antibiotic therapy with an extended-spectrum penicillin such as piperacillin-tazobactam or a carbapenem such as meropenem along with surgical debridement is required.

The bacteriology of the infected diabetic foot ulcer is similar to the infected pressure ulcer. (*See* also Chapter 22.) The most common isolates are *S. aureus*, streptococci, enterococci, anaerobes, *E. coli*, and *Proteus* spp *(16,17)*. Therapy consists of debridement of necrotic tissue and broad-spectrum antibiotic therapy.

REFERENCES

1. Magaziner, J., Tenney, J. H., DeForge, B., et al. (1991) Prevalence and characteristics of nursing home acquired infections in the aged. *J. Am. Geriatr. Soc.* **39,** 1071–1078.
2. Kauffman, C. A., Terpenning, M. S., He, X., et al. (1993) Attempts to eradicate methicillin-resistant Staphylococcus aureus from a long-term care facility with the use of mupirocin ointment. *Am. J. Med.* **94,** 371–378.

3. Baddour, L. M. and Bisno, A. L. (1984) Recurrent cellulitis after coronary artery bypass surgery. *JAMA*. **251**, 1049–1052.

4. Goldstein, E. J. C. (1992) Bite wounds an infection. *Clin. Infect. Dis.* **14**, 633–640.

5. Gold, W. L. and Salit, I. E. (1993) Aeromonas hydrophila infections of skin and soft tissue: report of 11 cases and review. *Clin. Infect. Dis.* **16**, 69–74.

6. Lineaweaver, W. C., Hill, M. K., Bunke, G. M., et al. (1992) Aeromonas hydrophila infections following use of medicinal leeches in reimplantation and flap surgery. *Ann. Plast. Surg.* **29**, 238–244.

7. Hill, M. K. and Sanders, C. V. (1998) Skin and soft tissue infections in critical care. *Crit. Care Clin.* **14**, 251–262.

8. Chuang, Y. C. (1992) Vibrio vulnificus infection in Taiwan: report of 28 cases and review of clinical manifestations and treatment. *Clin. Infect. Dis.* **15**, 271–276.

9. Reboli, A. C. and Farrar, W. E. (1989) Erysipelothrix rhuseopathiae: an occupational pathogen. *Clin. Microbiol. Rev.* **2**, 354–359.

10. Shea, K. W. and Cunha, B. A. (1996) Nodular lymphangitis. *Infect. Dis. Pract.* **20**, 22–23.

11. Heller, H. M. and Swartz, N. M. (1994) Nodular lymphangitis: clinical features, differential diagnosis and management, in *Current Clinical Topics in Infectious Diseases*, Vol. 14 (Remington, J. S. and Swartz, M. N., eds.) McGraw-Hill, New York, pp. 142–158.

12. Feingold, D. S. (1981) The diagnosis and treatment of gangrenous and crepitant cellulitis, in *Current Clinical Topics in Infectious Diseases*, Vol. 2 (Remington, J. S. and Swartz, M. N., eds.), McGraw-Hill, New York, pp. 259–277.

13. Sentochnik, D. E. (1995) Deep soft tissue infections in diabetic patients. *Infect. Dis. Clin. North Am.* **9**, 53–64.

14. Brandeis, G. H., Morris, J. N., Nash, D. J., et al. (1990) The epidemiology and natural history of pressure ulcers in elderly nursing home residents. *JAMA* **264**, 2905–2909.

15. Kertesz, D. and Chow A. W. (1992) Infected pressure and diabetic ulcers. *Clin. Geriatr. Med.* **8**, 835–852.

16. Louie, J. J., Bartlett J. G., Tally, F. P., et al. (1976) Aerobic and anaerobic bacteria in diabetic foot ulcers. *Ann. Intern. Med.* **85**, 461–463.

17. Smith, A. J., Daniels, T., and Bohnen, J. M. (1996) Soft tissue infections and the diabetic foot. *Am. J. Surg.* **2(Suppl 6A)**, 7S–12S.

14

Orofacial and Odontogenic Infections

Anthony W. Chow

1. EPIDEMIOLOGY AND CLINICAL RELEVANCE

Orofacial and odontogenic infections are diverse in etiology and clinical presentation. Elderly patients are particularly at risk because of poor oral health and relatively high prevalence of dental caries and periodontal disease. Such infections in the elderly may be localized and indolent, or invasive and life-threatening. Patients with systemic underlying diseases such as diabetes mellitus are also prone to more serious infections. The increasing need for valvular and joint replacements in the elderly also exposes this population to a greater risk for serious complications such as infective endocarditis or prosthetic infections from hematogenous seeding of odontogenic infections (1).

Virtually all infectious agents can present intraorally. Although bacterial and fungal infections of the oral mucosa usually result from direct inoculation of opportunistic pathogens from the external or resident microflora, viral infections of the oral mucosa generally arise by hematogenous dissemination or reactivation of a latent infection. Due to physiologic changes, such as blunted fever responses, chronic or coexisting diseases, and a tendency to underreport symptoms, the clinical presentation of odontogenic infections in the elderly may be atypical, and the diagnosis or severity of infection may be unrecognized or underestimated (2).

1.1. Prevalence of Dental Caries and Periodontal Disease in the Elderly

A survey among adults and senior citizens in the United States revealed that the fraction of individuals aged 65 yr or older who retained some or all of their natural teeth had risen from 40% in 1957 to 60% in 1986 and 72% in 1991 (3,4). These surveys document the notion that edentulism is no longer the norm in the aging population, and that oral health and dental care (including the appropriate diagnosis, management, and prevention of odontogenic infections) is an increasingly important issue in geriatric medicine.

In the 1988–1991 national survey, the prevalence of dental caries, particularly on root surfaces of the affected teeth, increased dramatically with age, from 47% in those 65–75 yr old to 56% in those 75 yr of age or older (5). Diseases of the periodontium are also extremely common in the elderly. In the same survey, 46% of individuals 65 yr or older suffered moderately severe gingival recession (more than 3 mm), and over 80 % experienced modest periodontal attachment loss (at least 3 mm) (6).

From: Infectious Disease in the Aging
Edited by: Thomas T. Yoshikawa and Dean C. Norman
© Humana Press Inc., Totowa, NJ

Longitudinal studies of oral health in the aging person are generally rare. Nordstrom and colleagues *(7)* conducted a 9-yr longitudinal study of dental and periodontal status in 70- and 79-yr-old city cohorts in northern Sweden. The frequency of reported annual dental visits increased in the younger but not in the older cohort during the 9-yr period. Clinical examination showed an increasing prevalence of tooth loss, root caries, and periodontal disease with advancing age. Among dentulous persons, 1.7 teeth per subject were lost from 1981 to 1990 in the younger cohort, compared with 2.6 teeth per subject in the older cohort. The number of good teeth decreased very little in the younger cohort (from 3.44–3.34) but did decrease more dramatically in the older cohort (from 3.47–2.65) during the 9-yr period. The frequency of surfaces with periodontal attachment loss exceeding 3 mm increased statistically from 1981–1990 in the older cohort. In general, subjects with annual dental visits had fewer oral problems.

The oral health of elderly patients in long-term care facilities was investigated during 1993 among 250 residents in a suburban community in Norway *(8)*. Results were compared with an identical examination of the residents in the same facilities in 1980. In general, the oral hygiene was poor. The mean number of remaining teeth per person was 11.7 (confidence interval [CI], 10.3–13.1). The mean number of filled teeth was (5.1 CI, 4.1–6.0), and the mean number of decayed teeth was 1.8 (CI, 1.4–2.2). The mean number of residual roots per person was 0.8 (CI, 0.5–1.1). Periodontal pockets exceeding 4 mm were observed in 5% of all teeth. Edentulousness had decreased from 80% in 1980 to 54% in 1993, and more remaining and filled teeth and fewer residual roots per person were observed in the 1993 population. These data underscore the need for resources to prevent periodontal disease and caries among elderly patients in long-term care facilities.

1.2. Microbial Etiology of Dental Caries and Periodontal Disease

Dental caries are caused by a variety of oral bacteria, particularly *Streptococcus mutans* and *Lactobacillus* spp., which colonize the tooth surface as a dental plaque *(9)*. The ingestion of carbohydrates, especially monosaccharides and disaccharides, results in the generation of acids on the tooth surface by these plaque bacteria, causing demineralization of the protective enamel coating and subsequent tooth decay. The tooth has at least three intrinsic mechanisms protecting it from carious decay: (1) constant flow of saliva of neutral pH that buffers and washes away bacterial acids, and supplies calcium and phosphate to remineralize and repair damaged tooth surfaces; (2) acquisition of an acellular, structureless, bacteria-free coating of salivary origin, known as the *acquired pellicle*, which acts as a surface barrier to dietary and bacterial damage; and (3) cleansing action of the tongue and buccal membranes that actively removes food particles from the proximity of the tooth. The saliva and its various constituents, such as lactoferrin, lysozyme, lactoperoxidase, β-lysin, and immunoglobulins, also possess important antimicrobial activity against dental plaque-associated bacteria. As well, the act of tooth brushing and flossing serves to remove food particles and bacterial plaques adherent to the tooth surface. However, with aging and poor dental hygiene, the acquired pellicle becomes colonized with bacteria, and is replaced by supragingival and subgingival bacterial plaques that ultimately progress to dental caries.

Unlike dental caries, diet does not appear to have a significant role in the pathogenesis of periodontal disease. Factors most commonly associated with gingivitis are inadequate oral hygiene and development of the supragingival or subgingival dental plaque. Plaques that accumulate above the gingival margin are composed mainly of Gram-positive facultative and microaerophilic cocci and bacilli; plaques that accumulate below the gingival margin are composed mainly of Gram-negative anaerobic bacilli and motile forms including spirochetes. Periodontal disease is mainly caused by microorganisms within the subgingival dental plaque, which penetrate the gingival epithelium and elicit an inflammatory host response. This ultimately results in destruction of the periodontium comprising the alveolar bone surrounding the root of the tooth, the periodontal membrane, and the gingiva *(10)*. This tissue destruction causes an apical migration of gingival tissues (gingival recession), loss of periodontal attachment, and an increase in the depth of the gingival crevice (periodontal pocket formation). The microflora associated with gingivitis is predominated by *Actinomyces viscosus* and *Bacteroides gingivalis*, whereas those closely associated with advanced periodontitis include *Actinobacillus actinomycetemcomitans*, *Porphyromonas gingivalis*, *Treponema denticola*, and *B. forsythus (11)*. A unifying hypothesis postulating the microbial shift from a plaque-free tooth surface and progression to supragingival and subgingival plaque organisms and various odontogenic infections is shown in Fig. 1.

1.3. Factors Predisposing to Orofacial and Odontogenic Infections in the Elderly

Several factors in the elderly may predispose to the development of dental caries and periodontal disease. These include difficulty in performing oral hygiene due to impaired manual dexterity or physical disability, inadequate fluoride exposure, frequent sugar consumption, gingival recession, and reduced sensory or motor function in the oral cavity and around the teeth *(12)*. Although individuals of all ages are susceptible to the development of dental plaque if daily oral care is withheld, older persons form dental plaques more rapidly than do younger people. Gingival recession, which is both common and more severe with advancing age, also renders the elderly more susceptible to the development of root caries by exposing the underlying tooth surfaces to subgingival dental plaques without the protection from enamel covers. Chronic medical illness, physical disability, and socioeconomic factors may also limit access to appropriate dental care in the elderly, either due to immobility, cost of transportation and treatment, or long-term care institutionalization *(13)*.

Salivary gland hypofunction with diminished salivary flow and the development of xerostomia, is an important contributor to poor oral hygiene in the elderly that ultimately leads to both dental caries and periodontal disease. Without an adequate volume or normal composition of saliva, chewing and swallowing becomes more difficult, and repeated irritation of the gingiva and other soft tissues results in gingivitis, mucositis, aphthous ulcers, and an increased rate of tooth decay. It is important to note that aging per se does not appear to lead to salivary hypofunction, and in healthy older adults there is no significant alteration either in the volume or composition of saliva produced *(13,14)*. The frequent finding of decreased salivary output and xerostomia is most likely caused by systemic diseases and their treatments rather than by the normal

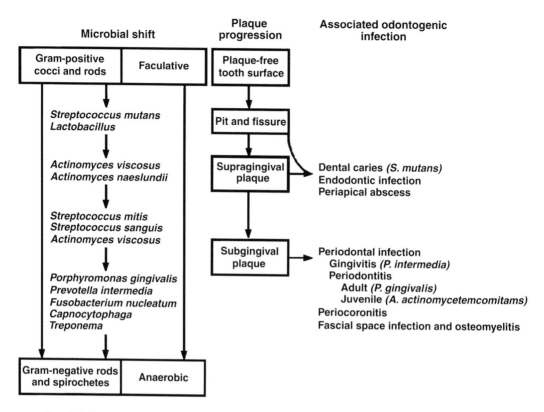

Fig. 1. Microbial etiology of odontogenic infections. A unifying hypothesis postulating the microbial shift from a plaque-free tooth surface and progression to supragingival and subgingival plaque organisms and various odontogenic infections. Modified with permission from ref. *24*.

biologic sequelae of aging. For example, agents used to manage urinary incontinence, hypertension, depression, and other major medical problems in the elderly, particularly anticholinergic drugs, are especially common causes of xerostomia *(15)*. In addition, several classes of medications frequently prescribed to older people, such as calcium channel blockers (e.g., diltiazem, verapamil, nifedipine), anticonvulsants (e.g., phenytoin), and immunosuppressants (e.g., cyclosporin), are associated with the development of gingival hyperplasia. If left untreated, this can also predispose to both dental caries and destructive periodontitis *(12)*.

2. CLINICAL MANIFESTATIONS

2.1. Orofacial Infections

The oral cavity of older adults, especially immunocompromised persons, are susceptible to a variety of bacterial, fungal, and viral infections. The lesions are often of protracted duration, and may not be associated with a clinically significant inflammatory reaction. Palpation and percussion of the oral structures are critical as tenderness may be the only abnormal finding.

2.1.1. Vesiculobullous Gingivostomatitis and Aphthous Ulcers

Vesiculobullous lesions of the oral mucosa and perioral region are commonly caused by viral agents, especially from reactivation of herpes simplex virus infection. Other viruses that may produce vesicular oral lesions include varicella-zoster, type A Coxsackie viruses, and cytomegalovirus (CMV). Oromucosal herpetic lesions typically occur on the gingiva, palate, or the tongue. The initial symptoms are sore throat, enlarged submandibular lymph nodes, and a burning sensation of the oral mucosa. This is rapidly followed by mucosal ulcers that may be small at first but often coalesce into large shallow lesions with serpiginous borders, and may become covered by a fibrinous, yellowish, firmly adherent membrane. The ulcer is very painful, and the patient is febrile and has considerable difficulty talking, eating, and swallowing.

Varicella-zoster, or shingles, occurs in the elderly at rates exceeding 10 per 1000 annually at age 80 yr *(13)*. Clinical manifestations include vesicular eruptions of the skin and mucous membranes in the areas following the distribution of ophthalmic, maxillary, or mandibular divisions of the trigeminal sensory nerves. Symptoms include fever, malaise, and pain and tenderness along the course of the involved sensory nerve. Postherpetic neuralgia may occur in 25–50% of patients older than age 60. CMV can manifest as mononucleosis-like symptoms with inflammatory sore throat, enlarged salivary glands, petechial hemorrhages, or persisting oromucosal ulcers. Dissemination is more likely in immunocompromised patients or organ transplantation recipients.

Coxsackie viral infection primarily affects the oropharynx (herpangina), although gingivostomatitis can occur in more severe cases. The onset is sudden, with relatively severe systemic reactions including fever, sore throat, dysphagia, vomiting, and abdominal pains. Small grayish papules and vesicles surrounded by red areolae develop on the tonsillar fauces, soft palate, uvula, tongue, and oropharynx; these rarely occur on the buccal mucosa or periodontium. The disease is usually self-limiting and lasts 3–4 d, followed by complete recovery.

Aphthous ulcers are among the most common causes of recurrent oral lesions, and must be distinguished from other conditions such as herpes simplex virus or Coxsackie virus infections, agranulocytosis, and Behçet's disease. The etiology of aphthous ulcers remains uncertain, although a number of infectious agents including viruses have been implicated. Three major clinical variants are recognized: (1) minor aphthous ulcers, (2) major aphthous ulcers, and (3) herpetiform aphthous ulcers. Minor aphthous ulcers appear as a number of small ulcers on the buccal and labial mucosa, the floor of the mouth, or the tongue. The palatal soft tissues, pharynx, and tonsillar fauces are rarely involved. A prodromal stage is usually present. The ulcers appear gray-yellow, often with a raised and erythematous margin, and are exquisitely painful. Lymph node enlargement is seen only with secondary bacterial infection. The course of ulceration varies from a few days to several weeks and is followed by spontaneous healing. Major aphthous ulcers are more protracted and may last up to several months. All areas of the oral cavity including the soft palate and tonsillar areas may be involved. Prolonged periods of remission may be followed by intervals of intense ulcer activity. Herpetiform aphthous ulcers are small and multiple, and characteristically affect the lateral margins and tips of the tongue. The ulcers are gray with a delineating erythematous border and are extremely painful. Despite its name, there is little clinical resemblance to an acute herpetic gingivostomatitis.

2.1.2. Oropharyngeal Candidiasis

Colonization of the oral cavity by *Candida* spp. increases in the elderly, although the frequency and intensity of carriage appears to be independent of denture use *(16)*. Clinical disease may be precipitated by the use of broad-spectrum antibiotics and inadequately cleaned or ill-fitting dentures. The most common oral manifestation is pseudomembranous candidiasis (thrush), which affects about 10% of the elderly population *(13)*. It is characterized by soft, white, slightly raised adherent plaques that can be wiped off leaving an erythematous or bleeding surface. Acute erythemic or atrophic candidiasis is characterized by painful erythematous mucosal lesions and a "bald" (depapillated) appearance of the tongue. Chronic atrophic candidiasis or denture-induced stomatitis is commonly found in denture wearers and elderly persons with diffuse inflammation of denture-bearing areas due to prolonged irritation. Chronic hyperplastic candidiasis is a leukoplakic or keratotoic lesion that cannot be removed by scraping, and is usually located on the anterior buccal mucosa.

2.1.3. Sialadenitis and Suppurative Parotitis

Sialadenitis, or infection of salivary tissue, is relatively common in the elderly, often from ductal obstruction caused by calculi, dehydration, sialogogic drugs, or general debility. In suppurative parotitis, there is a sudden onset of firm, erythematous swelling of the pre- and postauricular areas that extends to the angle of the mandible. This is associated with exquisite local pain and tenderness. Systemic findings of high fevers, chills, and marked toxicity are generally present. Progression of the infection may lead to massive swelling of the neck, respiratory obstruction, septicemia, and osteomyelitis of the adjacent facial bones. Staphylococci have been the predominant isolates, but Enterobacteriaceae, oral anaerobes, and other Gram-negative bacilli have also been reported.

2.1.4. Mucositis in the Severely Immunocompromised

Mucositis that complicates radiation or chemotherapy most commonly involves the nonkeratinized oral epithelium, including the buccal and labial mucosa, soft palate, oropharynx, floor of the mouth, and ventral and lateral surfaces of the tongue. Oral candidiasis, herpes simplex, varicella-zoster, and CMV infections are the most common manifestations. Bacteremia caused by viridans streptococci is particularly common in patients with severe mucositis associated with treatment for acute leukemia *(17)*. Ulceration and pseudomembrane formation are evident usually between 4 and 7 d after the initiation of chemotherapy, when the rate of destruction of the basal epithelium exceeds that of proliferation of new cells. The clinical manifestations may be quite variable. The lesions are often protracted in duration and may not be associated with an inflammatory reaction, thereby masking the usual symptoms and signs of infection. Pain or tenderness may be the only abnormal finding.

2.2. Odontogenic Infections

Odontogenic infections originate either in the dentoalveolar structures, the periodontium, or the pericoronal tissues. Complications include orofacial "space" infections and osteomyelitis. The unique features of their clinical manifestations in the elderly are emphasized as follows.

2.2.1. Dentoalveolar Infections

2.2.1.1. DENTAL CARIES

Both coronal and root caries are common in the elderly population. Coronal caries are more likely to present as recurrent lesions around existing restorations, which are more difficult to detect clinically than new carious lesions. The earliest findings are the presence of pits and fissures on the affected tooth surface that gradually becomes stained due to demineralization of enamel and dentine. Further destruction eventually leads to collapse of the overlying enamel. Because there are no cells or vascular elements in enamel or dentine except for the secondary odontoblasts lying on the pulpal surface, the diseased area is incapable of healing and replacement. The typical clinical presentation is a soft to rubbery textured and discolored defect on the tooth surface. Rapidly progressive caries tend to be soft and can be painful due to involvement of the pulp. Most coronal caries develop slowly as the infection must spread through highly calcified enamel and dentine, and hence the lesions are more likely to be long-standing, hard, and asymptomatic. The carious process progresses silently until the infection has invaded deeply enough into the pulp to cause pulpal reaction, and eventually the crown is destroyed. Root caries occur on the tooth surface where gingival recession has occurred and are characterized by discrete, well-defined, soft, discolored defects on the root surface or at the junction of the crown and the root. Root caries can be more difficult to diagnose than coronal caries as they tend to occur in the interproximal tooth surfaces that are particularly prone to decay due to retained food debris and their relative inaccessibility to brushing.

2.2.1.2. PULPITIS AND PERIAPICAL ABSCESS

Infection of the pulp can occur in one of three ways: (1) through a defect in the enamel and dentine due to extension of a carious lesion, traumatic fracture, or a dental procedure; (2) through the apical foramen or lateral canals (e.g., from a periodontal pocket or an adjacent tooth with a periapical abscess); and (3) through hematogenous seeding of the pulp that has been irritated mechanically. Once infected, the acute inflammatory reaction causes a rapid accumulation of pressure inside this rigid and unyielding space, compressing the blood vessels entering the pulp cavity through the apical foramen, and causing ischemia and necrosis of the pulp tissue. Pus may egress out of a cavity in the crown if one exists or may extrude apically into the surrounding periodontal tissue resulting in an *acute periapical periodontitis*. Alternately, the infected material may erode out of the apical foramen resulting in a *periapical* or *alveolar abscess*. The accumulation of pus causes loss of bone and periodontal tissue and may extend to involve other teeth. A more serious complication is lateral extension of the abscesses into planes of least resistance, resulting in deep fascial space involvement. The early and dominant symptom of an acute pulpitis is severe pain, which can be elicited by thermal changes, especially cold drinks. In addition, the involved tooth may be sensitive to palpation and percussion. As the disease progresses the pain becomes severe and continuous with increased intensity upon lying down. However, these symptoms may be less intense in older patients because of a more blunted inflammatory host response, and a predictable diminution with age in the number and viability of nerve fibers within the dental pulp. In addition, the disease is frequently more advanced in the elderly because of undue delays in seeking dental care. A more indolent form of pulpitis is *chronic pulpitis*, in which the inflammation is low grade with partial drainage of the infected material, and symptoms are characterized by a mild and dull intermittent pain that is not altered by thermal changes.

2.2.2. Periodontal Infections

2.2.2.1. GINGIVITIS

Mild gingivitis secondary to irritation from dental plaque, gingival bleeding, or calculus accumulation is relatively common in older adults. Clinically, there is swelling and bluish purple discoloration of the gingiva with a tendency for bleeding after eating or brushing. There is usually no pain but a mild fetor oris may be noticed. The inciting dental plaque may be difficult to observe until it has reached a certain thickness and becomes discolored or is calcified (calculus or tartar). The prevalence and extent of subgingival calculus increase directly with age and is found in 75% of individuals 65 yr or older. This is in contrast to supragingival calculus, which does not vary greatly with age, and is much less prevalent in the elderly (16% of individuals 65 yr or older) *(6)*. *Acute necrotizing ulcerative gingivitis*, also known as Vincent's disease or trench mouth, is relatively rare in the elderly. The patient typically experiences a sudden onset of pain in the gingiva, and the tissue appears eroded with superficial grayish pseudomembranes. There is halitosis and altered taste sensation in addition to fever, malaise, and lymphadenopathy.

2.2.2.2. PERIODONTITIS AND PERIODONTAL ABSCESS

Chronic adult periodontitis is characterized by gingival inflammation accompanied by loss of supportive connective tissues including alveolar bone, resulting in detachment of the periodontal ligament to the cementum. This leads to apical migration of the junctional epithelium (gingival recession), deepening of the gingival sulcus forming a "periodontal pocket" around the tooth, and mobility and eventual loss of the affected tooth. The destructive process is slow, likely from years of dental neglect and chronic gingivitis. Plaque and calculi are abundant both supra- and subgingivally, and frank pus may be present in the periodontal pockets. *Periodontal abscess* may be focal or diffuse and presents as a red, fluctuant swelling of the gingiva, which is extremely tender to palpation. These abscesses always communicate with a periodontal pocket from which pus can be readily expressed after probing.

2.2.3. Pericoronitis

Pericoronitis is an acute localized infection caused by food particles and microorganisms becoming trapped under the gum flaps of a partially erupted tooth or an impacted molar tooth. Most of these are associated with mandibular molars with extensive bone resorption. This causes the originally embedded tooth to become exposed intraorally. Prominent symptoms include pain and limitation of movement on opening the jaw, discomfort on mastication and swallowing, and facial swelling. Clinically, the pericoronal tissues are erythematous and swollen, and digital pressure can often express an exudate from under the infected flap. The masticator spaces are often involved and may manifest as trismus. Localized painful lymphadenopathy may be noted, and the breath is usually foul.

2.2.4. Orofacial "Space" Infections

Suppurative odontogenic infections may extend into potential fascial spaces in the orofacial area or deep in the head and neck *(18)*. Immunocompromised patients as well as the elderly are at particular risk for unhalted and spreading orofacial infections. Table 1 compares the salient clinical features of these "space" infections. However, fever may be blunted or absent in elderly patients even in the presence of severe infection *(19)*. The more superficial space infections of the face and oral cavity may involve the buccal, canine, masticator, submental, and infratemporal spaces. They serve as important clues to the precise location of the underlying infected tooth. If unrecognized and untreated, these infections are potentially life-threatening, as they may spread contiguously into the deeper fascial spaces of the head and neck such as the submandibular, lateral pharyngeal and retropharyngeal spaces, or into the carotid sheath *(18)*. Such infections may result in aspiration and airway obstruction, or may spread intracranially to cause purulent meningitis or subdural empyema, and caudally to result in fatal necrotizing mediastinitis.

2.2.5. Osteomyelitis

Odontogenic infections may also spread contiguously to cause osteomyelitis of the jaws. There is usually a predisposing condition such as compound fracture, irradiation, diabetes mellitus, or corticosteroid therapy. With initiation of infection, the intramedullary pressure markedly increases, further compromising blood supply and leading to bone necrosis. Pus travels through the haversian and perforating canals, accumulates beneath the periosteum, and elevates it from the cortex. If pus continues to accumulate, the periosteum is eventually penetrated, and mucosal or cutaneous abscesses and fistulas may develop. As the inflammatory process becomes more chronic, granulation tissue is formed. Spicules of necrotic and nonviable bone may become either totally isolated (sequestrum) or encased in a sheath of new bone (involucrum). Severe mandibular pain is a common symptom and may be accompanied by anesthesia or hypoesthesia on the affected side. In protracted cases, mandibular trismus may develop.

3. DIAGNOSTIC TESTS

3.1. Specimen Collection and Processing

Because most infections that originate from the oral cavity are polymicrobial in nature, care must be taken during specimen collection to avoid contamination by the resident oral flora. Aaerobic and anerobic blood cultures should always be obtained. In selected patients with pyogenic infections of the face and neck, particularly compromised hosts, needle aspiration of the spreading edge of the skin lesion (using a tuberculin syringe containing 0.5 mL nonbactericidal saline and a 23-gauge hypodermic needle) is a worthwhile procedure. For ulcerative oromucosal lesions, scrapings from the ulcer base should be obtained for Gram-stain, potassium hydroxide, and Tzanck preparations, and cytologic examination. The diagnosis of herpes simplex or varicella-zoster is readily confirmed by a positive Tzanck smear (prepared from scrapings of the

Table 1
Comparative Features of Odontogenic Deep Fascial Space Infections of the Head and Neck

Space Infections	Usual site of origin	Pain	Trismus	Swelling	Dysphagia	Dyspnea
Masticator						
Masseteric and Pterygoid	Molars (especially third)	Present	Prominent	May not be evident (deep)	Absent	Absent
Temporal	Posterior maxillary molars	Present	None	Face, orbit (late)	Absent	Absent
Buccal	Bicuspids, molars	Minimal	Minimal	Cheek (marked)	Absent	Absent
Canine	Maxillary canines, incisors	Moderate	None	Upper lip, canine fossa	Absent	Absent
Infratemporal	Posterior maxillary molars	Present	None	Face, orbit (late)	Occasional	Occasional
Submental	Mandibular incisors	Moderate	None	Chin (firm)	Absent	Absent
Parotid	Masseteric spaces,	Intense	None	Angle of jaw (marked)	Absent	Absent
Submandibular	2nd, 3rd mandibular molars	Present	Minimal	Submandibular	Absent	Absent
Sublingual	Mandibular incisors	Present	Minimal	Floor of mouth (tender)	Present if bilateral	Present if bilateral
Lateral pharyngeal						
Anterior	Masticator spaces, occasional	Intense	Prominent	Angle of jaw	Present	Occasional
Posterior	Masticator spaces, severe	Minimal	Minimal	Posterior pharynx	Present	Severe
Retropharyngeal (and danger)	Lateral pharyngeal space, distant via lymphatics	Present	Minimal	Posterior pharynx (midline)	Present	Present
Pretracheal	Retropharyngeal space, anterior esophagus	Present	None	Hypopharynx	Present	Severe

Clinical features

Reproduced with permission from ref. 25.

ulcer base), which demonstrates the presence of multinucleated giant cells with intranuclear inclusions. Cultures for bacterial, fungal, mycobacterial, and viral pathogens should be obtained where appropriate. Punch biopsy is also valuable for the investigation of chronic mucosal lesions and for the diagnosis of malignant or premalignant conditions. Immunofluorescence staining for antigen detection can also be performed for herpes simplex and varicella-zoster as well as papilloma viruses and other pathogens. Identification of potential pathogens by DNA amplification and hybridization techniques is a powerful tool that is increasingly being utilized to identify etiologic agents in suspected infections that are culture-negative.

3.2. Imaging Techniques

An orthopantomogram may reveal the true extent of advanced periodontitis or the presence of periapical abscess. Ultrasonography, radionuclide scanning, computed tomography (CT), and magnetic resonance imaging (MRI) are particularly useful for the localization of deep fascial space infections of the head and neck. A lateral radiograph of the neck may demonstrate compression or deviation of the tracheal air column or the presence of gas within necrotic soft tissues. In retropharyngeal infections, lateral radiographs of the cervical spine or CT scanning can help determine if the infection is in the retropharyngeal space or the prevertebral space. The former suggests an odontogenic source, whereas the latter suggests involvement of the cervical spine. Technetium bone scanning, used in combination with gallium- or indium-labeled white blood cells, is particularly useful for the diagnosis of acute or chronic osteomyelitis and for the differentiation of infection or trauma from malignancy.

4. THERAPY

Antimicrobial therapy of orofacial and odontogenic infections should be guided by the clinical history, careful physical examination, and associated or underlying medical conditions. Because the etiologic agents are remarkably diverse, every effort should be made to narrow down the differential diagnosis by pursuing a judicious but aggressive plan of investigation. Results of culture and susceptibility data, although important for establishing the etiologic diagnosis, are often not available. Thus, particularly in severely ill or immunocompromised patients, the initial choice of antimicrobial therapy is often empirical and designed to cover the most likely pathogens with broad-spectrum agents.

4.1. Dental Caries and Periodontitis

With the improvement of dental restorative materials such as bonding and fluoride-releasing agents, dental caries in older adults can be readily treated by restorative and prosthodontic treatment programs. Acute necrotizing ulcerative gingivitis should be treated with systemic antimicrobials such as metronidazole or penicillin. Certain types of severe periodontitis are amenable to systemic antimicrobials in conjunction with mechanical debridement (scaling and root planing) *(20)*. Double-blind clinical studies of advanced periodontitis in which systemic metronidazole (500 mg three times/day orally) or doxycycline (200 mg two times/d orally) for 1 or 2 wk used in conjunction with rigorous mechanical debridement was found to reduce the need for radical surgery by 80% compared with debridement plus placebo control. Oral antimicrobial rinses with

Table 2
Antimicrobial Agents Useful for Oromucosal and Odontogenic Infections

Systemic antibacterials for dental or periodontal infections
  Normal host
    Penicillin G, 1–4 MU IV q4–6 h; or ampicillin-sulbactam, 1.5–3 g IV q6 h
    Clindamycin, 450 mg PO or 600 mg IV q6–8 h
    Metronidazole, 500 mg PO or IV q8 h
    Levofloxacin, 400 mg PO or IV q24 h; or trovafloxacin[a] 200 mg PO or IV q24 h; or
    moxifloxacin, 400 mg PO of 24h
    Cefoxitin, 1–2 g IV q6 h; cefotetan, 2 g IV q12 h; or ceftizoxime, 1–2 g IV q8–12 h
  Compromised host
    (one of the following ± an aminoglycoside)
    Ceftizoxime, 4 g IV q8 h
    Cefotaxime, 2 g IV q6 h
    Piperacillin-tazobactam, 3 g IV q4 h
    Imipenem/cilastatin, 500 mg IV q6 h
    Trovafloxacin[a] 200 mg IV q24 h
Systemic antifungals
  Amphotericin B, fluconazole, ketoconazole, itraconazole
Systemic antivirals
  Acyclovir, valacyclovir, famcyclovir, gancyclovir, foscarnet
Topical medications:
  Antiseptics—chlorhexidine, povidone iodine
  Antibiotics—tetracycline, vancomycin, neomycin, bacitracin, polymyxin B,
    tobramycin lozenges.
  Antifungals—nystatin, amphotericin B, clotrimazole, miconazole, ketoconazole,
    itraconazole suspension, fluconazole suspension

MU, million units; IV, intravenous; PO, oral.
[a]Use of trofloxacin is restricted because of potential hepatotoxicity.

0.12% chlorhexidine is useful for the control of dental plaque bacteria that leads to gingivitis and periodontitis.

4.2. Suppurative Odontogenic Infections

The most important therapeutic modality for pyogenic odontogenic infections is surgical drainage and removal of necrotic tissue. Potentially involved fascial spaces should be carefully examined and incision and drainage performed at the optimal time. Premature incision into a poorly localized cellulitis can disrupt the normal physiologic barriers and cause further extension of infection. Antibiotic therapy is important in halting the local spread of infection and preventing hematogenous dissemination. Antimicrobial agents are generally indicated if fever and regional lymphadenitis are present. However, because fever may be blunted or absent in elderly patients, and immunocompromised patients including the elderly are particularly at risk for unhalted spread of severe orofacial infections, empiric antimicrobial therapy is usually warranted (*see* Table 2).

The initial choice of antibiotic regimens requires not so much the results of bacterial culture and sensitivity as knowledge of the indigenous organisms that colonize the teeth, gums, and mucus membranes. By far, most of these organisms, including both anaerobes and aerobes, are sensitive to penicillin. Thus, penicillin monotherapy in doses appropriate for the severity of infection remains a good choice. However, the problem of β-lactamase production among certain oral anaerobes, particularly pigmented *Prevotella* spp. and *Fusobacterium nucleatum* has been increasingly recognized, and treatment failure with penicillin due to β-lactamase-producing strains have been well documented. Ambulatory patients with less serious odontogenic infections may be treated with amoxicillin with or without a β-lactamase inhibitor, or with either penicillin or ciprofloxacin in combination with metronidazole. Penicillin-allergic patients may be treated with clindamycin, cefoxitin, cefotetan, or ceftizoxime. Erythromycin and tetracycline are not recommended because of increasing resistance among some strains of streptococci. Metronidazole, although highly active against anaerobic Gram-negative bacilli and spirochetes, is only moderately active against anaerobic cocci and is not active against aerobes, including streptococci. Except in acute necrotizing gingivitis and in advanced periodontitis, it should not be used as a single agent in odontogenic infections. In the compromised host, such as the patient with leukemia and severe neutropenia following chemotherapy, or the frail elderly, it is prudent to cover for facultative Gram-negative bacilli as well as oral anaerobes and streptococci. Agents with broad-spectrum activity against both aerobes and anaerobes, such as a third-generation cephalosporin, piperacillin-tazobactam, a carbapenem (imipenem or meropenem), or a new fluoroquinolone with enhanced activity against Gram-positive bacteria and anaerobes (e.g., moxifloxacin or trovafloxacin) are recommended (*see* Table 2).

4.3. Oromucosal Infections

For herpes labialis, 5% acyclovir topical ointment is only helpful if applied during the prodrome stage. In immunocompromised patients, systemic acyclovir (200 mg every 4 h for 7 d) or other antiviral agents (*see* Table 2) should be considered. Doses should be adjusted according to renal function in the elderly. Corticosteroids should be avoided. Severe complications of varicella-zoster can be treated with acyclovir (800 mg four times daily for 7–10 d) within 72 h of symptom onset. A tapered dose of 40–60 mg daily of prednisone for 2–3 wk has been suggested by some to decrease the risk of postherpetic neuralgia *(13)*. However, there are no data indicating the benefit of systemic corticosteroids in preventing postherpetic neruralgia *(21)*.

Treatment of candidiasis starts with improved oral hygiene, elimination of underlying local and systemic conditions, and topical or systemic antifungal agents. The most commonly used antifungal agents are nystatin oral suspension (100,000 units/mL with 5 mL rinse for 5 min and spit or swallow four times daily), and clotrimazole troches (10 mg four times daily for 7–10 d). If a patient has severely diminished salivary output, clotrimazole vaginal tablets should be recommended for oral use. Dentures must be soaked in solutions containing benzoic acid or 0.12% chlorhexidine to eliminate the organisms from the internal surface of the prosthesis. Antifungal creams should be placed in the dentures prior to use. For more severe oropharyngeal candidiasis, systemic antifungal agents (such as ketoconazole 200 mg daily or fluconazole 100 mg daily) are indicated.

In addition to topical and systemic antimicrobial agents, topical antiseptic (e.g., chlorhexidine) and anesthetic (e.g., benzydamine, viscous lidocaine, and the like) applications are often helpful to alleviate pain and discomfort from ulcerative lesions of the oral mucosa. Frequent saline rinses may reduce mucosal irritation, remove thickened secretions or debris, and increase moisture in the mouth. Coating agents such as milk of magnesia or aluminum hydroxide gel (amphogel) have been useful for symptomatic relief of painful oral lesions. Topical or oral cytoprotective agents (e.g., sucralfate) or nonsteroidal antiinflammatory analgesics (e.g., benzydamine, salicylates, etc.) may provide additional benefit.

4.4. Osteomyelitis

Treatment of osteomyelitis of the jaws is complicated by the presence of teeth and persistent exposure to the oral environment. Antibiotic therapy needs to be prolonged, often weeks to months. Adjuvant therapy with hyperbaric oxygen may prove beneficial in hastening the healing process. Surgical management including sequestrectomy, saucerization, decortication, and closed-wound suction irrigation may occasionally be necessary. Rarely in advanced cases, the entire segment of the infected jaw may have to be resected. However, in elderly patients with severe underlying disease, poor nutritional status or severe cognitive impairment, surgical intervention may not always be feasible.

5. PREVENTION

For both caries prevention and treatment of periodontitis in the elderly, the long-term goal must continue to be active promotion of oral hygiene and more ready accessibility to dental care and restorative prosthodontic treatment programs. Underlying diseases such as diabetes mellitus and conditions that predispose to salivary gland hypofunction should be rigorously treated. Medications that cause xerostomia or gingival hyperplasia should be avoided. Saliva substitutes, noncariogenic lozenges or gums, and vigorous brushing and flossing routines as well as dietary counseling should be provided. The diet should be scrutinized to eliminate or discourage frequent snacking of carbohydrate-rich foods or intake of sugar-containing beverages. Behavioral modification of corisk factors such as cessation of tobacco smoking and promotion of regular visits to dental care professionals are equally important preventative measures.

Meticulous attention must be paid to oral hygiene with fluoride-containing dentifrices and rinses (e.g., sodium fluoride 1.1% or stannous fluoride 0.4%) and dental flossing after each meal. Individuals with physical or mental limitations who cannot adequately perform oral hygiene by themselves should receive daily oral hygiene by care providers. Topical fluorides and oral antimicrobial rinses such as chlorhexidine are indicated for high-risk patients. More frequent visits to dentists and use of electrical toothbrushes should be considered in these patients. The prospect for an effective and safe vaccine against dental caries, such as the use of various immunogens derived from *S. mutans*, remains remote and unlikely to be available for clinical application in the near future *(22)*.

Finally, dental sources of bacteremia in the elderly is of increasing concern for those undergoing prosthetic heart valve implantation or artificial joint replacement. Routine preoperative dental assessment should be performed for all patients undergoing valvular operations, and appropriate therapeutic intervention should be initiated whenever possible before prosthetic implantations. The value of prophylactic antibiotics during dental procedures for the prevention of infective endocarditis has remained controversial *(23)*. The routine use of prophylactic antimicrobials in the healthy host for the prevention of postoperative infections is unwarranted, since the risk of such infections is less than 1% *(24)*.

REFERENCES

1. Bartzokas, C. A., Johnson, R., Jane, M., et al. (1994) Relation between mouth and haematogenous infection in total joint replacements. *Brit. Med. J.* **309,** 506–508.
2. Norman, D. C. and Toledo, S. D. (1992) Infections in elderly persons—an altered clinical presentation. *Clin. Geriatr. Med.* **8,** 713–719.
3. Meskin, L. and Brown, J. (1988) Prevalence and patterns of tooth loss in U. S. adult and senior populations. *Int. J. Oral Implantol.* **5,** 59–60.
4. Marcus, S. E., Drury, T. F., Brown, L. J., et al. (1996) Tooth retention and tooth loss in the permanent dentition of adults: United States, 1988–1991. *J. Dent. Res.* **75,** 684– 695.
5. Winn, D. M., Brunelle, J. A., Selwitz, R. H., et al. (1996) Coronal and root caries in the dentition of adults in the United States, 1988–1991. *J. Dent. Res.* **75,** 642–651.
6. Brown, L. J., Brunelle, J. A., and Kingman, A. (1996) Periodontal status in the United States, 1988–91: prevalence, extent, and demographic variation. *J. Dent. Res.* **75,** 672–683.
7. Nordstrom, G., Bergman, B., Borg, K., et al. (1998) A 9-year longitudinal study of reported oral problems and dental and periodontal status in 70- and 79-year-old city cohorts in northern Sweden. *Acta Odontol. Scand.* **56,** 76–84.
8. Jokstad, A., Ambjornsen, E., and Eide, K. E. (1996) Oral health in institutionalized elderly people in 1993 compared with in 1980. *Acta Odontol. Scand.* **54,** 303–308.
9. Chow, A. W. (1998) Odontogenic infections in the elderly. *Infect. Dis. Clin. Pract.* **6,** 587–596.
10. Loesche, W. J. (1993) Bacterial mediators in periodontal disease. *Clin. Infect. Dis.* **16(Suppl 4),** S203–S210.
11. Johnson, T. C., Reinhardt, R. A., Payne, J. B., et al. (1997) Experimental gingivitis in periodontitis-susceptible subjects. *J. Clin. Periodontol.* **24,** 618–625.
12. Shay, K. and Ship, J. A. (1995) The importance of oral health in the older patient. *J. Am. Geriatr. Med.* **43,** 1414–1422.
13. Ship, J. A. and Lin, B. P. J. (1996) Oral medical problems in older persons. Part 1. Infectious diseases. *Clin. Geriatr. Med.* **4,** 23–49.
14. Wu, A. J., Baum, B. J., and Ship, J. A. (1995) Extended stimulated parotid and submandibular secretion in a healthy young and old population. *J. Gerontol. (Med. Sci.)* **50A,** M45–M48.
15. Atkinson, J. C. and Wu, A. J. (1994) Salivary gland dysfunction: causes, symptoms, treatment. *J. Am. Dent. Assoc.* **125,** 409–416.
16. Lockhart, S. R., Joly, S., Vargas, K., et al. (1999) Natural defenses against *Candida* colonization breakdown in the oral cavities of the elderly. *J. Dent. Res.* **78,** 857–868.
17. Epstein, J. B. and Chow, A. W. (1999) Oral complications associated with immunosuppression and cancer therapies. *Infect. Dis. Clin. North Am.* **13,** 901–923.
18. Chow, A. W. (1998) Life-threatening infections of the head, neck, and upper respiratory tract, in *Principles of Critical Care*, 2nd ed. (Hall, J. B., Schmidt, G. A. and Wood, L. D. H., eds.), McGraw-Hill, New York, pp. 887–902.
19. Norman, D. C. and Yoshikawa, T. T. (1996) Fever in the elderly. *Infect. Dis. Clin. North Am.* **10,** 93–96.
20. Loesche, W. J., Giordano, J., Soehren, S., et al. (1996) Nonsurgical treatment of patients with periodontal disease. *Oral Surg. Oral Med. Oral Pathol. Oral Radiol. Endod.* **81,** 533–543.

21. Chao, P. W., Galil, K., Donahue, J. G., et al. (1997) Risk factors for postherpatic neuralgia. *Arch. Intern. Med.* **15,** 1217–1224.
22. Bowen, W. H. (1996) Vaccine against dental caries—a personal view. *J. Dent. Res.* **75,** 1530–1533.
23. Hall, G., Hedstrom, S. A., Heimdahl, A., et al. (1993) Prophylactic administration of penicillins for endocarditis does not reduce the incidence of postextraction bacteremia. *Clin. Infect. Dis.* **17,** 188–194.
23. Loesche, W. J. (1996) Antimicrobials in dentistry: with knowledge comes responsibility. *J. Dent. Res.* **75,** 1432–1433.
24. Chow, A. W. (1987) Odontogenic infections, in *Infections of the Head and Neck* (Schlossberg, D., ed.), Springer, New York, p. 148.
25. Megran, D. W., Scheifele, D. W., and Chow, A. W. (1984) Odontogenic infections. *Ped. Infect. Dis.* **3,** 256–265.

15

Otitis Externa, Otitis Media, and Sinusitis

Vinod K. Dhawan

1. OTITIS EXTERNA

1.1. Epidemiology and Clinical Relevance

Otitis externa, an inflammatory condition involving the superficial layer of the external auditory canal, may be acute or chronic. Acute otitis externa in the elderly is generally a benign disorder, which may be localized or generalized. Chronic otitis externa is caused by the irritation due to the drainage from the middle ear in patients with chronic suppurative otitis media. An uncommon form of external otitis called "malignant otitis externa" is an invasive, necrotizing infection that spreads from the squamous epithelium of the ear canal to the periauricular soft tissue, blood vessels, cartilage, and bone (1–3).

Otitis externa is observed in the summer months more frequently, as the maceration of the skin lining the externa auditory meatus is facilitated by heat, humidity, and perspiration. Swimming may lead to otitis externa (swimmer's ear) by introducing moisture into the ear canal. Malignant otitis externa is typically seen in elderly diabetics in whom chronic hyperglycemia, tissue hypoperfusion due to microangiopathy, altered cell-mediated immunity, and impaired phagocytic function all play a pathogenetic role. Occasionally, malignant otitis externa has been noted after the syringing of the ear canal (4) and in patients infected with human immunodeficiency virus (HIV) (5). Complications that may be life threatening could result from the spread to the temporal bone, sigmoid sinus, jugular bulb, base of the skull, meninges, and the brain.

Otitis externa is generally caused by organisms such as *Staphylococcus aureus* and *Pseudomonas aeruginosa*. Malignant otitis externa is almost always due to *P. aeruginosa* (*see* Table 1). Only rare cases of malignant otitis externa due to *S. aureus* (6), *Proteus mirabilis* (7), and *Aspergillus fumigatus* (8) have been reported. Rare causes of chronic otitis externa include tuberculosis, fungal infections, syphilis, yaws, leprosy, and sarcoidosis. Fungal otitis externa may be part of a general or local fungal infection; *Aspergillus* spp. are responsible for the most cases (9).

1.2. Clinical Manifestations

Acute otitis externa causes pain in the ear that may be quite severe due to the limited space for expansion of the inflamed tissue. The movement of the external ear and sometimes of the jaw aggravates the pain. The patients may experience itching of the

From: Infectious Disease in the Aging
Edited by: Thomas T. Yoshikawa and Dean C. Norman
© Humana Press Inc., Totowa, NJ

Table 1
Salient Features of Malignant Otitis Externa in the Elderly

Predisposing factors	Diabetes mellitus
	Immunocompromise
Microbiology	Usually due to *P. aeruginosa*
Complications	Cranial nerve palsies (facial, glossopharyngeal, vagus, spinal accessory, hypoglossal, abducens, and trigeminal)
	Jugular venous thrombosis
	Cavernous sinus thrombosis
	Meningitis
Therapy	Aminoglycoside + antipseudomonal penicillin (piperacillin, ticarcillin etc.) OR
	Aminoglycoside + ceftazidime OR
	Quinolones: ciprofloxacin, ofloxacin

ear. The infection typically starts at the junction of the cartilage and bone in the external meatus. Speculum examination of the canal reveals the skin to be edematous and erythematous. There may be an accumulation of moist debris in the canal. The tympanic membrane may be difficult to visualize and may be mildly inflamed but is normally movable on insufflation. Acute localized otitis externa may occur as a pustule or furuncle associated with the hair follicles; *S. aureus* is generally the causative organism in these patients. Infection due to group A streptococcus may cause erysipelas of the concha and the canal. Examination may reveal hemorrhagic bullae in the ear canal or on the tympanic membrane, and regional lymphadenopathy may be noted.

Most episodes of otitis externa in the elderly resolve completely within 5–7 d. Failure of resolution of otitis externa should lead to suspicion of malignant otitis externa especially in elderly diabetics. Such patients have unremitting otalgia, tenderness of the tissues around the ear and mastoid, and purulent drainage from the canal. Examination of the ear canal reveals granulation tissue at the osseous-cartilaginous junction. The progression of malignant otitis externa along Santorini's fissure into the mastoid may lead to facial nerve palsy. The infection may further spread to the jugular foramen at the base of skull and involve the glossopharyngeal, vagus, and spinal accessory nerves. Similarly, extension of infection into the hypoglossal canal may involve the hypoglossal nerve, and involvement of the petrous apex may lead to the abducens and trigeminal nerves palsies. Other potential complications of malignant otitis externa include jugular venous thrombosis, cavernous sinus thrombosis, and meningitis.

1.3. Diagnostic Tests

The white blood cell count may be elevated in acute otitis externa, but this finding is nonspecific. The erythrocyte sedimentation rate is usually very high in patients with malignant otitis externa and may be useful in monitoring therapy *(10)*. Cultures from the granulation tissue or the involved bone will reveal the organism. Plain film radiography is inadequate for the evaluation of malignant otitis externa. The extent of damage to the soft tissue and bone may be identified and monitored by use of computed tomographic (CT) and magnetic resonance image (MRI) scans *(3,11)*. Technetium 99 bone scans and gallium 67 scans are very sensitive but not very specific *(12,13)*. Bone scans may remain positive long after the microbiologic cure of this condition and therefore are not very useful in monitoring the response to therapy.

1.4. Therapy

The therapy of otitis externa consists of the gentle cleansing of the external auditory canal to remove debris and the instillation of appropriate topical antibiotics *(14)*. The ear canal may be irrigated with hypertonic saline (3%) or cleansed with mixtures of alcohol (70–95%) and acetic acid. Inflammation of the canal may be reduced with hydrophilic solutions such as 50% Burrow solution. Eardrops of topical antibiotics (including neomycin and polymyxin), combined with a corticosteroid preparation, diminish the local inflammation. The placement of a wick in the ear canal may facilitate the delivery of antibiotic drops into the ear canal. Incision and drainage of the furuncle may be necessary to relieve severe pain. Systemic antibiotic therapy is reserved for significant tissue infection and systemic toxicity. Malignant otitis externa is treated with local debridement of the canal and topical treatment with antipseudomonal antibiotics combined with corticosteroids. Additionally, systemic therapy directed at *P. aeruginosa* should be used for 4–6 wk. The combination of a ceftazidime or an antipseudomonal penicillin (ticarcillin or piperacillin) with an aminoglycoside (gentamicin or tobramycin) should be considered for synergy. Oral quinolones with activity against *P. aeruginosa*, such as ciprofloxacin and ofloxacin, are also generally effective *(15–18)*. Some consider ciprofloxacin to be the drug of choice due to its high concentration in the bone and cartilage, ease of oral administration, and low toxicity *(19)*.

1.5. Prevention

Prevention of excessive moisture in the ear canal may favorably impact on the incidence of otitis externa. Use of a blow dryer after swimming to dry the ear canal has been suggested as a preventive measure. Aggressive cleansing of the ear canal should be avoided as the resulting disruption of its lining and subsequent invasion by resident bacterial flora may lead to infection. Prompt recognition of malignant otitis externa and its aggressive therapy will minimize its devastating complications.

2. OTITIS MEDIA

2.1. Epidemiology and Clinical Relevance

Acute otitis media has been best studied in children in whom the disease is particularly common *(20–23)*. Few studies have addressed the epidemiology of middle ear infections in the elderly. In 1990, there were an estimated 24.5 million visits made to offices of physicians in the United States at which the principal diagnosis was otitis media *(24)*. The peak incidence occurs in the first three years of life and is increased in the absence of breastfeeding for three or more months *(25)* and the presence of passive smoking *(26)*. Acute otitis media occurs more often in the males than in the females and likely has a genetic susceptibility. Native Americans, Alaskan and Canadian Eskimos, and Australian aborigines have an extraordinary incidence and severity of otitis media. The single-most frequently recognized cause of acute otitis media is a viral upper respiratory tract infection. Others have anatomic changes (cleft palate, cleft uvula, submucous cleft), alteration of normal physiologic defenses (patulous Eustachian tube), and congenital or acquired immunologic deficiencies including acquired immunodeficiency syndrome (AIDS).

Although otitis externa is infrequent among the elderly, infection of the middle ear may be the cause of fever, significant pain, and impaired hearing. Acute otitis media or inflammation of the middle ear is defined by the presence of fluid in the middle ear accompanied by the symptoms or signs of illness. The simple presence of fluid in the middle ear without clinical symptoms or signs of active infection is referred to as otitis media with effusion. Acute otitis media is considered to be recurrent when three new episodes of acute otitis media have occurred in 6 mo or four episodes within 12 mo. The term "chronic otitis media" refers to a prolonged duration of middle ear effusion usually resulting from a previous episode of acute infection. The epithelial lining of the middle ear contains ciliated cells, mucus-secreting goblet cells, and cells capable of secreting local immunoglobulins. The middle ear secretions drain into the nasopharynx through the Eustachian tube. The pathogenesis of otitis media involves interactions among host characteristics, virulence factors of viral and bacterial pathogens, and environmental factors. Conditions resulting in obstruction of the Eustachian tube, including congestion of the mucosa during viral infections, play a critical role in the development of otitis media. Bacterial pathogens may infect the middle ear secretions accumulated behind the obstruction leading to otitis media.

The most frequent etiological agents recovered from patients with acute otitis media are *Streptococcus pneumoniae*, nontypable *Haemophilus influenzae*, *Moraxella catarrhalis*, and group A streptococcus (*see* Table 2). Otitis media may be caused by type B *H. influenzae* in approx 10% of patients. *M. catarrhalis* is less commonly isolated from the middle ear fluids of with acute otitis media (*27*). Most strains produce β-lactamase and are resistant to penicillin G, ampicillin, and amoxicillin. Viruses isolated from patients with acute otitis media include respiratory syncytial virus, influenza virus, enteroviruses, and rhinoviruses. The bacterial flora isolated from the elderly patients with chronic otitis media is a polymicrobial mixture of aerobes (*P. aeruginosa*, predominating) and anaerobes (*Peptostreptococcus* predominating). Uncommon varieties of otitis include tuberculous otitis, otitis due to *Mycobacterium chelonae*, or Wegener's granulomatosis.

2.2. Clinical Manifestations

The elderly with acute otitis media may present with ear pain, ear drainage, or hearing loss. Vertigo, nystagmus, and tinnitus may occur at times. Other nonspecific manifestations include fever and lethargy. On examination the tympanic membrane may be erythematous and obliteration of its landmarks may occur due to its inflammation and the fluid in the middle ear. Perforation of the tympanic membrane is frequent but usually not a serious complication. With proper treatment most perforations heal uneventfully within a couple of weeks. The middle ear fluid may resolve rather slowly

Table 2
Bacterial Pathogens in Acute Otitis Media

Pathogen	Mean %	Range %
Streptococcus pneumoniae	39	27–50
Haemophilus influenzae	30	17–50
Moraxella catarrhalis	10	6–27
Streptococcus pyogenes	3	2–6

despite effective antimicrobial therapy. Serous otitis media may cause mild discomfort, but when it is bilateral the patient may complain of significant hearing loss. Cholesteatoma is a complication that can lead to bony erosion and requires surgical management. Mastoiditis, a rare complication of otitis media, should be suspected in the presence of mastoid tenderness or edema. Intracranial complications, such as epidural abscess or lateral sinus thrombosis, are noted uncommonly.

2.3. Diagnostic Tests

The presence of middle ear fluid, the hallmark of otitis media, can be ascertained by several tests. Fluid or high negative pressure in the middle ear dampens the mobility of the tympanic membrane, a useful sign demonstrated by pneumatic otoscopy. Tympanometry, a technique using an electroacoustic impedance bridge to record compliance of the tympanic membrane and middle ear pressure, presents objective evidence of the status of the middle ear and the presence or absence of fluid. Acoustic reflectometry measures sound reflectivity from the middle ear and is able to distinguish an air- or fluid-filled space.

There are no diagnostic laboratory tests for acute otitis media; the white blood cell count may be elevated nonspecifically. A blood culture is positive in only about 3% of febrile patients with acute otitis media but should be performed if the patient is toxic. Needle aspiration of the middle ear effusion (tympanocentesis) to define the microbiology should be considered in selected patients: the critically ill, those not responding to initial antimicrobial therapy in 48–72 h, and patients with altered host defenses. Imaging studies are not routinely useful for the evaluation of acute otitis media, but radiographs of the mastoid air cells may be helpful in patients suspected to have complicating mastoiditis.

2.4. Treatment

Antibiotic therapy of acute otitis media must be initiated without the knowledge of the exact organism and therefore must be aimed at *S. pneumoniae* and *H. influenzae*, organisms responsible for the vast majority of these infections. Organisms recovered less frequently in otitis media of the elderly, i.e., *M. catarrhalis*, group A streptococcus, and *S. aureus*, need not be considered in the initial therapeutic decision. However, Gram-negative enteric bacilli must be considered in the immunocompromised hosts.

Amoxicillin, at a dose of 60–90 mg/kg/d, is the current drug of choice for initial therapy. The current incidence of ampicillin-resistant *H. influenzae* and *M. catarrhalis* in acute otitis media of the elderly is not high enough to require a change in this recommendation. With appropriate antimicrobial therapy, most patients with acute otitis media are significantly improved within 48–72 h. The therapy should be switched to β-lactamase-stable agents, such as amoxicillin-clavulanate, cefaclor, cefuroxime axetil, cefixime, cefprozil, cefpodoxime proxetil, loracarbef, and trimethoprim-sulfamethoxazole, if symptoms persist or worsen after 3 d. Treatment for a 10-d period is generally considered adequate. Clinical resolution may occur in some patients without the use of antimicrobial agents as the contents of the middle ear are discharged through the Eustachian tube or through a spontaneous perforation of the tympanic membrane. However, acute otitis media should be treated with appropriate antimicrobial agents to prevent the suppurative complications. Appropriate antipyretics and analgesics should be offered for symptomatic relief. Oral decongestants, antihistamines, and corticosteroids, although commonly prescribed, have no proven benefit *(28)*.

Surgical management of the persistent effusion of the middle ear includes the use of myringotomy and the placement of tympanostomy tubes. Currently, myringotomy is recommended for the relief of intractable ear pain, hastening resolution of mastoid infection, and drainage of the persistent middle ear effusion. Tympanostomy tubes are placed for persistent middle ear effusions unresponsive to adequate medical treatment over a period of 3 mo. Hearing improves dramatically after placement of the ventilating tubes. The tubes have also been of value in patients who have difficulty maintaining ambient pressure in the middle ear such as would occur due to barotrauma in airline personnel. The risks inherent in the placement of tubes include those of anesthesia associated with the procedure, persistent perforation, scarring of the tympanic membrane, development of cholesteatoma, and otitis media caused by swimming with ventilating tubes in place.

2.5. Prevention

The use of chemoprophylaxis (antimicrobial agents) and immunoprophylaxis (pneumococcal vaccine) should be considered for the prevention of recurrent episodes of acute otitis media. The currently available 23-type pneumococcal polysaccharide vaccine protects against the most common types of *S. pneumoniae* found in otitis media. Intermittent antibiotic prophylaxis (during the period of upper respiratory tract infections), using a once-a-day regimen of amoxicillin or sulfisoxazole, has been shown to be protective in children with recurrent middle ear infection. A similar approach may be helpful in the elderly with recurrent disease.

3. SINUSITIS

3.1. Epidemiology and Clinical Relevance

It is estimated that sinusitis affects 16% of the United States population annually, leading to approx 16 million office visits and a yearly expenditure of approx 2 billion dollars on its medical therapy *(29)*. Sinusitis, an infection of one or more of the paranasal sinuses, usually begins as a complication of viral upper respiratory tract infection in the elderly population. Obstruction of sinus drainage and retention of secretions are the fundamental events in sinus infection. Geriatric patients may be predisposed to sinusitis by several conditions that compromise the integrity of the sinus ostia, thereby interfering with aeration of the sinuses and creating a closed space that is susceptible to bacterial infection. Sinusitis is, therefore, more likely in the elderly with allergic rhinitis, nasal septal deviation, nasal fractures, nasal polyps or tumors. About 5–10% of cases of bacterial maxillary sinusitis are secondary to dental root infection. Sinusitis is generally subdivided into acute sinusitis (symptoms less than 3 wk), subacute sinusitis (symptoms lasting 3 wk–3 mo) and chronic sinusitis (symptoms lasting longer than 3 mo). Sinusitis may potentially cause serious intracranial suppurative complications such as meningitis, brain abscess, epidural abscess, and subdural empyema.

Acute bacterial sinusitis is commonly due to *S. pneumoniae* and *H. influenzae*. Less frequently isolated organisms include *Streptococcus pyogenes*, α-hemolytic streptococci, *S. aureus*, and *M. catarrhalis (30)*. The β-lactamase production by most strains of *M. catarrhalis* and a variable proportion of *H. influenzae* strains may lead to therapeutic failure of β-lactam agents such as amoxicillin in treating sinusitis due to these organisms. Over 200 viruses associated with the common cold have been implicated in acute sinusitis *(31)*. Ventilator-associated sinusitis is most frequently caused by *S. aureus*, followed by *P. aeruginosa*, enteric Gram-negative bacilli, and various *Streptococcus* spp. *(32)*. The risk of developing bacterial sinusitis on a ventilator increases both with the duration of nasal canulation and the size of the cannula *(33)*. Among patients who have been ventilator-treated for ≥1 wk, the occurrence of bacterial sinusitis is approximately 10% *(32)*. Chronic sinusitis, on the other hand, is caused by *H. influenzae* (in approx 60%), *S. aureus*, and anaerobes. *P. aeruginosa* may be the causative agent in patients with nasal polyps and cystic fibrosis. Fungal organisms such as mucor should be considered in the setting of diabetes mellitus and an immunocompromised host.

3.2. Clinical Manifestations

Acute sinusitis is usually preceded by a viral infection of the upper respiratory tract; an estimated 0.5% of common colds evolve into acute sinusitis. No single clinical finding is predictive of acute sinusitis. Three symptoms (maxillary toothache, poor response to decongestants, and history of colored nasal discharge) and two signs (purulent nasal secretion and abnormal transillumination) are the best clinical predictors of acute sinusitis. Sinusitis should be considered when purulent nasal or pharyngeal discharge and cough persist for over a week following a cold. The elderly may complain of headache, facial pain or tightness over the involved sinus, nasal obstruction, nasal quality of voice, and a fever *(34)*. Nasal examination may reveal mucosal hyperemia and mucopurulent discharge. Purulent secretion from the middle meatus is highly predictive of maxillary sinusitis. Direct inspection of the posterior pharynx or use of a pharyngeal mirror may reveal posteriorly draining purulent secretions. Tenderness over the maxillae or the frontal bone suggesting an underlying sinusitis occurs much less commonly. Transillumination may be used to evaluate the maxillary and frontal sinuses, but its value is controversial. In chronic sinusitis, persistent nasal drainage, postnasal drip, persistent cough, foul breath, and altered taste may be noted. Neglected sinusitis may exacerbate an underlying chest disease leading to increased morbidity in the elderly *(35)*. Sinusitis should be distinguished from several disease entities such as those listed in Table 3.

Table 3
Differential Diagnosis of Sinusitis in the Elderly

Viral upper respiratory infection

Rhinitis medicamentosa (topical decongestant use)

Drug-induced rhinitis (e.g., reserpine, prazosin,

    ACE inhibitors, guanethidine, cocaine abuse, etc.)

Allergic rhinitis

Sinus tumors

Sarcoidosis

Nasal foreign body

Midline granuloma

Wegner's granulomatosis

Rhinoscleroma

ACE, angiotensin-converting enzyme.

3.3. Diagnostic Tests

Radiologic studies are not routinely performed for the evaluation of sinus infection. Basic radiographic examination of the paranasal sinuses includes four views: the Waters view (occipitomental), to evaluate the maxillary sinuses; the Caldwell view (angled posteroanterior), to evaluate the ethmoid and frontal sinuses; the lateral view, to evaluate the sphenoid sinuses and to confirm disease in the paired maxillary, ethmoid, and frontal sinuses; and the submentovertex view, to evaluate the sphenoid and ethmoid sinuses. This last view is also useful for examining the lateral walls of the maxillary sinuses. All radiographs are done with the patient erect in order to evaluate air-fluid levels. Most studies have demonstrated that sinusitis involves the maxillary sinuses in approx 90% of cases. Therefore, most cases of sinusitis would be diagnosed using only the Waters view. Radiographic evidence of acute sinusitis consists of sinus opacification, mucosal thickening of >5 mm, and the presence of air-fluid level in the affected sinus. A computed tomographic (CT) scan is more sensitive than sinus radiography for evaluating sinus disease and is particularly helpful in delineating the osteomeatal complex (36). The CT scan appears to be more sensitive than plain radiography for detecting sinus abnormalities, particularly in the sphenoid and ethmoid sinuses. However, due to its cost and poor specificity, which is around 60%, CT scanning of sinuses is not indicated for patients with uncomplicated acute bacterial sinusitis. In one study, 40% of asymptomatic patients and 87% of patients with colds had sinus abnormalities on CT scanning (37). This study should be reserved for patients with recurrent disease,

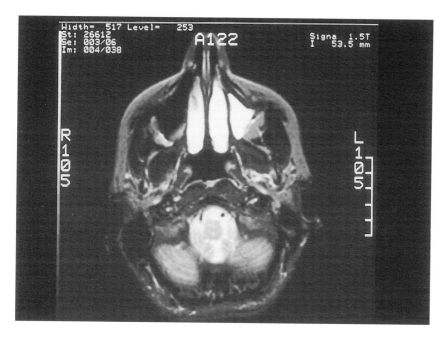

Fig. 1. MRI scan showing a left maxillary sinusitis (white, triangle-shaped area).

orbital or central nervous system complications, or when surgical intervention is contemplated due to a protracted sinus disease. The use of MRI scan may be helpful in select patients in distinguishing soft-tissue tumors from inflammatory lesions (*see* Fig. 1).

Surface colonization of the nasal passage makes the nasal purulence or the sinus exudate obtained by rinsing through the natural sinus ostium unsuitable for microbiologic diagnosis. Sinus puncture and quantitative cultures of the aspirated exudates remain the gold standard for reliable microbiologic diagnosis. However, such a procedure is not performed in an average case due to its invasive nature and the rather predictable bacteriology of acute sinusitis. Sinus puncture is reserved for patients with unusually severe disease, those responding inadequately to medical therapy or suspected of having intracranial extension, and when sinusitis occurs in an immunocompromised individual.

3.4. Therapy

The management of sinusitis has been recently reviewed *(38–40)*. Because the distinction between viral and bacterial etiology of acute sinusitis is difficult based on clinical findings, patients with acute sinusitis are generally treated for a presumed bacterial etiology. The antimicrobial therapy is directed at *S. pneumoniae* and *H. influenzae*. The commonly prescribed antimicrobial agents and their recommended dosages are listed in Table 4. The antibiotic therapy is generally administered for 14 d. Many clinicians are reluctant to prescribe amoxicillin or ampicillin for therapy due to the increasing frequency of β-lactamase-producing *H. influenzae* and *M. catarrhalis* in acute sinusitis. Quinolones with limited activity against *S. pneumoniae*, e.g., ciprofloxacin, should not be used for therapy of acute sinusitis. Fungal sinusitis, such as mucor, requires aggressive surgical debridement and appropriate antifungal therapy for cure.

Table 4
Antimicrobial Therapy of Acute Sinusitis in the Elderly

Antimicrobial agent	Commonly prescribed dose
Amoxicillin	500 mg q6 h
Ampicillin	500 mg q8 h
Amoxicillin-clavulanate	500/125 mg q8 h
Trimethoprim-sulfamethoxazole	160 mg/800 mg bid
Cefaclor	500 mg q6 h
Cefuroxime axetil	250 mg q12 h
Clarithromycin	500 mg q12 h
Azithromycin	500 mg day 1, and 250 mg qd, days 2–5.
Levofloxacin	500 mg qd

bid, twice a day; qd, once a day; q8 h, once every 8 hours.

The nasal spray decongestants such as phenylephrine hydrochloride (0.5%) and oxymetazoline hydrochloride (0.05%) are frequently used to treat acute sinusitis. However, there are no published placebo-controlled studies proving their role or efficacy. Rebound vasodilatation may occur in patients who use such agents frequently or for longer periods. Oral decongestants (pseudoephedrine and phenylpropanolamine) are α-adrenergic agonists that reduce nasal blood flow. Theoretically, oral preparations can penetrate the ostiomeatal complex, where topical agents may not penetrate effectively. The use of oral decongestants has been shown to improve nasal patency. These agents can increase the functional diameter of the maxillary ostium. Some oral decongestants are available in combination with mucoevacuants, which may help to thin secretions and facilitate drainage. The antihistamines have not proven to be effective in the management of acute sinusitis. Their use may be counterproductive as the dryness of mucous membranes caused through their anticholinergic action may interfere with the clearance of purulent mucous secretions. Topical corticosteroid preparations have not shown convincing benefit in the treatment of sinusitis. There have been no controlled clinical trials of systemic glucocorticosteroid therapy for acute sinusitis.

Surgery may be necessary to facilitate drainage of the involved sinus and to remove the diseased mucosa. In acute bacterial sinusitis, surgical intervention is reserved for its complications, or lack of appropriate response to medical therapy. Functional endoscopic sinus surgery has revolutionized the surgical approach to sinus disease. With this approach, the affected tissue is removed and the normal tissue is left in place. Functional endoscopic sinus surgery can surgically correct anatomic obstructions and has been shown to result in moderate to complete relief of symptoms in 80–90% of patients.

3.5. Prevention

Annual immunization with the influenza and pneumococcal vaccines, aggressive management of upper respiratory infections, and the prevention or treatment of upper respiratory allergies may reduce the incidence of sinusitis in the elderly. A high index of suspicion of sinusitis and its prompt therapy may prevent complications. Corrective surgery for nasal abnormalities to establish sinus drainage reduces the risk of sinusitis.

Good dental hygiene and prompt treatment of maxillary tooth root infection will prevent the onset of maxillary sinusitis as its complication.

REFERENCES

1. Evans, P. and Hoffman, L. (1994) Malignant otitis externa: a case report and review. *Am Fam. Phys.* **49,** 427–431.
2. Doroghazi, R. M., Nadol, J. B., Hyslop, N. E., et al. (1981) Invasive external otitis. *Am. J. Med.* **71,** 603–613.
3. Rubin, J. and Yu, V. L. (1988) Malignant external otitis: Insights into pathogenesis, clinical manifestations, diagnosis, and therapy. *Am. J. Med.* **85,** 391–398.
4. Ford, G. R. and Courtney-Harris, R. G. (1990) Another hazard of ear syringing: malignant external otitis. *Laryngol. Otol.* **104,** 709–710.
5. Wernorth, S. E., Schessel, D., and Tuazon, C. U. (1994) Malignant otitis externa in AIDS patients: case report and review of the literature. *Ear Nose Throat J.* **73,** 772–778.
6. Bayardelle, P., Jolivet-Granger, M., and Larochelle, D. (1982) Staphylococcal external otitis. *Can. Med. Assoc. J.* **126,** 155–156.
7. Coser, P. L., Stamm, A. E. C., Lobo, R. C., et al. (1980) Malignant external otitis in infants. *Laryngoscope* **90,** 312–316.
8. Petrak, R. M., Pottage, J. C., and Levin, S. (1985) Invasive external otitis caused by Aspergillus fumigatus in an immunocompromised patient. *J. Infect. Dis.* **15,** 196–196.
9. Phillips, P., Bryce, G., and Shepherd, J. (1990) Invasive external otitis caused by Aspergillus. *Rev. Infect. Dis.* **12,** 277–281.
10. Johnson, M. P. and Ramphal, R. (1990) Malignant external otitis: report on therapy with ceftazidime and review of therapy and prognosis. *Rev. Infect. Dis.* **12,** 173–180.
11. Rubin, J., Curtin, H. D., Yu, V. L., et al. (1990) Malignant otitis externa. Utility of CT in diagnosis and follow up. *Radiology* **174,** 391–394.
12. Levin, W. J., Shary, J. H., Nichols, L. T., et al. (1986) Bone scanning in severe external otitis. *Laryngoscope* **96,** 1193–1195.
13. Parisier, S. C., Lucente, F. E., Som, P. M., et al. (1992) Nuclear scanning in necrotizing progressive"malignant" external otitis. *Laryngoscope* **92,** 1016–1020.
14. Boustred, N. (1999) Practical guide to otitis externa. *Aust. Fam. Phys.* **28,** 217–221.
15. Hickey, S. A., Ford, G. R., O'Connor, A. F., et al. (1989) Treating malignant otitis with oral ciprofloxacin. *Br. Med. J.* **299,** 550–551.
16. Lang, R. L., Goshen, K., Kitzes-Cohen, R., et al. (1990) Successful treatment of malignant otitis externa with oral ciprofloxacin: report of experience with 23 patients. *J. Infect. Dis.* **161,** 537–540.
17. Gehanno, P. (1994) Ciprofloxacin in the treatment of malignant otitis externa. *Chemotherapy* **1,** 35–40.
18. Rapoport, Y., Shalit, I., Redianu, C., et al (1991) Oral ofloxacin therapy for invasive external otitis. *Ann. Otol. Rhinol. Laryngol.* **100,** 632–637.
19. Levenson, M. J., Parisier, S. C., Dolitsky, J., et al. (1991) Ciprofloxacin: drug of choice in malignant external otitis. *Laryngoscope* **101,** 821–824.
20. Bluestone, C. D. and Klein, J. O. (eds.) (1987) *Otitis Media in Infants and Children,* Saunders, W. B., Philadelphia, PA.
21. Berman, S. (1995) Otitis media in children. *N. Engl. J. Med.* **332,** 1560–1565.
22. Karver, S. B. (1998) Otitis media. *Primary Care: Clin. Office Pract.* **25,** 619–632.
23. Klein, J. O. (1994) Otitis media. *Clin. Infect. Dis.* **19,** 823–833.
24. Schappert, S. M. (1992) Office visits for otitis media: United States, in *Vital and Health Statistics of the Centers for Disease Control/National Centers for Health Statistics,* Atlanta, Centers for Disease Control and Prevention. **214,** 3–18.

25. Teele, D. W., Klein, J. O., and the Greater Boston Collaborative Study Group. (1981) Use of pneumococcal vaccine for prevention of recurrent acute otitis media in infants in Boston. Rev. Infect. Dis. **3(Suppl),** 113–119.

26. Etzel, R. A., Pattishall, E. N., Haley, N. J., et al. (1992) Passive smoking and middle ear effusion among children in day care. *Pediatrics* **90,** 228–223.

27. Van Hare, G. F., Shurin, P. A., Marchant, C. D., et al. (1987) Acute otitis media caused by Branhamella catarrhalis: Biology and therapy. *Rev. Infect. Dis.* **9,** 16–27.

28. Bluestone, C. D., Connell, J. T., Doyle, W. J., et al. (1988) Symposium: questioning the efficacy and safety of antihistamines in the treatment of upper respiratory infection. *Pediatr. Infect. Dis. J.* **7,** 15–42.

29. Benson, V. and Marano, M. A. (1994) Current estimates from the national health interview survey, 1992. *Vital Health Stat.* **189,** 1–269.

30. Gwaltney, J. M. J. (1996) Acute community-acquired sinusitis. *Clin. Infect. Dis.* **23,** 1209–1223.

31. Yonkers, A. J. (1992) Sinusitis—inspecting the cause and treatment. *Ear Nose Throat J.* **71,** 258–262.

32. Westergren, V., Lundblad, L., Hellquist, H. B., et al. (1998) Ventilator-associated sinusitis: a review. *Clin. Infect. Dis.* **27,** 851–864.

33. Pedersen, J., Schurizek, B. A., Melsen, N. C., et al. (1991) The effect of nasotracheal intubation on the paranasal sinuses: a prospective study of 434 intensive care unit patients. *Acta. Anaesth. Scand.* **35,** 11–13.

34. Dingle, J. H., Badger, G. F., and Jordan, W. S., Jr. (1964) *Illness in the Home: A Study of 25,000 Illnesses in a Group of Cleveland Families,* Press of Western Reserve University, Cleveland, OH, p. 292.

35. McMahan, J. T. (1990) Paranasal sinusitis—geriatric considerations. *Otolaryngol. Clin. N. Am.* **23,** 1169–1177.

36. McAlister, W. H., Lusk, R., and Muntz, H. R. (1989) Comparison of plain radiograph an CT scan in infants and children with recurrent sinusutis. *Am. J. Roentgenol.* **153,** 1259–1264.

37. Gwaltney, J. M. J., Phillips, C. D., Miller, R. D., et al. (1994) Computed tomographic study of the common cold. *N. Eng. J. Med.* **330,** 25–30.

38. Evans, K. L. (1998) Recognition and management of sinusitis. *Drugs* **56,** 59–71.

39. Fagnan, L. J. (1998) Acute sinusitis: a cost-effective approach to diagnosis and treatment. *Am. Fam. Phys.* **58,** 1795–1806.

40. Poole, M. D. (1999) A focus on acute sinusitis in adults: changes in disease management. *Am. J. Med.* **106,** S38–S52.

16
Ocular Infections

Charles W. Flowers, Jr. and Richard S. Baker

Age-related degenerative ocular and adnexal changes predispose the elderly to eye infections. The reduction in host defenses associated with age-related degenerative changes significantly compromises the capacity of eyes of elderly people to withstand prolonged exposure to microbial pathogens. Consequently, the elderly tend to have higher rates of eye infection and poorer treatment outcomes. The poorer treatment outcomes are, in part, due to delays in diagnosis as well as delays in presentation.

1. EYELID INFECTIONS

1.1. Epidemiology and Clinical Relevance

1.1.1. Blepharitis

Inflammatory disorders of the eyelid constitute a major class of external eye infections affecting the elderly. The eyelid, particularly the lid margin, is a common site of ocular adnexal infection in the elderly. Staphylococcal blepharitis is by far the most common lid infection encountered. As with other forms of blepharitis, staphylococcal blepharitis is a chronic condition that has periodic exacerbations, which often leads the patient to seek medical attention.

1.1.2. Hordeola

Hordeola are infections of the lid margin sebaceous glands and manifest in two clinical forms: external (stye) and internal. These two forms are differentiated by the particular group of sebaceous glands infected. An external hordeolum (stye) is an infection of the glands of Zeis, which extend along the base of the eyelash hair follicle. It is by far the most common type of hordeolum, and *Staphylococcus aureus* is the predominant microbial pathogen.

1.1.3. Chalazion

A lid lesion that is often confused with an internal hordeolum is a chalazion. A chalazion is a sterile granulomatous reaction to inspissated and impacted meibomian gland secretions. Meibomian gland orifices often become plugged as a result of lid margin inflammation produced by chronic blepharitis. Consequently, meibomian gland secretions build up within the gland and eventually leak out into the surrounding lid connective tissue. These lipid secretions are highly inflammatory and incite a granulomatous inflammatory reaction, which leads to the formation of a chalazion.

From: Infectious Disease in the Aging
Edited by: Thomas T. Yoshikawa and Dean C. Norman
© Humana Press Inc., Totowa, NJ

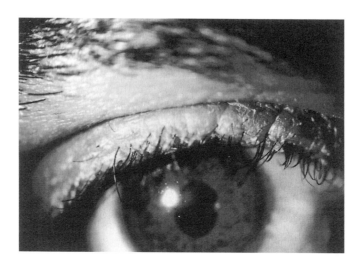

Fig. 1. Staphylococcal blepharitis. Notice the lid margin crusting and the dandruff-like flakes adherent to the lashes. (Reprinted with permission from ref. *19.*)

1.2. Clinical Manifestations

1.2.1. Blepharitis

Patients with blepharitis usually complain of bilateral eye redness, irritation, burning, and tearing. In general these symptoms constitute no more than an annoyance, but can become incapacitating during acute exacerbations. The predominant clinical findings include bilateral lid margin crusting, the accumulation of dandruff-like flakes at the base of the lashes, and lid margin hyperemia (*see* Fig. 1). Over time, because of the chronic nature of this condition, many patients sustain permanent structural changes to the lid margin, consisting of lid margin thickening, loss of lashes (madarosis), and misdirected lashes.

Meibomitis, which is generally considered a manifestation of blepharitis, is an associated finding in almost every case. Meibomitis specifically refers to inflammation of the meibomian glands, which supply the lipid layer of the tear film. The lipid layer of the tear film is most superficial layer and retards tear evaporation. Inflammation of the meibomian glands disrupts the production and secretion of the tear film lipid layer and consequently, leads to rapid tear evaporation and ocular surface drying. Thus, in addition to the symptoms noted above, patients will complain of a sandy-gritty foreign body or dry eye sensation as result of ocular surface drying.

To view inflammation of the meibomian glands, it requires the magnification of the slitlamp biomicroscope; the lesion manifests as pouting and dilation of the orifices, which lie just posterior to the lashes, and inspissation of the meibomian secretions. Several of the orifices will also display complete occlusion as a result of plugging by congealed meibomian secretions.

1.2.2. Hordeola

Because of the association with the lash follicle, an external hordeolum, or stye, manifests primarily at the base of an eyelash, with redness, swelling, and microabscess formation being the predominant clinical features.

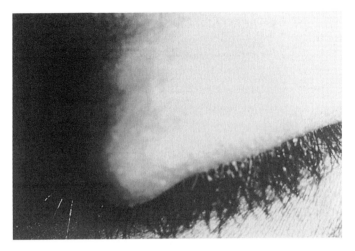

Fig. 2. Chalazion. Note the large well-circumscribed lid mass above the lid margin. An internal hordeolum would look similar, except show more intense signs of acute inflammation and manifest exquisite tenderness. (Reprinted with permission from ref. *20.*)

Internal hordeola arise as a result of infections within the meibomian glands. *Staphylococcus* aureus is the major microbial pathogen in this condition as well. Internal hordeola typically manifest as red swollen large discrete nodules in the lid a clear distance away from the lid margin. Additionally, these lesions are generally more tender than styes and point toward the conjunctival surface instead of the external lid surface. The overlying conjunctiva will show marked hyperemia.

1.2.3. Chalazion

Chalazia clinically manifest as large discrete nontender nodules within the lid a fixed distance away from the lid margin (*see* Fig. 2). Although these lesions look similar to internal hordeola clinically , there are some important differentiating features. Whereas an internal hordeolum represents an acute infectious process, a chalazion is a chronic noninfectious process. Therefore, internal hordeola develop over a much shorter time period (days versus weeks), manifest signs of acute inflammation such as redness, swelling, and tenderness, and require systemic antibiotic therapy for effective treatment. In contrast, chalazia develop over a period of weeks to months, are nontender, have minimal to no associated inflammatory signs, and are effectively treated with lid hygiene and warm compresses in most instances.

1.3. Diagnostic Tests

The diagnosis of all of these infectious processess of the lid is made clinically; consequently, no laboratory or radiological tests exist to aid in the diagnosis of these conditions.

1.4. Therapy

1.4.1. Blepharitis

Treatment of blepharitis consists of lid hygiene and a short course of antistaphylococcal antibiotic therapy. Lid hygiene is performed with dilute baby shampoo dissolved in warm water (one or two drops of baby shampoo in a bottle cap full of warm water) and a cotton tip applicator or wash cloth two to three times daily. Commercially prepared eyelid cleansing kits are available over the counter but are generally more expensive. Lid hygienic therapy does not completely eradicate this disease process but simply brings it under control such that patients are symptom free. Consequently, patients must undergo prolonged courses of lid hygiene, usually over several months, and require lifetime maintenance therapy thereafter for disease control. Two to 3 wk courses of topical antistaphylococcal antibiotic therapy should be reserved for acute flareups or severe, previously untreated disease and should be combined with lid hygiene. Bacitracin or erythromycin ophthalmic ointments are the agents of choice. Systemic tetracycline has been shown to be quite effective in bringing advanced cases of meibomitis under control.

1.4.2. Hordeola

External hordeola, or styes, often sharply localize and rupture spontaneously within a matter of days after forming and thus, warm compresses four to six times a day more than suffices for treating this condition. Resolution can be hastened if the localizing lesion is decompressed with a fine sterile needle. Antibiotic therapy is of questionable value for a single lesion and is often not indicated. In the case of recurrent or multiple styes, topical antistaphyloccocal antibiotic therapy in the form of bacitracin or erythromycin ophthalmic ointment is warranted along with lid hygiene, and depending on the severity, systemic antistaphylococcal antibiotics may be required.

Unlike styes, internal hordeola usually do not rupture and drain spontaneously, and require warm compresses in conjunction with systemic antistaphyloccocal antibiotics. If the lesions do not respond to this regimen, incision and drainage is indicated, and the patient should be referred to an ophthalmologist.

1.5. Prevention

Lid hygiene is the key to prevention for each of the lid infectious processes. Patients who present with recurrent lid infections should be advised to incorporate twice daily lid cleansing into their daily personal hygiene regimen.

2. LACRIMAL SYSTEM INFECTIONS

2.1. Epidemiology and Clinical Relevance

Lacrimal system infections commonly affecting the elderly predominantly involve the lacrimal outflow system. The lacrimal outflow system is composed of the puncta, which are present on the medial aspect of the upper and lower lid margins; the upper and lower canaliculi, the nasolacrimal sac, and the nasolacrimal duct (*see* Fig. 3). Infections of the lacrimal gland (dacryoadenitis) are uncommon and will not be discussed here.

2.1.1. Canaliculitis

A number of organisms have been found to infect the canaliculi including bacteria (i.e., *Actinomyces israelii*, *Propionibacterium* spp., *Nocardia*, and *Bacteroides*), viruses (i.e., herpes simplex and varicella-zoster), and fungi (i.e., *Candida* and *Aspergillus* spp.).

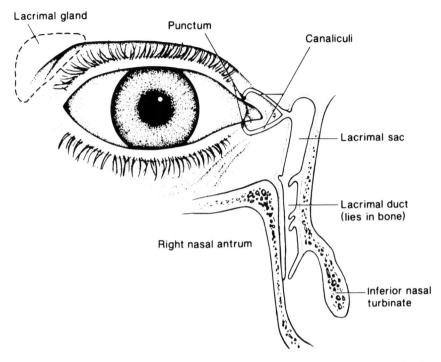

Fig. 3. Nasolacrimal system anatomy. (Reprinted with permission from ref. *21*.)

Despite this seeming variety of potential infectious agents, *A. israelii* causes the overwhelming majority of canalicular infections.

2.1.1. Dacryocystitis

Dacryocystitis refers to an infection of the nasolacrimal sac that often develops as a result of blockage of the nasolacrimal duct. Nasolacrimal duct obstruction causes tear stasis, which leads to ascending bacterial colonization and infection of the nasolacrimal system from the nasopharynx *(1)*. The cause of acquired lacrimal drainage obstruction may be primary or secondary. Primary acquired nasolacrimal duct obstruction results from inflammation of unknown cause that eventually leads to occlusive fibrosis. Secondary acquired lacrimal drainage obstruction may arise from a wide variety of infectious, inflammatory, neoplastic, traumatic, or mechanical causes. In the elderly, the primary acquired form predominates.

2.2 Clinical Manifestations

2.2.1. Canaliculitis

Canaliculitis clinically manifests with the patient complaining of excessive tearing (epiphora). In addition to the symptom of tearing, the patient will exhibit conjunctival injection, particulary in the nasal area, along with punctal dilation and hyperemia. Digital pressure applied to the medial canthal area will often lead to punctal expression of a yellow-green exudate or yellowish "granules," which is highly characteristic of *A. israelii* infections.

2.2.2. Dacryocystitis

Dacryocystitis may manifest as either an acute or chronic infectious process. The acute infectious process presents with localized pain, swelling, and erythema in the medial canthal area, representing an inflamed and distended nasolacrimal sac. Digital pressure applied to the skin overlying the nasolacrimal sac usually results in the expression of purulent material from the eyelid puncta. Patients will often complain of excessive tearing as well as eye redness and purulent discharge. The most common microbial pathogens in adults are staphylococcal and streptococcal species.

Chronic dacryocystitis typically manifests subtly with patients complaining of chronic or recurrent bouts of excessive tearing. The skin over the lacrimal sac usually appears normal, but digital pressure applied to the medial canthal area often results in the expression of purulent material from the puncta. Additionally, patients may also report intermittent episodes of conjunctivitis in the eye ipsilateral to the chronic dacryocystitis. The conjunctivitis results from the reflux of the bacterial pathogens infecting the nasolacrimal sac into the eye through the puncta. Because of the low-grade activity of this disease process, many patients tolerate the symptoms for an extended period of time before seeking medical attention.

2.3. Diagnostic Tests

2.3.1. Canaliculitis

In cases of canaliculitis, diagnostic confirmation of *Actinomyces* can be obtained by Gram-staining the expressed material, which will demonstrate delicate Gram-positive branching filaments.

2.3.2. Dacryocystitis

The diagnosis of dacryocystitis is generally made clinically, but culturing any expressed discharge can be helpful in precisely targeting antibiotic therapy to the causative organism.

2.4. Therapy

2.4.1. Canaliculitis

Treatment of canaliculitis consists of mechanical expression of the exudative or granular material from the canaliculi combined with probing and irrigation of the nasolacrimal system with either a 10% sulfacetamide solution or a penicillin G (100,000 units/mL) eyedrop solution. Patients should be referred to an ophthalmologist for definitive therapy of this condition.

2.4.2. Dacryocystitis

Systemic antibotic therapy is required in all cases of dacryocystitis and empiric therapy with an antibiotic with good Gram-positive coverage, such as oral dicloxacillin or cephalexin is usually started while culture specimens are being processed.

Although systemic antibiotics can be curative in acute disease, they are of little benefit in chronic disease. These patients have total nasolacrimal duct obstruction and require surgical decompression for disease eradication. Irrigating the nasolacrimal sac through the puncta with an antibiotic solution, similar to that used to treat canaliculitis, is a good temporizing measure worth instituting in those patients who cannot undergo immediate surgical drainage. Definitive therapy ultimately rests with the ophthalmologist.

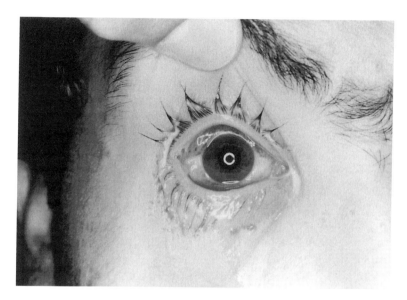

Fig. 4. Bacterial conjunctivitis. Note the copious purulent discharge. (Reprinted with permission from ref. *19*).

2.5. Prevention

Currently, there are no known preventive measures that patients can take to avert either of these condition.

3. CONJUNCTIVAL INFECTIONS

3.1. Epidemiology and Clinical Relevance

Infectious conjunctivitis is primarily caused by bacteria and viruses, with viruses being the more common offending agent in the United States. Bacterial conjunctivitis may be classified as hyperacute, acute, or chronic depending on the rapidity of onset and disease progression. Hyperacute bacterial conjunctivitis is characterized by a very rapid onset (a matter of hours), copious purulent discharge, and intense conjunctival swelling and redness. This form of conjunctivitis is primarily caused by *Neisseria gonorrhoeae* and is uncommon among the elderly population.

3.2. Clinical Manifestations

3.2.1. Bacterial Conjunctivitis

Acute bacterial conjunctivitis, unlike hyperacute bacterial conjunctivitis, evolves over a matter of days and induces a less severe inflammatory response. Patients will manifest a purulent discharge, which is the hallmark feature of all bacterial conjunctivitides, diffuse conjunctival injection, and crusting along the lid margins (*see* Fig. 4). Patients will usually complain of ocular irritation and pain, and experience a decrease in vision due to reflex tearing and the purulent discharge. Staphylococcal and streptococcal species cause the majority of acute bacterial conjunctivitis in adults. Gram-negative bacteria are rare causes of conjunctivitis.

Chronic bacterial conjunctivitis is typically seen in conjunction with one of two conditions: chronic blepharitis and chronic dacryocystitis. Chronic bacterial conjunc-

Table 1
Commercially Available Antibiotic Eyedrops and Ophthalmic
Ointments Commonly Used to Treat Bacterial Conjunctivitis

Antibiotic	Trade Name[a]
Bacitracin ointment	AK-TRACIN™[a]
Ciprofloxacin	Ciloxan™
Ofloxacin	Ocuflox™
Erythromycin ointment	—
Sulfacetamide	Bleph-10™, AK-SULF™[a]
Tetracycline ointment	Achromycin™[a]
Trimethoprim, polymyxin B	Polytrim™

[a]The trade name(s) listed are not all-inclusive.

tivitis associated with blepharitis is primarily caused by *S. aureus* and *Moraxella lacunata*. These infections cause prominent lid margin erythema, scaling, and thickening in addition to purulent discharge, which is usually minimal, and conjunctival injection. Lid margin ulcerations may also develop during acute exacerbations. Because of the associated blepharitis, these patients will undoubtedly have some degree of meibomian gland dysfunction resulting in a compromised tear film. The tear film abnormality may intensify the ocular irritation these patients experience, as well as predispose them to corneal epithelial breakdown.

Chronic bacterial conjunctivitis arising from chronic dacryocystitis is predominantly caused by staphylococcal and streptococcal species. These infections cause many of the symptoms and signs noted, but in addition patients will complain of chronic or recurrent bouts of excessive tearing; digital compression of the medial canthal area will result in the expression of purulent material from the puncta.

3.3. Diagnostic Tests

Culture and sensitivity testing of the conjunctival sac should be performed prior to the initiation of antibiotic therapy in every case of a suspected bacterial conjunctivitis. Gram staining of the purulent exudate should also be attempted. The information obtained from either diagnostic maneuver seldom alters the course of therapy; however, in the case of an infection not responding to the standard therapeutic regimen, this diagnostic information proves invaluable.

3.4. Therapy

The standard therapy for acute bacterial conjunctivitis consists of topical application of antibiotic drops every 2–4 h or antibiotic ointment every 4–6 h for 7–10 d. Repeated saline lavage of the conjunctival sac along with lid hygiene is helpful in rinsing away the bacterial pathogens and removing purulent debris. Cultures should be obtained prior to initiating antibiotic therapy to ensure that the causative organism is sensitive to the empiric antibiotic therapy. Empiric antibiotic therapy should be targeted toward Gram-positive organisms, as they are the predominant cause of acute bacterial conjunctivitis (*see* Table 1). In general, aminoglycosides (gentamicin, neomycin, and tobramycin) should be avoided unless culture and sensitivity results indicate that these agents are the most efficacious. Topical aminoglycosides, particularly gentamicin and neomycin, have been found to induce a toxic reaction in a significant percentage of patients.

Treatment for chronic bacterial conjunctivitis in the setting of chronic blepharitis involves combining lid-margin hygiene with topical antibiotic therapy. The antibiotics used for chronic bacterial conjunctivitis are no different from those used to treat the acute condition; however, antibiotic ointments are preferred over drops, because they can be easily applied to the lid and conjunctiva simultaneously, as well as aid in combating the ocular surface drying associated with meibomian gland dysfunction. The treatment of dacryocystitis-induced bacterial conjunctivitis involves the same topical antibiotic regimen outlined; however, these patients require surgical intervention for definitive therapy and thus, should be promptly referred to an ophthalmologist (*see* discussion).

3.5. Prevention

Hand-to-eye contact is the primary route of ocular contamination leading to acute bacterial conjunctivitis. Therefore, patients should be encouraged to avoid frequent eye rubbing and to engage in diligent handwashing when they come in contact with individuals with red eyes ("pinkeye"). Moreover, definitive treatment of blepharitis or dacryocystitis will avert the secondary bacterial conjunctivitis that can develop in association with these conditions.

4. VIRAL CONJUNCTIVITIS

4.1. Epidemiology and Clinical Relevance

Adenovirus is by far the most common cause of viral conjunctivitis and tends to be the most virulent. Herpes simplex virus (HSV) (usually type 1) primarily causes conjunctivitis in children and usually produces a mild inflammatory response. Other viral pathogens, which can cause viral conjunctivitis in the elderly, include enterovirus, coxsackievirus, and varicella-zoster.

4.2. Clinical Manifestations

Viral conjunctivitis classically produces a clear watery discharge, a follicular conjunctival reaction, and preauricular lymphadenopathy. A purulent discharge may be seen on occasion but is usually more characteristic of a bacterial conjunctivitis. Conjunctival follicles represent lymphoid germinal follicles within the conjunctiva and appear as translucent cobblestones or pebbles with small blood vessels arborizing over the surface. Follicles are highly characteristic of viral infections, although they can also be seen in chlamydial infections of the conjunctiva. It should also be pointed out that due to the highly contagious nature of viral infections, the majority of patients present with bilateral eye involvement, whereas bacterial conjunctival infections typically present unilaterally.

Epidemic keratoconjunctivitis (EKC) is caused by adenovirus types 8 and 19 and is characterized by severe eye pain, photophobia, diffuse punctate corneal epithelial defects, and conjunctivitis. The inflammatory reaction produced by this viral organism can be so intense that inflammatory membranes or pseudomembranes and subepithelial corneal infiltrates develop. True membranes are differentiated from pseudomembranes by the presence of bleeding on removal of true membranes. The corneal subepithelial infiltrates do not occur in every patient but typically manifest 10–14 d after the onset of symptoms. These infiltrates are sterile and represent an immune reaction to viral antigens. They usually resolve spontaneously without visual sequelae, but it may take several months for complete resolution. During the acute infiltrative phase, patients may experience a temporary reduction in vision.

EKC typically lasts for 2–4 wk with contagious viral shedding occurring during the first 2 wk from the onset of symptoms. Therefore, patients must be quarantined during this infectious period. The virus is extremely contagious and can remain viable on inanimate objects such as equipment, doorknobs, and other fomites for up to 2 mo *(2)*. Adenovirus has also been found to be common cause of severe outbreaks of viral conjunctivitis in chronic care facilities *(3)*.

4.3. Diagnostic Tests

The diagnosis of viral conjunctivitis is generally made on clinical findings; however, culture and sensitivity testing does prove useful in identifying cases of EKC and excluding a concurrent bacterial conjunctivitis.

4.4. Therapy

As with all forms of viral conjunctivitis, there is no specific treatment for adenoviral conjunctivitis. Thus, therapy is aimed at palliation and limiting complications. The use of cool compresses, artificial tears, and analgesics are typically very helpful in easing patients' discomfort. Antibiotics are not indicated, unless the patient develops signs of a superimposed bacterial infection. Topical corticosteroids should be avoided.

4.5. Prevention

Hand-to-eye contamination is the primary route of transmission of viral conjunctivitis. Thus, precautions regarding hand-to-eye contact and handwashing should be adhered to regarding this condition. As stated earlier, it is also important to note that adenovirus types 8 and 19 remain infectious for up to 2 mo after being deposited on environmental surfaces *(2,4)*. Therefore, contracting EKC does not require direct contact with an infected individual.

5. CORNEAL INFECTIONS

5.1. Bacterial Keratitis

5.1.1. Epidemiology and Clinical Relevance

Infectious keratitis constitutes a sight-threatening ocular emergency and requires prompt recognition and immediate referral to an ophthalmologist. Bacterial keratitis results from a breakdown in the corneal epithelial barrier and subsequent bacterial invasion of the corneal stroma. Bacterial invasion and white cell infiltration of the cornea leads to tissue destruction and may even lead to perforation if therapy is not instituted in a timely manner. Because of the destructive nature of this disease process

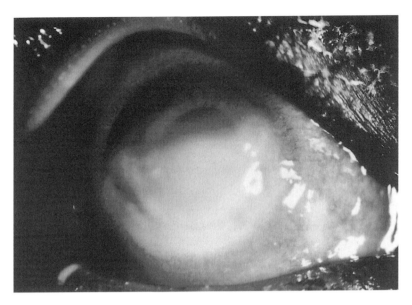

Fig. 5. Bacterial Keratitis. The white corneal opacity represents white cell infiltration into the corneal stroma. (Reprinted with permission from ref. *19.*)

and the cornea's fragile composition, all bacterial infections of the cornea result in some degree of corneal scarring and opacification, regardless of how soon therapy is instituted. Therefore, the amount of corneal scarring and the extent to which vision is affected is largely determined by the time interval between disease onset and disease control. Staphylococcal and streptococcal species are the predominant corneal pathogens.

The risk factors that appear to be the most important in the elderly include dry eye disease, involutional lid abnormalities, diabetes mellitus, and surgical trauma. All of these conditions predispose the elderly patient to corneal epithelial breakdown and corneal bacterial invasion.

5.1.2. Clinical Manifestations

Patients generally complain of a unilateral decrease in vision, eye redness, pain, light sensitivity (photophobia), tearing, and mucoid discharge. Clinically the eye will manifest marked conjunctival injection, a moderate amount of purulent discharge, corneal clouding, and a well-demarcated corneal white cell infiltrate, which appears as a dense white opacity on direct illumination with a penlight (*see* Fig. 5). There may also be a visible layering of pus in the anterior chamber (hypopyon), which is usually a sterile inflammatory response. Fluorescein staining will demonstrate the size and location of the corneal epithelial defect.

5.1.3. Diagnostic Tests

As it was pointed out earlier, prompt antibiotic therapy is crucial for limiting the extent of corneal tissue damage; however, an attempt should be made to obtain diagnostic cultures prior to initiating antibiotic therapy. Treatment should not be withheld, however, if culturing materials are not readily available. Recent studies have found no significant increase in adverse outcomes when diagnostic scraping and culture are not performed at the outset of therapy *(5,6)*.

5.1.4. Therapy

Although Gram-positive organisms cause the majority of community-acquired non-contact lens-related bacterial keratitis, broad-spectrum topical antibiotics are the mainstay of therapy. Most ophthalmologists prescribed specially formulated high concentration antibiotic eyedrops (i.e., cefazolin, 50 mg/mL and tobramycin 14 mg/mL) with an instillation frequency of every 30–60 min around the clock for the first 24–72 h. The primary care physician's role in these cases will often be to institute temporizing measures, while the patient is enroute to the ophthalmologist for definitive therapy. Commercially available fluoroquinolone eyedrops (Ciloxan™ or Ocuflox™) provide the best form of temporizing therapy because of their broad spectrum of antimicrobial activity. Additionally, these agents have been shown to effectively treat bacterial keratitis at their commercially available concentrations *(7)*. Both agents require very frequent instillation (i.e., every 15–30 min for the first 2 h) at the onset of therapy to provide adequate tissue loading of the antibiotic. Beyond the tissue-loading period, the instillation frequency can be reduced to every hour.

5.1.5. Prevention

Effective prevention for this condition entails ensuring that at-risk individuals are receiving appropriate ophthalmic management of their predisposing conditions. In the elderly, dry eye disease and involutional lid malpositions are the most common predisposing risk factors for the development of infectious keratitis. Both predisposing conditions constitute age-related degenerative changes affecting the eye and thus, have a high prevalence among the elderly. The prevalence of dry eye disease, for example, steadily increases with age, with prevalence rates increasing from 2% in individuals 45 yr of age up to 16% in individuals 80 yr of age *(8)*. Similarly, the generalized lid laxity and diminution of muscle tone associated with aging result in structural eyelid malpositions that almost exclusively affect the elderly. It is also important to note that several common systemic conditions and a number of over-the-counter and prescription medications predispose elderly patients to developing dry eye disease. Rheumatoid arthritis, Sjogren's syndrome, sarcoidosis, and other autoimmune/collagen-vascular disorders all produce a decrease in tear production as a result of autoimmune-mediated destruction of conjunctival-based lacrimal gland tissue. The systemic medications that adversely affect tear production include β-adrenergic inhibitors and diuretics used to treat hypertension, tricyclic antidepressants, anti-parkinsonian agents, and over-the-counter cold or hay fever preparations.

5.2. Viral Keratitis

5.2.1. Epidemiology and Clinical Relevance

Herpes simplex and varicella-zoster are the two most common corneal viral pathogens. HSV is the most common cause of infectious keratitis in the United States, causing an estimated 500,000 cases of infectious keratitis each year *(9)*. Herpes zoster ophthalmicus is the term given to the herpes zoster occurring in the first division of the trigeminal nerve, which innervates the ocular surface. Involvement of the ophthalmic

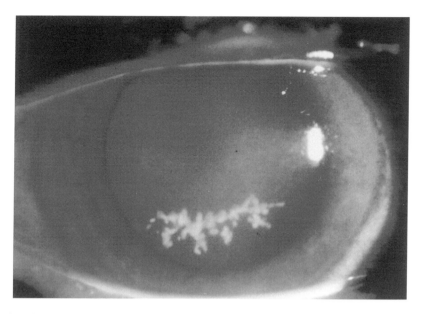

Fig. 6. HSV keratitis showing dendritic ulcer highlighted with fluorescein staining. (Reprinted with permission from ref. *19*).

division of the trigeminal nerve accounts for 9–16% of cases of varicella-zoster occurring annually in the United States and is associated with severe, chronic ocular complications *(11)*. Unlike bacterial keratitis, viral keratitis does not require a breach in the corneal epithelial layer to become established.

5.2.2. Clinical Manifestations

The epithelial keratitis produced by HSV is characterized by thin branching dendritic ulcerations, which are best seen with fluorescein staining (*see* Fig. 6). The lesions are usually centrally or paracentrally located and each linear branch of the dendritic ulcer terminates in bulblike conglomerations commonly referred to as "terminal bulbs." This infection is predominantly unilateral, with bilateral involvement only rarely seen. Patients will typically report symptoms of sharp eye pain, light sensitivity, tearing, and blurring of vision. It is interesting to note that although most patients complain of eye pain, objective testing of corneal sensitivity in the area of the dendritic lesion will demonstrate decreased or absent corneal sensitivity.

Varicella-zoster virus (VZV) epithelial keratitis clinically appears very similar to HSV epithelial keratitis but has several important distinguishing features. First, VZV keratitis is usually accompanied by a vesicular eruption involving the periorbital skin in a dermatomal pattern (*see* Fig. 7). The epithelial keratitis and the rash typically appear together. However, ocular involvement can be delayed, and it is important to note that ocular involvement does not occur in every case of VZV facial dermatitis. Ocular involvement occurs in approximately 50–72% of patients with periocular zoster *(11)*. A vesicular eruption extending to the tip of the nose indicates involvement of the nasociliary nerve, which is a branch of the ophthalmic division of the trigeminal nerve. This clinical finding, known as "Hutchinson's sign," has an 85% predictability of the

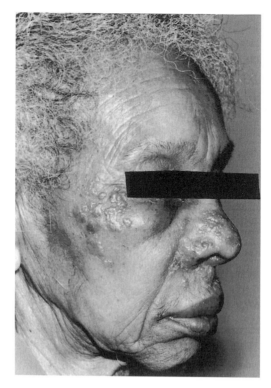

Fig. 7. Herpes zoster ophthalmicus. Note the dermatomal pattern of the vesicular eruption. Also note the tip of the nose involvement, "Hutchinson's sign." (Reprinted with permission from ref. *19*).

eye being involved *(12)*. Other differentiating features of VZV epithelial keratitis include the absence of terminal bulbs, smaller and less branching dendrites, more profound corneal anesthesia, and the lack of recurrences. HSV has been found to recur in approximately 33% of patients within 2 yr of the initial episode *(13)*.

5.2.3. Diagnostic Tests

The diagnosis of HSV and VZV keratitis is generally made clinically. Because of their unique features, both conditions can be diagnosed in the majority of cases based on the clinical appearance of the lesions, the history of present illness, and the patient's symptomatology. When necessary, confirmation of the diagnosis can be made by culturing a swab or scrape of the corneal epithelium. Alternatively, fluorescent immunoassay of corneal epithelial cells reacting with HSV monoclonal antigen, polyclonal recombinant polymerase chain reaction amplification, and Southern blot analysis of HSV or VZV genomic sequences may be used for diagnosis confirmation.

5.2.4. Therapy

The management of HSV epithelial keratitis consists of the topical administration of antiviral eyedrops. Several agents have been shown to be efficacious in treating this condition; however, at present, only one agent, trifluridine (Viroptic™ 1%) has been shown to have a greater than 90% cure rate. The recommended dosing regimen is one drop every 2 h, but no more than nine times a day for the first 3–5 d. The frequency of administration should be decreased to five times a day once the epithelium heals or the fifth day is reached. Topical therapy should be continued for at least 2 wk, but no more than 3 wk, because of the risk of drug toxicity. The drop frequency should continue to be tapered over the remainder of the treatment period.

Currently, there are no topical antiviral agents that have been shown to be effective in treating VZV-related epithelial keratitis. Treatment for this condition is aimed at preventing ocular complications and consists of oral acyclovir, 800 mg five times a day for 10 d, if within 72 h of the appearance of the skin lesions. The epithelial disease is benign and usually resolves spontaneously.

5.3. Fungal Keratitis

5.3.1. Epidemiology and Clinical Relevance

Fungal keratitis is one of the most devastating ocular infections encountered in ophthalmic clinical practice. The destructive nature of these infections is largely due to the lack of effective topical antifungal agents and the organisms' ability to resist host defenses. This fact, coupled with the innate virulence of fungal organisms, makes early detection an absolute requisite for achieving therapeutic success. Fungi, like bacteria, require a breach in the corneal epithelium in order to penetrate the cornea and produce tissue destruction. Fungal infections have been primarily associated with corneal trauma due to vegetable or organic material (e.g., tree branch, nylon lawn trimmer).

The leading corneal pathogens include *Fusarium*, *Aspergillus*, and *Candida*. These organisms cause the overwhelming majority of corneal fungal infections and appear to have climate specificity. *Fusarium* is the predominant corneal pathogen in the warmer southern United States, whereas *Candida* is the predominant corneal pathogen in the cooler northern United States. *Aspergillus* is found both in the northern and southern United States. *Candida* corneal infections are notable for occurring mainly in the setting of a compromised ocular surface (i.e., prolonged topical corticosteroid use, hypesthetic cornea from HZV, severe dry eye disease, and the like).

5.3.2. Clinical Manifestations

Fungal keratitis classically presents as an indolent infection with the infectious process evolving over a matter of days to weeks. In most infections, symptoms and signs typically develop within 1 or 2 d of inoculation, but because of the less fulminant evolution, patients are not motivated to seek medical attention until days or weeks later. The characteristic clinical appearance of a fungal keratitis consists of a gray-white stromal infiltrate with feathery or fluffy borders usually accompanied by several satellite lesions adjacent to the primary focus of infection. The corneal surface often appears to have a dry coarse texture and the epithelium at the margins of the ulcer tends to be heaped up. Keratomycosis is also frequently associated with sterile hypopyon formation.

5.3.3. Diagnostic Tests

The diagnostic evaluation involves culturing for both bacteria and fungi using blood and chocolate agar plates for bacterial isolation and Sabouraud agar for fungal isolation. Smears for Gram and Giemsa stains and potassium hydroxide preparation are obtained as well. Patients should be referred immediately to an ophthalmologist to have definitive culturing performed. If initial cultures are negative, patients often require corneal biopsy and special fungal staining of the biopsied tissue.

5.3.4. Therapy

The treatment of fungal keratitis requires a prolonged course of medical therapy. The antifungal agents currently available are primarily fungistatic and have poor penetration into the cornea. Therefore, protracted courses of therapy are necessary in order to achieve adequate antifungal tissue levels for a sufficient period of time to eradicate the organism. It is generally recommended that therapy for fungal keratitis be continued for at least 12 wk. Empiric therapy is usually started with natamycin (5%) eyedrops, which is the only ocular antifungal preparation commercially available in the United States. Natamycin belongs to the polyene class of antifungal agents and has been shown to be most effective against filamentous fungi, such as *Aspergillus* and *Fusarium*. This agent is administered every 30–60 min around the clock for the first 24–72 h. Unfortunately, natamycin has poor corneal penetration and therefore, has limited efficacy in those cases in which the organism lies deep within the corneal stroma. Amphotericin B is the drug of choice for treating fungal keratitis produced by yeasts, such as *Candida*. Topical preparations of amphotericin B can be made by a hospital pharmacy. The recommended concentration is 0.15%. Oral flucytosine (150 mg/kg) is often used in combination with amphotericin in treating *Candida* corneal infections, because of the demonstrated synergistic effects. Other antifungals commonly used to treat fungal keratitis include clotrimazole 1% vaginal cream, miconazole 1% fabricated from the intravenous preparation, oral fluconazole (400–800 mg/d), and oral ketoconazole (200–400 mg/d). Fungal infections unresponsive to medical therapy require corneal transplantation for disease eradication.

5.3.5. Prevention

Because corneal trauma is the predominant risk factor for the development of fungal keratitis, patients should be strongly encouraged to wear protective eyewear when they are performing yard work. Moreover, patients with severe dry eye disease or hypesthetic corneas require frequent follow-up with an ophthalmologist to monitor the status of their ocular surface.

6. RETINAL AND VITREOUS INFECTIONS

6.1. Endophthalmitis

6.1.1. Epidemiology and Clinical Relevance

Postoperative endophthalmitis is the most significant retinal-vitreal infection encountered among the geriatric population. Endophthalmitis is defined as inflammation of the intraocular contents and develops as a result of microbial pathogens or chemical toxins gaining intraocular access. Although several etiologic mechanisms exist for the development of this infection (i.e., penetrating ocular trauma, or hematogenous spread from another infectious site), postsurgical infection is the predominant mechanism among the elderly, who undergo the majority of intraocular surgery. Fortunately, it is a rare complication of intraocular surgery. The relative incidence of postoperative

Table 2
Incidence of Endophthalmitis Following Intraocular Surgery

Procedure	Incidence %
Cataract surgery	0.13
Corneal transplantation surgery	0.11
Glaucoma surgery	0.061
Retinal-vitreous surgery	0.051

Adapted from refs. *14* and *15*.

endophthalmitis for each of the commonly performed intraocular surgical procedures is listed in Table 2 *(14,15)*.

Studies have shown that postoperative endophthalmitis is primarily caused by organisms that colonize the eyelids, conjunctiva, and nose, with 90% of culture-positive postoperative endophthalmitis cases caused by Gram-positive organisms, of which coagulase-negative staphylococci are the most common *(16,17)*. The major host risk factors for the development of postoperative endophthalmitis include bacterial blepharitis, nasolacrimal duct infections, nasolacrimal duct obstruction, active nonocular infections, diabetes mellitus, and immunosuppression from any cause.

6.1.2. Clinical Manifestations

Postoperative endophthalmitis can manifest early or late in the postoperative period. Early postoperative endophthalmitis typically occurs within the first week after surgery. Patients will typically present complaining of severe ocular pain and decreased vision. On examination, these patients will show intraocular and periocular inflammation in excess of the normal postoperative inflammatory response. Depending on the severity of the infection, patients may also demonstrate frank purulence at the surgical wound site, purulent conjunctival discharge, or a hypopyon in the anterior chamber. It is important to note that most cases of endophthalmitis following cataract extraction occur early. In the Endophthalmitis Vitrectomy Study (EVS), for example, the median time to presentation was 6 d and about 80% of patients presented within 2 wk of cataract surgery *(16)*.

Late or delayed-onset postoperative endophthalmitis can occur days to weeks and even years after surgery. The type of surgery appears to play a definite role in the development of these late infections, with glaucoma surgery being more frequently associated with late-onset postoperative endophthalmitis. Late infections can present very subtly or in a fulminant suppurative manner. The type of presentation is primarily determined by the virulence of the infecting organism. The subtle presentation of postoperative endophthalmitis is most commonly associated with postcataract surgery cases. This form of endophthalmitis usually manifests as persistent low-grade postoperative inflammation well beyond the expected time period for normal postoperative inflammation. Patients will complain of persistent photophobia and blurred vision. These patients will typically not manifest any signs of frank purulence and the eyes will often appear white and quiet. The etiologic mechanism underlying this form of endophthalmitis has been shown to be colonization of the intraocular lens implant by *Propionibacterium acnes* and coagulase-negative staphyloccocal species.

The fulminant presentation of late postoperative endophthalmitis is more frequently associated with streptococcal species and Gram-negative organisms, which cause the majority of late endophthalmitis. Glaucoma filtration surgery is the most frequently associated surgical procedure. Patients with this form of the disease will present in similar fashion to patients with acute postoperative endophthalmitis, i.e., severe pain, decreased vision, and marked intraocular and periocular inflammation. Given the strong association of late postoperative endophthalmitis with glaucoma filtration surgery, it is recommended that patients who have undergone glaucoma surgery and present with conjunctivitis be placed on topical antibiotic therapy immediately and referred to an ophthalmologist for a more in-depth evaluation.

6.1.3. Diagnostic Tests

The diagnosis of endophthalmitis is exclusively made clinically. Diagnostic needle taps of the anterior chamber or vitreous cavity may be performed to confirm the clinical diagnosis and identify the infecting organism.

6.1.4. Therapy

The prognosis for postoperative endophthalmitis is largely dependent on the virulence of the infecting organism and the length of time between the onset of infection and the initiation of therapy. The delicate intraocular structures cannot withstand prolonged exposure to destructive bacterial pathogens and inflammatory cells and therefore, early diagnosis and rapid therapy implementation are the keys to treatment success for this condition. The treatment of endophthalmitis involves intraocular antibiotic injections along with frequent application of topical fortified antibiotics and topical corticosteroids. The antibiotics most commonly used for intraocular injection are amikacin (400 µg) and vancomycin (1 mg). In advanced cases, a vitrectomy is performed in conjunction with the above measures to debulk the infectious debris. One of the key findings of the EVS was that immediate vitrectomy was of use only in patients who presented with visual acuity of light perception or worse *(16)*. Most retinal surgeons will also place patients on a short course of oral corticosteroids following vitrectomy. Diagnostic specimens of the aqueous and vitreous humors are obtained at the time of intraocular antibiotic injection or vitrectomy.

6.1.5. Prevention

Given the strong association with lid flora, patients with active blepharitis must be adequately treated prior to undergoing any form of ocular surgery. To further combat this problem ophthalmic surgeons instill preoperative prophylactic broad-spectrum antibiotics in the operative eye. In addition, some surgeons infuse antibiotics in the eye during surgery.

7. ORBITAL INFECTIONS

7.1. Preseptal Cellulitis

7.1.1. Epidemiology and Clinical Relevance

Preseptal cellulitis represents a superficial cellulitis of the eyelid skin and subcutaneous tissue. This infection can arise from one of three sources: paranasal sinus infections, direct extension from a localized infection of the eyelid or adjacent tissues (i.e., acute dacryocystitis or hordeola), and periorbital trauma (i.e., infected cuts or abrasions to the periorbital facial area). This infectious process is confined to the lid because the orbital septum has not been violated. The orbital septum is a fibrous extension of the bony periosteum attached to the orbital rim that inserts into the upper and lower eyelids and serves as a barrier to the spread of infection from the eyelid posteriorly into the orbit.

7.1.2. Clinical Manifestations

The predominant clinical manifestations of this disease process are lid edema and erythema. There may be associated reactive conjunctival injection, but the ocular globe and visual function are otherwise unaffected. Patients maintain normal visual acuity, normal pupillary responses, and good ocular motility, and proptosis does not develop.

7.1.3. Diagnostic Tests

The diagnostic evaluation includes a good history, which specifically ascertains information regarding sinus disease, sinus surgery, trauma, or excessive tearing. In addition, computed tomographic (CT) scans of the orbit and sinuses are important for determining the extent and possible etiology of the disease.

7.1.4. Therapy

Effective therapy is usually obtained with a 10–14 d course of oral antibiotics. Empiric therapy with dicloxacillin or cephalexin is more than adequate in the majority of cases.

7.1.5. Prevention

Localized lid infections and sinus infections should be promptly treated to prevent preseptal cellulitis from developing.

7.2. Orbital Cellulitis

7.2.1. Epidemiology and Clinical Relevance

Orbital or postseptal cellulitis, unlike preseptal cellulitis, is a sight-threatening emergency. Harmful infectious pathogens entering the orbital space have access to the optic nerve, the extraocular muscles, and the principal vasculature of the eye. If left untreated, this condition will surely result in blindness or severe visual impairment.

7.2.2. Clinical Manifestations

Patients present with dull aching pain, eyelid swelling and erythema, decreased vision, proptosis, conjunctival swelling and injection, and ocular motility disturbances. In addition, the patients frequently have constitutional symptoms of fever and malaise. Paranasal sinus infections constitute the most common source of orbital cellulitis, with ethmoid sinusitis being the principal source. Other important sources include dacryocystitis, dental abscess, and trauma, as well as risk factors such as systemic debilitation. Patients debilitated from advanced diabetic disease, septicemia, systemic malignancy, human immunodeficiency virus disease, chronic diarrhea, and prolonged immunosuppression are particularly at risk for developing fungal orbital infections.

7.2.3. Diagnostic Tests

As with preseptal cellulitis, CT scans of the orbits and sinuses are obtained to determine the extent of disease and look for the presence of orbital abscesses. The presence of an orbital abscess and/or multiple sinus disease is an indication for immediate surgical drainage. Nasopharynx cultures can be helpful in identifying the causative organism, although orbital cellulitis in adults tends to be polymicrobial. It is also important to note that in the elderly intraocular and extraocular tumors can masquerade as orbital cellulitis. Intraocular melanoma extending through the sclera, for example, has been found to induce a significant orbital inflammatory response similar to what one may see with orbital cellulitis *(18)*.

7.2.4. Therapy

Patients diagnosed with orbital cellulitis require hospitalization and the initiation of broad-spectrum intravenous antibiotics. Empiric therapy with ceftriaxone is a regimen frequently employed. Urgent ophthalmology and otolaryngology consultation should be obtained as well.

7.2.5. Prevention

Orbital cellulitis is an infectious process that arises secondarily from extension of a primary infection in a periorbital structure. Thus, appropriate treatment of the primary infectious process will prevent the development of orbital cellulitis in most cases.

REFERENCES

1. Lundsgard, K. K. K. (1927) The Doyne Memorial lecture. Pneumococcus in connection with ophthalmology. *Trans. Ophthalmol. Soc. UK.* **47**, 294–312
2. Dawson, C. R. and Darrell, D. (1963) Infections due to adenovirus type 8 in the United States. An outbreak of epidemic keratoconjunctivitis originating in physician's office. *N. Engl. J. Med.* **268**, 1031–1034.
3. Buffington, J., Chapman, L. E., Stobierski, M. G., et al. (1993) Epidemic keratoconjunctivitis in a chronic care facility: risk factors and measures for control. *J. Am. Geriatr. Soc.* **41**, 1177–1181.
4. Wegman, D. H., Guinee, V. F., and Millian, S. J. (1970) Epidemic kertaconjunctivits. *Am. J. Public Health* **60**, 1230–1237
5. Kowal, V. O. and Mead, M. D. (1992) Community acquired corneal ulcers: the impact of culture on management. *Invest. Ophtahlmol. Vis. Sci.* **33**, 1210
6. McLeod, S. D., LaBree, L., Tayyanipour, R., et al. (1995) The importance of initial management in the treatment of severe infectious corneal ulcer. *Ophthalmology* **102**, 1943–1948.
7. Leibowitz, H. M. (1991) Clinical evaluation of ciprofloxacin 0.3% ophthalmic solution for treatment of bacterial keratitis. *Am. J. Ophthalmol.* **112**, 34S–47S.
8. Schein, O. D., Munoz, B., Tielsch, J. M., et al. (1997) Prevalence of dry eye among the elderly. *Am. J. Ophthalmol.* **124**, 723–728
9. Mader, T. H. and Stulting, R. D. (1992) Viral keratitis. *Infect. Dis. Clin. North Am.* **6**, 831–849.
10. Ragozzino, M. W., Melton, L. L., 3rd, Kerland, L. T., et al. (1982) Population-based study of herpes zoster and its sequelae. *Medicine* **61**, 310–316.
11. Chang, E. J. and Dreyer, E. B. (1996) Herpesvirus infection of the anterior segment. *Int. Ophthalmol. Clin.* **36**, 17–28.
12. Jones, D. B. (1974) Herpes zoster ophthalmicus, in *Ocular Inflammatory Disease* (Golden, B. ed.), Charles C. Thomas, Springfield, IL, pp. 198–209.
13. Shuster, J. J., Kaufman, H. E., and Nesburn, A. B. (1981) Statisitcal analysis of the rate of recurrence of herpes virus ocular epithelial disease. *Am. J. Ophthalmol.* **91**, 328–331.
14. Kattan, H. M., Flynn, H. M., Pflugfelder, S. C., et al. (1991) Nosocomia endophthalmitis survey: current incidence of infection after intraocular surgery. *Ophthalmology* **98**, 227–238.
15. Powe, N. R., Schein, O. D., Gieser, S.C., et al. (1994) Synthesis of the literature on visual acuity and complications following cataract extraction with intraocular lens implantation. *Arch. Ophthalmol.* **112**, 239–252.

16. Endopthalmitis Vitrectomy Study Group. (1995) Results of the endophthalmitis vitrectomy study. *Arch. Ophthalmol.* **113,** 1479–1496.
17. Speaker, M. G., Milch, F. A., Shah, M. K., et al. (1991) Role of external bacterial flora in the pathogenesis of acute postoperative endophthalmitis. *Ophthalmology* **98,** 639–650.
18. Rumelt, S. and Rubin, P. A. D. (1996) Potential sources for orbital cellulitis. *Int. Ophthalmol. Clin.* **36,** 207–221.
19. Flowers, C. W. (1988) Managing eye infections in older adults. *Infect. Dis. Clin. Pract.* **7,** 447–458.
20. Berson, F. G. (1993) The red eye, in *Basic Ophthalmology for Medical Students and Primary Care Residents* (Berson, F. G., ed.), San Francisco, CA: American Academy of Ophthalmology, pp. 57–74.
21. Barza, M. and Baum, J. (1983) Ocular infections. *Med. Clin. N. Am.* **67,** 131–152.

17

Prosthetic Device Infections

Steven Berk and James W. Myers

Fortunately, infection is a rare complication of prosthetic devices. Despite the presence of infection, removal of these devices is not always possible or necessary. The introduction of foreign material enhances the pathogenicity of known pathogens and increases the potential of less virulent microorganisms to cause damage. Thus, *Staphylococcus epidermidis* is a very common organism in patients with prosthetic devices as compared with the normal healthy population. Fibronectin promotes adherence of staphylococci to chronically implanted devices. An extracellular substance called "glycocalyx" has been associated with coagulase-negative staphylococci including *S. epidermidis*. A polysaccharide "adhesin" facilitates adherence of staphylococci to foreign material and functions as an antiphagocytic capsule. The function of polymorphonuclear leukocytes is also impaired in the presence of foreign bodies. There is deficient superoxide production, which leads to impaired killing of microorganisms. Also, recent data suggest a role for small colony variants (SCV) of staphylococci that may cause persistent and recurrent infections as a result of their capacity to survive within, but not lyse, whole cells. When these bacteria adhere to foreign bodies, they undergo dramatic metabolic changes such as slower growth, decreased metabolism, and enhanced resistance to antibiotics. These organisms can be difficult to detect in the microbiology laboratory and also difficult to treat with conventional antibiotics *(1)*.

1. SHUNT INFECTIONS

1.1. Epidemiology and Clinical Relevance

The most common indication for central nervous system (CNS) shunts has been to divert fluid in patients with hydrocephalus. Another indication for insertion of a CNS prosthetic device is to monitor intracranial pressure in patients who have had a variety of cerebral insults. The prevalence of infection ranges from 1.5–15%. Shunt infections often lead to an extension of the hospital stay by 2–3 wk and often require additional surgery. Risk factors for shunt infections appear to be extremes of age, especially infants and the elderly. Elderly patients have an incidence of shunt infection of 16.8% versus 6.8% for younger adults. A history of revision of a previous shunt or a prior external drainage device also increases the risk of having a shunt infection. Most shunts are either ventricular peritoneal (VP) or ventricular atrial (VA) devices. It is unclear whether the infection rate varies among the types of shunts; however, the presentation

From: *Infectious Disease in the Aging*
Edited by: Thomas T. Yoshikawa and Dean C. Norman
© Humana Press Inc., Totowa, NJ

may differ between the devices in that "shunt nephritis"and infective endocarditis are much more common with a VA shunt.

1.2. Clinical Manifestations

There are different mechanisms by which a shunt may become infected (2,3). The primary mechanism is colonization during surgery. Infection may also ascend from the distal end of the shunt with a VP shunt, or the route of infection may be hematogenous, particularly with a VA shunt. One third of these infections occur during hospitalization, and the majority occur within 2 mo of surgery. The patient may present with headache, vomiting, and fever. As mentioned previously, shunt nephritis and infective endocarditis may also be a manifestation of VA shunt infections. VP shunt infections may be associated with abdominal complaints.

1.3. Diagnostic Tests and Microbiology

The diagnosis of shunt infections is usually made by ordering a computed tomographic (CT) scan and performing a shunt aspiration for cerebrospinal fluid (CSF). A cranial CT scan will show hydrocephalus or an abdominal CT scan may show a cyst or abscess around the ventricular peritoneal catheter. Lumbar punctures are not useful. Blood cultures are positive in 90% of VA shunt infections but only positive in less than 25% of other types of shunt infections (2,3). Clinicians should not ignore "skin contaminants" isolated on culture of CSF, particularly when managing a VA shunt. The CSF protein may be elevated. The CSF cellular reaction is usually modest, averaging approx 15 white blood cells per mm^3. The presence of more than 100 white blood cells per mm^3 correlates with a positive culture 90% of the time.

The primary organisms involved with shunt infections are S. epidermidis and S. aureus (2,3). Coagulase-negative staphylococci cause 50% or greater of infections in the postoperative period. S. aureus accounts for approx 20%, and streptococci for another 10% of infections. Gram-negative bacilli and diphtheroids have been isolated in approx 5–10% of infections. As mentioned previously, the presence of skin contaminants such as diphtheroids should not be disregarded when evaluating a shunt infection.

1.4. Treatment

The management of shunt infections varies between individuals and surgeons. Upon clinical suspicion of a CNS shunt infection, a Gram stain and culture of CSF should be obtained from the shunt reservoir and blood cultures should also be obtained. Cultures should be held for at least 7 d. In practice there are three options for treatment of a shunt infection. The first requires removing the shunt, utilizing an external drainage device, and instituting systemic antibiotics. The second involves removal of the infected shunt and replacing it immediately with a new indwelling device and instituting antibiotic therapy. The third alternative is to leave the shunt in place and treat with systemic and/or intraventricular antibiotics. A review of studies of management alternatives noted that 94% of infections that were treated with shunt removal and insertion of an external drainage device were cured compared with 71% of patients that were treated with immediate shunt replacement (2,3). Usually after removal of the entire shunt components, the surgeon places an external ventricular drainage device. This might also be accomplished by externalizing the distal end of a VP shunt. A period of effective systemic and/or intraventricular antibiotics are given. Usually after cultures have been documented to be sterile for 3–5 d, the external device is removed, and the new shunt is replaced at a different site. Continuation of systemic antibiotics for >10 d is then prescribed after removal of the infected shunt. A 21-d total course of antibiotics might be required depending upon the organism, particularly if a new shunt is reimplanted at the same time as removal of the infected shunt. If the shunt is not removed, 3–6 wk of treatment is generally advised. Empiric therapy is generally with vancomycin and perhaps a third-generation cephalosporin. Rifampin may be added under some circumstances. Specific therapy is guided by isolation of an organism. If vancomycin or gentamicin is given intraventricularly, a "preservative-free" preparation should be used. If vancomycin is given intraventricularly, usually 10 mg is an appropriate starting dose. Vancomycin levels should be monitored as the drug can accumulate. The literature is unclear regarding the use of prophylactic antibiotics before placement of an intraventricular shunt. Options include a 2-d course of trimethoprim-sulfamethoxazole, a single 10 mg intraventricular dose of vancomycin, or perhaps intravenous cefazolin *(2,3)*. Patients with VA shunts might require antibiotic prophylaxis while undergoing dental or other bacteremia-causing procedures.

2. PERITONITIS ASSOCIATED WITH CONTINUOUS AMBULATORY PERITONEAL DIALYSIS

2.1. Clinical Relevance and Microbiology

The rate of peritonitis associated with continuous ambulatory peritoneal dialysis (CAPD) is decreasing, down from 2.8 to 0.8 episodes per year *(4)*. *S. aureus* and coagulase-negative staphylococci account for 50–80% of CAPD peritonitis cases. Streptococci cause approx 10%, of these infections and Gram-negative bacilli are isolated in another 20% of cases. Infections with mycobacteria and fungi are rare but cause serious complications. Sources of peritonitis associated with CAPD include contamination of the catheter during implantation, manipulation of the dialysate tubing, the dialysate fluid itself, and possible bowel perforation. Most often, the peritoneum is infected by organisms that invade along the catheter tract. Lack of proper sterile technique is a major risk factor.

2.2. Clinical Manifestations, Diagnostic Tests, and Treatment

The clinical diagnosis of peritonitis associated with CAPD is suggested by abdominal pain (78%), a cloudy effluent (98%), vomiting (25%), nausea, fever (50%), and an elevated peripheral white blood cell count with a left shift. The Gram stain is positive in only 10–40% of cases. There should be more than 100 polymorphonuclear cells per mm^3 in the examined fluid. If blood culture bottles are used to culture the dialysate fluid, then the yield of positive cultures is increased (80%). Bacteremia is unusual. An ultrasonogram may reveal pericatheter fluid collections as well.

The Advisory Committee on Peritonitis Management of the International Society for Peritoneal Dialysis has published guidelines for treatment of these infections on the Internet. These are available at http://www.ispd.org/guidelines.php3. *See* Tables 1 and 2 for specific therapy. Cefazolin and tobramycin are regarded as appropriate initial therapy *(4,5)*. Because of the potential for emergence of vancomycin resistance, van-

Table 1
Treatment of Peritonitis Associated with Chronic Ambulatory Peritoneal Dialysis

Initial empiric therapy
> Cefazolin—500 mg/L loading dose, maintenance 125 mg/L ip and tobramycin
> or gentamicin or netilmicin—0.6 mg/kg B.W. ip once daily or amikacin 2.0 mg/kg
> B.W. ip once daily
> Because of the emergence of vancomycin-resistant organisms, vancomycin is reserved
> for the following: methicillin-resistant *S. aureus,* β-lactam-resistant organisms
> or serious peritonitis in patients allergic to other antibiotics

Enterococci
> Stop cephalosporin, continue aminoglycosides, add ampicillin 125 mg/L
> and continue therapy for 14 d.

S. aureus
> Discontinue aminoglycoside, continue cephalosporin, and consider rifampin 600 mg/d
> p.o.; continue therapy for 21 d, and reevaluate. If no improvement by 96 h,
> consider other antibiotics or catheter removal

Coagulase-negative staphylococci
> Discontinue aminoglycoside and continue cephalosporin for 14 d if susceptible.

Single Gram-negative organism (other than *P. aeruginosa*)
> Adjust antibiotics according to sensitivity patterns (usually sensitive to an
> aminoglycoside).

P. aeruginosa
> Tobramycin or gentamicin or netilmicin - 0.6 mg/kg B.W. ip once daily
> or amikacin 2.0 mg/kg B.W. ip once daily for 21–28 d
> with another anti-*Pseudomonal* agent.

Multiple organisms
> Consider surgical intervention
> Add metronidazole 500 mg every 8 h iv po, or rectally; continue therapy up to 21 d

B.W., body weight; ip, intraperitoneal; po, oral; iv, intravenous.

Table 2
Fungal and Tuberculous Peritonitis

Fungal
> Fluconazole 150 mg/ip every second d and flucytosine (loading dose 2000 mg po,
> maintenance 1000 mg po) or amphotericin B 25 mg/d iv and flucytosine as above.
> Note: duration of therapy 4–6 wk or longer

Tuberculous
> Early diagnosis and treatment is crucial. Catheter removal appears to be mandatory.
> Mycobacterial DNA in peritoneal fluid, using polymerase chain reaction appears
> to offer the fastest diagnosis, but culture and smear should be done as well.
> Laparoscopy and biopsy may be necessary for diagnosis. Triple drug therapy
> (isoniazid, rifampin, and pyrazinamide) is the mainstay of therapy, but local
> drug sensitivities should be considered.

ip, intraperitoneal; po, oral; iv, intravenous.

comycin is reserved for methicillin-resistant *S. aureus*, β-lactam-resistant organisms or serious peritonitis in patients allergic to other antibiotics. If the patient is culture negative after 2–3 d and clinically improved, the aminoglycoside may be discontinued and the cephalosporin continued for 14 d. Intraperitoneal antibiotics are as effective as systemic in most cases.

2.3. Prevention

In patients with peritoneal catheters, prophylaxis for invasive procedures such as dentistry and colonoscopy could follow the American Heart Association Guidelines for Prevention of Endocarditis. However, no control studies have ever been performed. Many patients with Tenchoff catheters are carriers of *S. aureus*. Intranasal mupirocin and oral rifampin may reduce the frequency of exit site infections due to *S. aureus*.

3. PROSTHETIC JOINT INFECTION

3.1. Epidemiology and Clinical Relevance

The prevalence of infection of prosthetic hip joints is 0.5–1.3%. Prosthetic knee joints have a prevalence of infection of 1.3–2.9%. Elbows have an infection rate of approx 9%, whereas that of shoulders, wrist, and ankles is approx 1–2%. From 35–50% of the patients with an infected joint present within 3 mo of surgery with increasing pain both at rest and with activity *(6)*. Another 30–35% of the patients present from 3–24 mo postoperatively with joint pain. Infection also may spread hematogenously from a distant focus to the joint as well. The average age of patients with an infected prosthetic hip is 67 yr. Elderly patients frequently have rheumatoid or degenerative joint disease *(7)*. Pressure ulcers and urinary tract infections are particularly likely to occur in the elderly and serve as sources of transient bacteremia, which can seed a prosthetic joint.

3.2. Clinical Manifestations

Elderly patients often require prosthetic joints because of degenerative or rheumatoid arthritis, or fractures. Patients often present complaining of pain (>90%) or altered mobility. Signs of systemic toxicity or fever are often absent. Only 40–45% of elderly patients with prosthetic joint infection may have fever *(7)*. Drainage or erythema may be present at the site of the incision, but infections can be quite indolent *(8)*.

3.3. Diagnostic Tests and Microbiology

Radiographic signs of loosening of the prosthesis are seen in two thirds of late infections but in less than 50% of early infections. Arthrography (after hip aspiration) may be helpful for determining loosening of the cemented components by showing penetration of the dye between cement and bone. Radiographic and bone scans may fail to distinguish between a low-grade infection and aseptic loosening of the prosthesis. A bone scan following hip surgery may take as long as 6 mo to become normal in the area of the lesser trochanter. The area around the acetabulum and the tip of the prosthesis may show increased activity for up to 2 yr. Infection on bone scan generally shows a more diffuse pattern of abnormality along the prosthetic shaft, and it is usually positive on the two early phases of the scan. False-positive scans may occur in up to 40% and false-negative findings in 5–10% of cases. A gallium scan would suggest osteomyelitis by a focal uptake. However, any inflammatory bone process may cause increased uptake. White blood cell scans are more specific for making a definitive diagnosis of infection but may be less sensitive *(9)*.

The erythrocyte sedimentation rate (ESR) may be elevated in greater than 85% of the patients with infection. If 30–35 mm/h is used as the threshold for infection, then the sensitivity rate will range from 61–88%. With ESR below 30 mm/h, those infections are unlikely and the specificity rate will range from 96–100%. However, ESRs may not accurately diagnosis those patients with an infection in the early postoperative period *(8)*. The C-reactive protein (CRP) is an acute phase protein that can be used to follow the course of acute infections. It rises and falls faster than the ESR. If 10 mg of CRP are used as the threshold for a total hip infection, the specificity and sensitivity for CRP are both about 90%. The CRP should return to normal in about 2–3 wk after hip replacement. The fluid obtained for culture usually has visible organisms on Gram stain in about 30% of cases, and pathogens are recovered by culture in about 85–98% of cases, depending on whether or not the patient had previously received antibiotics. The criteria for infection on histology or frozen section is that there must be 5–10 white blood cells per high-powered field. The sensitivity is about 85% using this criteria, and the specificity is 99% when 10 white blood cells per high powered field are noted. Staphylococci are isolated from about 50% percent of patients with infected prosthetic joints with *S. aureus* as the most common pathogen in most series, particularly if hematogenous infections are included. In a series of elderly patients only, coagulase-negative staphylococci and *S. aureus* were isolated in nearly equal frequency; enterococci were isolated as the third most common isolate *(7)*. Gram-negative bacteria, including *Pseudomonas*, can occasionally be present. Other fastidious bacteria or mycobacteria can be present and cause indolent infections *(8)*.

3.4. Treatment

To eradicate infection, usually removable of the prosthesis is required *(7,8)*. This may be difficult, as elderly patients are often poor surgical candidates for repeated prosthetic joint procedures. Debridement and retaining of the components can have a high success rate (>50%) in well selected patients, i.e., those in whom the interval between onset of symptoms and surgical intervention is short (2–5 d) *(10)*. Following debridement, antibiotics should be continued for at least 6 wk. If a one-stage reimplantation procedure is performed, it is essential that all foreign material be removed. Many surgeons choose to implant the femoral component with antibiotic-laden cement *(11)*. Prolonged antibiotic therapy should be considered if one-stage procedures are chosen. More often, a two-stage procedure, in which a new prosthesis is implanted after 4–6 wk of antibiotics are given, is chosen *(8)*. Success rates vary from 70–100% for hips, and 85–90% for knees. If a virulent organism such as a Gram-negative bacilli has been isolated, some clinicians advise the delay of up to 1 yr before implanting a new hip prosthesis. As stated earlier, the original prosthesis can be salvaged by debridement and intensive antibiotic therapy in select cases *(8,10,12)*. This approach is successful only when the infection has been diagnosed early (<2 wk), the prosthesis remains securely fixed, and the bone–cement interface is not disrupted by infection.

When removal of an infected prosthesis is not possible, chronic suppressive oral antibiotic therapy has occasionally been successful (8,12). The use of oral agents such as ciprofloxacin combined with rifampin has recently been shown to be beneficial in some cases of prosthetic joint infection (13). The functional outcomes for elderly patients are poor with the majority unable to walk without assistance (7), and 40% may show persistent or recurrent infection (14).

3.5. Prevention

The use of antibiotic prophylaxis for high-risk procedures for patients who have prosthetic joint infections is somewhat controversial. For patients undergoing dental procedures, perhaps prophylaxis might be beneficial for patients who are immuno-compromised or immunosuppressed *(15)*. Other patients who could possibly benefit are patients who have diabetes mellitus, those with a history of a previous prosthetic joint infection, hemophiliac patients, and perhaps patients during the first 2 yr follow-ing joint placement *(16)*. Recommendations regarding dental prophylaxis for those patients with prosthetic joints can be found on the Internet at http://www.ninthdistrict.org/pro-01.html. Preoperative antibiotics are generally given prior to the placement of a prosthetic joint. Usually a first-generation cephalosporin is chosen. The value of "ultra-clean" rooms in decreasing infections is somewhat controversial.

4. PROSTHETIC HEART VALVES

4.1. Epidemiology and Microbiology

The accumulative rate of prosthetic valve endocarditis (PVE) is 1.5–3% within 1 yr after valve surgery. This increases to 5.7% after 5 yr *(17)*. Coagulase-negative staphylo-cocci are the predominant agent of PVE during the initial 2 mo of surgery and, in fact, are the most common organisms throughout the first year after a valve replacement. Thereafter, viridans streptococci, enterococci, *S. aureus*, and fastidious Gram-negative coccobacilli increase in prevalence. Gram-negative bacilli and fungal etiologies of pros-thetic valve endocarditis are most common in the initial 2 mo after surgery.

4.2. Clinical Manifestation

The clinical features of PVE are similar to those of native valve endocarditis except that new murmurs are more frequent among those infected with prosthetic valves. Patients with PVE may develop congestive heart failure and systemic emboli. These symptoms are common in the general elderly population but should alert the clinician to the possibility of PVE. Any prolonged fever in a patient with a prosthetic valve should be viewed as possible PVE *(17,18)*. Elderly patients often have less pronounced clinical symptoms than younger patients.

4.3. Diagnosis and Microbiology

The new Duke criteria enable the clinician to make the diagnosis of infective endo-carditis more accurately *(19)*. Definite diagnosis of infective endocarditis can be made by pathological criteria. (See chapter, "Infective Endocarditis," Tables 2 and 3.)

The use of transesophageal echocardiograms (TEE) has greatly improved the diag-nosis of both native valve and prosthetic valve endocarditis. Kemp and colleagues

Table 3
Indications for Transesophageal Echocardiography
for Suspected Infective Endocarditis

Prosthetic cardiac valves
Left-sided infective endocarditis (IE)
S. aureus IE
Fungal IE
Previous IE
Prolonged clinical symptoms (3 mo) consistent with IE
Cyanotic congenital heart disease
Patients with systemic to pulmonary shunts
Poor clinical response to antimicrobial therapy for IE

reviewed the use of TEE in diagnosing PVE and found a range of sensitivity from 77–100%, and a negative predictive value of 90% *(20)*. Table 3 illustrates conditions for which TEE might be especially helpful diagnostically.

4.4. Treatment

Treatment for PVE often involves prolonged therapy (Table 4) *(17,21)*. In elderly patients who are taking coumadin, there may be drug interactions with rifampin. Also, nephrotoxicity with gentamicin is increased in the elderly and in patients taking concurrent nephrotoxins. Guidelines for therapy for infective endocarditis may be found on the Internet at http://www.americanheart.org. As many as 65% of patients with PVE may be candidates for surgical valve replacement *(22,23)*. The need for cardiac surgery is increased in patients who have moderate to severe heart failure due to dysfunction of the prosthesis. Uncontrolled bacteremia, fever persisting for more than 10 d during appropriate antibiotic therapy, recurrent arterial emboli, and relapse after appropriate antimicrobial therapy are other indications for surgery. In addition, infections caused by fungi, *S. aureus* and Gram-negative bacteria often require surgical intervention.

4.5. Prevention

Prosthetic valves may become infected because of bacteremia resulting from invasive procedures *(24)*. Elderly patients often have dental, gastrointestinal (GI), or genitourinary (GU) procedures that may cause a transient bacteremia. Table 5 reviews the dental procedures for which endocarditis prophylaxis including PVE is recommended. The indications for endocarditis prophylaxis for GI procedures are noted in Table 6 and the indications for PVE prophylaxis for GU (and respiratory) procedures are noted in Table 7. Note that prophylaxis is considered "optional" for some procedures but might be useful for high-risk patients such as those with prosthetic valves, a previous history of infective endocarditis, cyanotic congenital heart disease, ventricular septal defect, aortic valve disease, and mitral regurgitation. Moderate-risk cardiac conditions include mitral valve prolapse with regurgitation, tricuspid valve disease, mitral stenosis, and degenerative valve disease of the elderly. The regimens used for prophylaxis for patient allergic to penicillin may include clindamycin or azithromycin. (See chapter "Infective Endocarditis," Tables 5–7 [this chapter] for specific antibiotic regimens for oral and respiratory tract, and gastrointestinal and genitourinary tracts procedures, respectively).

Table 4
Prosthetic Valve Endocarditis Treatment

Streptococci
 Highly penicillin-susceptible viridans streptococci or *S. bovis* (MIC ≤ 0.1 μg/mL)
  In patients whose infection involves prosthetic valves or other prosthetic materials,
  a 6-wk regimen of penicillins recommended together with gentamicin for at least
  the first 2 wk.

Streptococci with an MIC >0.1 μg/mL
 It may be desirable to administer the aminoglycoside for more than 2 wk (4–6 wk).
  Vancomycin can be used in penicillin allergic patients

Enterococci and nutritionally variant streptococci
 Ampicillin or vancomycin plus gentamicin or streptomycin for 6–8 wk.

Methicillin-sensitive *S. aureus*
 Nafcillin (or a first-generation cephalosporin or vancomycin if allergic) plus rifampin
  for 6 wk plus gentamicin for 2 wk. Rifampin plays a unique role in the eradication
  of staphylococcal infection involving prosthetic material; combination therapy
  is essential to prevent emergence of rifampin resistance

Methicillin-resistant *S. aureus*
 Vancomycin plus rifampin for 6 wk plus gentamicin for 2 wk

Coagulase-negative staphylococci
 Vancomycin plus rifampin for 6 wk plus gentamicin for 2 wk

HACEK
 Third-generation cephalosporin for 6 wk
 Ampicillin plus gentamicin for 6 wk

For culture-negative or empiric treatment
 Vancomycin plus gentamicin plus ceftriaxone or ampicillin-sulbactam plus gentamicin

---

MIC, minimum inhibitory concentration; HACEK, *Haemophilus* spp., *Actinobacillus actinomycetam-comitans, Cardiobacterium hominis, Eikenella* spp., *Kingella kingae.*

5. VASCULAR GRAFT INFECTIONS

5.1. Epidemiology and Microbiology

The frequency of graft infections ranges from 1–5%. The majority of infections are thought to occur at the time of implantation. Staphylococci are the most common microorganism. Early infections are usually caused by *S. aureus*, whereas later infections are usually caused by coagulase-negative staphylococci. Rarely, Gram-negative bacilli may also cause infections of grafts.

5.2. Clinical Manifestations and Diagnostic Tests

Graft infections, especially those involving coagulase-negative staphylococci, may not become evident for months to years. The majority of graft infections present as localized wound infections. Blood cultures are usually positive in less than 50% of patients. Graft thrombosis may suggest a graft infection. Graft infection may also manifest itself as an aortoenteric fistula with gastrointestinal bleeding. Needle aspiration of

Table 5
Endocarditis Prophylaxis and Dental Procedures

Endocarditis prophylaxis recommended[a]
    Dental extractions
    Periodontal procedures including surgery, scaling and root planing, probing,
       and recall maintenance
    Dental implant placement and reimplantation of avulsed teeth
    Endodontic (root canal) instrumentation or surgery only beyond the apex
    Subgingival placement of antibiotic fibers or strips
    Initial placement of orthodontic bands but not brackets
    Intraligamentary local anesthetic injections
    Prophylactic cleaning of teeth or implants where bleeding is anticipated

Not recommended
    Restorative dentistry[b] (operative and prosthodontic) with or without retraction cord[c]
    Local anesthetic injections (nonintraligamentary)
    Intracanal endodontic treatment; post placement and buildup
    Placement of rubber dams
    Postoperative suture removal
    Placement of removable prosthodontic or orthodontic appliances
    Taking oral impressions
    Fluoride treatments
    Orthodontic appliance adjustment
    Shedding of primary teeth

[a]Prophylaxis is recommended for patients with high- and moderate-risk cardiac conditions (*see* text for definitions).
[b]This includes restoration of decayed teeth (filling cavities) and replacement of missing teeth.
[c]Clinical judgment may indicate antibiotic use in selected circumstances that may create significant bleeding.

Table 6
Endocarditis Prophylaxis and Gastrointestinal Procedures

Indicated[a]
    Sclerotherapy for esophageal varices
    Esophageal stricture dilation
    Endoscopic retrograde cholangiography with biliary obstruction
    Biliary tract surgery
    Surgical operations that involve intestinal mucosa

Not indicated
    Transesophageal echocardiography
    Endoscopy with or without gastrointestinal biopsy (prophylaxis is optional
       for high-risk patients such as prosthetic valves)

[a]For moderate- to high-risk cardiac conditions (see text for definitions).

para graft collections under ultrasonographic or CT guidance can provide additional information. CT scans or white blood cell scans may also be helpful in diagnosing graft infections.

Table 7
Prosthetic Valve Endocarditis Prophylaxis and Respiratory
and Genitourinary Procedures

Respiratory
    Indicated[a]
        Tonsillectomy and/or adenoidectomy
        Surgical operations that involve respiratory mucosa
        Bronchoscopy with a rigid bronchoscope
    Not indicated
        Endotracheal intubation
        Bronchoscopy with a flexile bronchoscope, with or without biopsy[b]
        Tympanostomy tube insertion

Genitourinary
    Indicated[a]
        Prostatic surgery
        Cystoscopy
        Urethral dilation
    Not indicated
        Vaginal hysterectomy[b]
        Vaginal delivery[b]
        Cesarean section
        In uninfected tissue
        Urethral catheterization
        Uterine dilation and curettage
        Sterilization procedures
        Insertion or removal of intrauterine devices

[a]Recommended for moderate- to high-risk cardiac conditions.
[b]Prophylaxis is optional for high-risk conditions (*see* text for definitions).

5.3. Treatment

For management of graft infections, the infected prosthetic needs to be removed and then revascularization considered after an appropriate course of antibiotics *(25,26)*. Generally, patients with graft infections are treated with a minimum of 6 wk of parenteral therapy; depending on the microorganisms, a longer course of antibiotics may be required. If the newly implanted graft appears to have been contaminated at the anastomotic site or the if the arterial stump was closed proximal to the infected site, the clinician may need to consider lengthy, perhaps lifelong, suppressive regimens of oral antibiotics. Generally, surgical management includes excision of the affected graft followed by revascularization *(25)*. An extra-anatomic bypass (EAB) such as an axillary–femoral artery conduit is often employed. Occasionally, *in situ* replacement of the infected graft is attempted. Mortality in the course of reconstructive efforts can be 25% or greater.

5.4. Prevention

For prevention of infection of a vascular graft, regimens similar to infective endocarditis prophylaxis could be considered. However, data are inadequate at this time to make firm recommendations. Nevertheless, clinicians may consider using pro-phylaxis especially during the first 4 mo postoperatively when the graft would be more susceptible to bacteremic seeding *(24)*.

6. PACEMAKER INFECTIONS

6.1. Epidemiology and Clinical Relevance

A pacemaker consists of essentially two components. The pulse generator is the power source that is used to deliver the electrical stimulus. This is linked to a pacing electrode, either an endocardial or epicardial lead. Elderly patients seem to be especially prone to pacemaker infections. The average age of patients with pacemaker endocardi-tis is 72 yr.

Pacemaker infections may appear as either a localized infection and/or abscess in the pulse–generator pocket *(27)*. There may be erosion of the skin in the pacing system with subsequent infection. There may be fever with positive blood cultures in the patient who has a pacemaker and no obvious focus of infection. Generally, pulse–generator pocket infections result from contamination at the time of implantation of the pace-maker. Those infections involving the conducting system may occur secondary to bacteremic spread. There is an approximate prevalence of 0.13–12% of pacemaker infections reported in the literature *(27)*. It has been demonstrated that endothelialization of the leads become evident at 6–8 wk.

6.2. Clinical Manifestations and Microbiology

The clinical manifestations of pacemaker infections are those related complications such as erosion of the pulse–generator pocket, sepsis, pericarditis, or even mediastini-tis *(27)*. Generally, bacteremia from a pacemaker infection is from infection of the pacer pocket or related to extension of infection along the wire into the vascular sys-tem. Hematogenous colonization of the pacemaker conducting system resulting from bacteremia from a distant source has been documented but is fortunately rare. Both *S. aureus* and coagulase-negative staphylococci account for greater than 75% of pacemaker infections. Rarely, Gram-negative bacilli and fungi may be involved as well *(27)*.

6.3. Treatment

The management of the pacemaker infection varies according to the clinical sce-nario *(28)*. Most patients require at least 4 wk of antibiotic therapy. If the infectious process has been clearly demonstrated to ride in the pulse–generator pocket only, the generator should be removed and another one implanted at a distant site. The situation becomes more complicated if the conducting system or leads are infected. It is gener-ally necessary to try to remove the entire pacemaker system at that point. This may be somewhat difficult in elderly patients who may have a limited life expectancy and may have a very high operative risk. The failure to remove an infected lead can result in mortality as high as 65%. If the lead is retained after infection of the pacemaker wire, there can be complications in as high as 50% of patients. The various techniques for lead extraction have been described in detail in the literature *(27)*. Under some circum-stances, cardiopulmonary bypass must be used to remove the infected material *(28)*.

6.4. Prevention

There have been no well-controlled studies that allow firm conclusions regarding prevention of infection during pacemaker replacement or implantation. In general, it is felt that there is no need for infective endocarditis prophylaxis in patients with pacemakers.

REFERENCES

1. Chuard, C., Vaudaux, P. E., Proctor, R. A. et al. (1997) Decreased susceptibility to antibiotic killing of a stable small colony variant of *Staphylococcus aureus* in fluid phase and on fibronectin-coated surfaces. *J. Antimicrob. Chemother.* **39(5),** 603–608.
2. Gardner, P., Leipzig, T. J., and Sadigh, M. (1988) Infections of mechanical cerebrospinal fluid shunts. *Curr. Clin. Top. Infect. Dis.* **9,**185–214.
3. Gardner, P., Leipzig, T., and Phillips, P. (1985) Infections of central nervous system shunts. *Med. Clin. North Am.* **69(2),** 297–314.
4. Keane, W. F., Alexander, S. R., Bailie, G. R., et al. (1996) Peritoneal dialysis-related peritonitis treatment recommendations: 1996 update. *Perit. Dial. Int.* **16(6),** 557–573.
5. Tzamaloukas, A. H. (1996) Peritonitis in peritoneal dialysis patients: an overview. *Adv. Ren. Replace. Ther.* **3(3),** 232–236.
6. Stecklberg, J. M. and Osmon, D. R. (1994) Prosthetic joint infections, in *Infections Associated With Indwelling Medical Devices* (Bisno, A. L. and Waldvogel, F. A., eds.), 2nd ed., American Society for Microbiology, Washington, DC, pp. 259–290.
7. Powers, K. A., Terpenning, M. S., Voice, R. A., et al. (1990) Prosthetic joint infections in the elderly. *Am. J. Med.* 88, 5-9N–5-13N.
8. Gillespie, W. J. (1997) Prevention and management of infection after total joint replacement. *Clin. Infect. Dis.* **25(6),** 1310–1317.
9. Nijhof, M. W., Oyen, W. J., van Kampen, A., et al. (1997) Hip and knee arthroplasty infection. In-111-IgG scintigraphy in 102 cases. *Acta. Orthop. Scand.* **68(4),** 332–336.
10. Tattevin, P., Cremieux, A.-C., Pottier, P., et al. (1999) Prosthetic joint infection: when can prosthesis salvage be considered? *Clin. Infect. Dis.* **29,** 292–295.
11. Wininger, D. A. and Fass, R. J. (1996) Antibiotic-impregnated cement and beads for orthopedic infections. *Antimicrob. Agents Chemother.* **40(12),** 2675–2679.
12. Segreti, J., Nelson, J. A., and Trenholme, G. M. (1998) Prolonged suppressive antibiotic therapy for infected orthopedic prostheses. *Clin. Infect. Dis.* **27(4),** 711–713.
13. Zimmerli, W., Widmer, A. F., Blatter, M., et al. (1998) Role of rifampin for treatment of orthopedic implant-related staphylococcal infections: a randomized controlled trial. Foreign-Body Infection (FBI) Study Group. *JAMA* **279(19),** 1537–1541.
14. Norman, D. C. and Yoshikawa T. T. (1994) Infections of the bone, joint, and bursa. *Clin. Geriatr. Med.* **10(4),** 703–718.
15. American Dental Association; American Academy of Orthopaedic Surgeons. (1997) Advisory statement. Antibiotic prophylaxis for dental patients with total joint replacements. *J. Am. Dent. Assoc.* **128(7),** 1004–1008.
16. Berbari, E. F., Hanssen, A. D., Duffy, M. C., et al. (1998) Risk factors for prosthetic joint infection: case-control study. *Clin. Infect. Dis.* **27(5),** 1247–1254.
17. Karchmer, A. W. and Gibbons, G. W. (1994) Infections of prosthetic heart valves and vascular grafts, in *Infections Associated With Indwelling Medical Devices*, 2nd ed. (Bisno, A. L. and Waldvogel, F. A., eds.), American Society for Microbiology, Washington, DC, pp. 213–249.
18. Bayer, A. S. (1993) Infective endocarditis. *Clin. Infect. Dis.* **17,** 313–320.
19. Durack, D. T., Lukes, A. S., and Bright, D. K. (1994) New criteria for diagnosis of infective endocarditis: utilization of specific echocardiographic findings: Duke Endocarditis Service. *Am. J. Med.* **96,** 200–209.

20. Kemp, W. E., Jr., Citrin, B., and Byrd, B. F., III (1999) Echocardiography in infective endocarditis. *South. Med. J.* **92,** 744–754.

21. Wilson, W. R., Karchmer, A. W., Dajani, A. S., et al. (1995) Antibiotic treatment of adults with infective endocarditis due to streptococci, enterococci, staphylococci, and HACEK microorganisms: American Heart Association. *JAMA* **274,** 1706–1713.

22. Moon, M. R., Stinson, E. B., and Miller, D. C. (1997) Surgical treatment of endocarditis. *Prog. Cardiovasc. Dis.* **40,** 239–264.

23. Vlessis, A. A., Hovaguimian, H., Jaggers, J., et al. (1996) Infective endocarditis: ten-year review of medical and surgical therapy. *Ann. Thorac. Surg.* **61,** 1217–1222.

24. Dajani, A. S., Taubert, K. A., Wilson, W., et al. (1997) Prevention of bacterial endocarditis: recommendations by the American Heart Association. *JAMA* **277,** 1794–1801.

25. Yeager, R. A. and Porter, J. M. (1996) The case against the conservative nonresectional management of infected prosthetic grafts. *Adv. Surg.* **29,** 33–39.

26. Earnshaw, J. J. (1996) Conservative surgery for aortic graft infection. *Cardiovasc. Surg.* **4(5),** 570–572.

27. Waldvogel, F. (1994) Pacemaker infections, in *Infections Associated With Indwelling Medical Devices*, 2nd ed. (Bisno, A. L. and Waldvogel, F. A., eds.), American Society for Microbiology, Washington, DC, pp. 251–258.

28. Vogt, P. R., Sagdic, K., Lachat, M., et al. (1996) Surgical management of infected permanent transvenous pacemaker systems: ten year experience. *J. Card. Surg.* **11(3),** 180–186.

18
Fungal Infections

Carol A. Kauffman

1. INTRODUCTION

Serious fungal infections can be separated into the opportunistic mycoses, including candidiasis, cryptococcosis, aspergillosis, and mucormycosis (zygomycosis), and the endemic mycoses, comprised of histoplasmosis, blastomycosis, and coccidioidomycosis. The fungal infections represented in these broad groups differ with respect to the characteristics of the organisms causing infection, their epidemiology, the clinical manifestations, the approach to diagnosis, and the principles guiding therapy.

Not only are there differences in the organisms in these two groups, but host defense mechanisms in response to these infections differ. In regard to the opportunistic mycoses, serious infection with these ubiquitous organisms is rare except in immunocompromised hosts. In contrast, the endemic mycoses are true pathogens in that they cause disease in any host, healthy or compromised. The extent of infection with these fungi, however, is determined in part by the host's response.

2. OPPORTUNISTIC FUNGAL INFECTIONS

2.1. Epidemiology and Clinical Relevance

Opportunistic fungal infections have increased dramatically in recent years as the number of immunocompromised patients has risen. In the last decade, the elderly appear to be at increasing risk for infections with the opportunistic fungi. There are several reasons for this enhanced risk. First, with increasing realization that older adults with cancer should not be excluded because of age from intensive chemotherapeutic treatment regimens, there are more immunosuppressed older cancer patients. Second, solid organ transplantation is now more common in patients over the age of 60, as evidence for the efficacy and safety of transplantation in this population has accrued. Third, immunosuppressive regimens are now routine in the management of rheumatologic and dermatologic conditions often found in older adults. Fourth, and possibly the most important risk factor for older adults, is the increasing role of treatment in intensive care units with the use of life-support systems, catheters, and broad-spectrum antibiotics.

From: *Infectious Disease in the Aging*
Edited by: Thomas T. Yoshikawa and Dean C. Norman
© Humana Press Inc., Totowa, NJ

2.1.1. Candidiasis

The increase in opportunistic infections in elderly patients is primarily due to infections with *Candida* species. The spectrum of disease varies from localized infections (e.g., oropharyngeal candidiasis) to candidemia and disseminated infection.

Factors that predispose older patients to the development of oropharyngeal candidiasis include xerostomia, broad-spectrum antibiotics, inhaled corticosteroids, and dentures *(1,2)*. Age alone does not appear to be an independent risk factor for the development of oropharyngeal candidiasis. In older adults, the presence of systemic diseases and a multiplicity of medications frequently lead to xerostomia, which then enhances *Candida* colonization of the mucosa *(1)*. Denture stomatitis due to *Candida* species is very common. Patients who do not remove their dentures at night and those who have poor oral hygiene are more likely to have this manifestation of candidiasis.

In contrast to other *Candida* infections, *Candida* vulvovaginitis is unusual in older women *(3)*. Without estrogen stimulation, the vaginal epithelium becomes thin and atrophic, glycogen production decreases, vaginal pH rises, and colonization by *Candida* decreases. However, with the increasing use of estrogen replacement therapy to prevent osteoporosis, heart disease, and menopausal vasomotor symptoms, *Candida* vulvovaginitis may emerge as a more common problem in older women.

A recently reported multicenter surveillance study noted that the mean age of patients with candiduria was 64.5 yr, and patients had one or more of the following risk factors: diabetes mellitus, obstructive uropathy or neurogenic bladder, indwelling urinary catheters, and prior antibiotic therapy *(4)*.

Candida spp. are now the fourth most common cause of nosocomial bloodstream infections. Several studies have found that those over 60 constitute the majority of patients with candidemia and also have the highest mortality rates *(5,6)*. *C. albicans* is the species most commonly found causing candidemia, but other species, especially *C. glabrata*, appear to be increasing. Elderly patients at the highest risk are those in an intensive care unit, who are on broad-spectrum antibiotics, have an indwelling central venous catheter in place, are receiving total parental nutrition, and have had a surgical procedure on the gastrointestinal (GI) tract.

2.1.2. Cryptococcosis

Cryptococcosis is increased modestly in older persons. Approximately 25% of non-acquired immunodeficiency syndrome (AIDS) patients with cryptococcal meningitis are over age 60. The usual underlying conditions are lymphoma, organ transplantation, corticosteroids or cytotoxic drugs, and cirrhosis. However, from 25–30% of patients have no overt underlying immunosuppressive disease, and many of these patients are elderly. Mortality appears to be increased in older patients who have cryptococcal meningitis *(7)*.

2.1.3. Aspergillosis

There are a huge number of *Aspergillus* species that are ubiquitous in the environment; however, very few cause infection in humans. The most common pathogenic species are *A. fumigatus* and *A. flavus*. Infection ensues when conidia (spores) are inhaled into the alveoli or upper respiratory tract of a susceptible host. *Aspergillus* is common enough in the environment that a discrete point source leading to exposure is not obvious for most patients. However, nosocomial *Aspergillus* infections are not uncommon and are usually traced to hospital construction. A wide spectrum of infections can occur, depending almost entirely on the immune response of the host. Although less common than candidiasis, *Aspergillus* infections are usually life threatening in immunosuppressed patients. Several forms, specifically chronic necrotizing pulmonary aspergillosis and sino-orbital infection, are seen more often in older adults *(8,9)*.

2.1.4. Mucormycosis

Mucormycosis or zygomycosis, more often caused by *Rhizopus* than *Mucor* species, is the least common of the major opportunistic fungal infections. Age, per se, is not a risk factor; however, underlying diseases, such as diabetes mellitus, that are associated with increasing age, increase the risk for mucormycosis *(10)*. Other risk factors include hematologic malignancies with neutropenia and chelation therapy given for iron overload, as found in older patients with myelodysplasia *(11)*.

2.2. Clinical Manifestations

2.2.1. Candidiasis

White plaques on the buccal, palatal, or oropharyngeal mucosa that can easily be removed are typical of oropharyngeal candidiasis. Angular cheilitis and diffuse erythema, often present beneath upper dentures, are also manifestations of oropharyngeal candidiasis. Because typical plaques are absent, the diagnosis may be easily overlooked *(2)*.

Candida vaginitis usually presents with pruritus and vaginal discharge that may range from "cottage cheese-like" to thin and watery. When cheesy material is absent, *Candida* vulvovaginitis must be differentiated from atrophic vaginitis.

Most patients with candiduria are asymptomatic, and most are probably merely colonized *(4)*. Fewer than 5% of patients have dysuria and frequency, and even fewer have symptoms of upper tract infection. Rarely, obstructive symptoms and renal failure have been noted secondary to fungus balls composed of masses of fungi.

The manifestations of systemic infection with *Candida* are quite varied (*see* Table 1). After entering the bloodstream, either from an intravenous catheter or the GI tract, the organism disseminates widely causing microabscesses in many organs, including eye, kidney, liver, spleen, myocardium, and brain. Patients with candidemia usually have fever and chills, and appear "toxic." However, in some patients, the symptoms of candidemia are more subtle, and the patient presents weeks later with decreased vision secondary to *Candida* endophthalmitis or back pain secondary to *Candida* osteomyelitis. Skin lesions occurring during the course of candidemia are usually tiny pustular lesions on an erythematous base (*see* Fig. 1).

2.2.2. Cryptococcosis

Although the major manifestation of infection with *C. neoformans* is meningitis, the pathogenesis of infection begins with inhalation of the organism from the environment and subsequent pulmonary infection. The chest radiograph may show nodular infiltrates, a pleural-based mass, cavitary lesions, or diffuse infiltrates *(12)* (*see* Fig. 2). However, most often, the pulmonary infection is asymptomatic, and clinical manifestations of cryptococcosis occur only after the organism has spread to the central nervous system. Elderly patients may not have the usual symptoms of fever, headache, and cranial nerve palsies but instead may present solely with confusion without fever, nuchal rigidity, or focal neurologic findings (*see* Table 1).

Table 1
Systemic Opportunistic Fungal Infections in Older Adults

Fungal infection	Risk factors	Usual clinical manifestations
Candidiasis	Neutropenia, hematologic malignancy, corticosteroids, transplant; ICU, antibiotics, IV catheters, TPN, GI surgical procedure	Fever, pustular skin rash, hypotension; later may have bone pain, visual loss, eye pain
Cryptococcosis	Lymphoma, transplant, cirrhosis, corticosteroids; ~25% have no risk factor identified	Headache, fever, cranial nerve palsy, confusion; cough, dyspnea, sputum production
Aspergillosis	Neutropenia, hematologic malignancy, corticosteroids, transplant	Fever, pleuritic chest pain, cough, hemoptysis; eye/sinus pain, proptosis. ophthalmoplegia, visual loss
Mucormycosis	Diabetes mellitus with ketoacidosis, hematologic malignancy, neutropenia, deferoxamine chelation therapy	Eye/sinus pain, necrotic eschar (palate, nares) cavernous sinus thrombosis; fever, pleuritic chest pain, cough, hemoptysis

ICU, intensive care unit; IV, intravenous; TPN, total parenteral nutrition; GI, gastrointestinal.

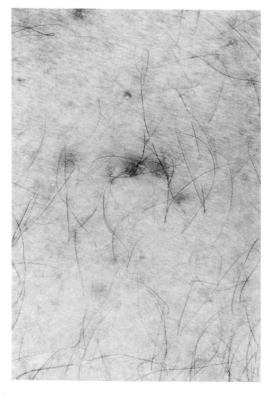

Fig. 1. Typical skin lesions seen in patients with disseminated candidiasis.

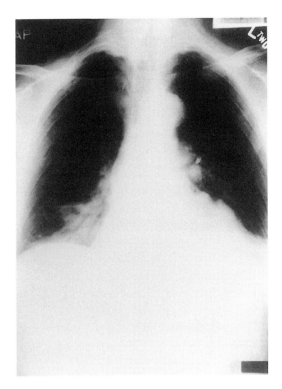

Fig. 2. Right lower lobe infiltrate due to cryptococcosis in a 67-yr-old man who was on corticosteroids and who had confusion, headache, and fever. Sputum and cerebrospinal fluid yielded *C. neoformans.*

2.2.3. Aspergillosis

Aspergillus invasion of the upper respiratory tract leads to sinusitis and may proceed to subsequent invasion of the orbit. In patients with neutropenia, the acute onset of pain, erythema, fever, serosanguinous drainage, and proptosis is seen. In older patients who are not immunosuppressed, but who may have been on corticosteroids or are diabetic, *Aspergillus* causes subacute infection with pain, proptosis, ophthalmoplegia, and loss of vision due to invasion of the apex of the orbit *(8)*. Most patients are thought to have a retro-orbital tumor until biopsy reveals hyphae and inflammatory debris *(13)*.

Acute pulmonary aspergillosis in immunosuppressed patients presents with fever, pleuritic chest pain, hemoptysis, and dyspnea (*see* Table 1). Chronic necrotizing pulmonary aspergillosis, occurring mostly in middle-aged to elderly men with chronic obstructive pulmonary disease, is a subacute illness. Low-dose corticosteroids and broad-spectrum antibiotics are predisposing factors. Patients have fever, cough, purulent sputum, weight loss, and pleuritic chest pain. Multilobar involvment is common, cavity formation is usual, and extension to the pleura is frequent (*see* Fig. 3). Progressive pneumonia with death is the rule unless the diagnosis is made and appropriate therapy given.

2.2.4. Mucormycosis

Patients with mucormycosis are quite ill. Diabetics with acidosis most often have the rhinocerebral form. A black eschar is seen on the palate or around the orbit, and serosanguinous material can be found in the sinuses (*see* Table 1). Orbital invasion

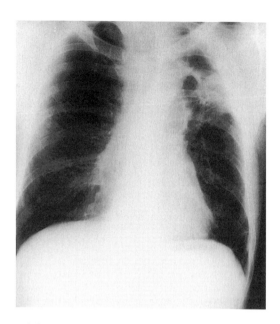

Fig. 3. Chronic necrotizing pulmonary aspergillosis in a middle-aged man with no known risk factors other than chronic obstructive pulmonary disease.

progresses rapidly to cavernous sinus thrombosis, and cerebral infarction often ensues *(10)*. In patients with pulmonary mucormycosis, the chest radiograph shows wedge-shaped or nodular infiltrates, which tend to cavitate *(11)* (*see* Fig. 4). Localized cutaneous and GI forms occur and generally carry a better prognosis than the rhinocerebral or pulmonary forms of infection.

2.3. Diagnostic Tests

Diagnosis of systemic opportunistic fungal infection must be made promptly because of the life-threatening nature of these infections. Growth of opportunistic fungi is rarely difficult; cultures are usually positive within a few days. The major complicating issue is that organisms as ubiquitous in the environment as *Aspergillus* or *Rhizopus* can easily contaminate specimens. Therefore, growth in culture must be carefully assessed as to whether it truly reflects infection. Confounding the diagnosis of candidiasis is the fact that *Candida* are normal flora in the GI and genitourinary (GU) tracts and on skin, and thus, growth from samples taken from nonsterile body sites often means only colonization. However, growth of *Candida* from blood or normally sterile body fluids is obviously significant. In contrast to the other opportunists, *C. neoformans* is neither common in the environment nor part of the normal flora, and thus growth of this organism in culture almost always reflects infection.

Especially in immunocompromised patients who are acutely ill, histopathologic demonstration of fungi in tissues is the most important diagnostic tool. For cryptococcosis, examination of cerebrospinal fluid (CSF) with an India ink preparation that highlights the large capsule of *C. neoformans* is a quick and reliable test.

Antibody and antigen assays for aspergillosis and candidiasis have not yet proved to be clinically useful. The only rapid antigen test with excellent sensitivity and specificity is the latex agglutination test for cryptococcal polysaccharide antigen.

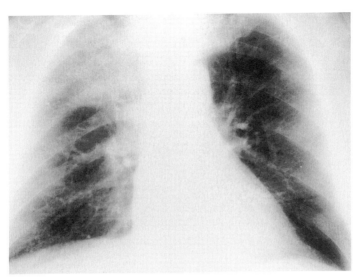

Fig. 4. Right upper lobe mucormycosis in an elderly man who had myelodysplasia leading to dependence on transfusions and treatment with deferoxamine chelation.

2.4. Treatment

2.4.1. Candidiasis

Treatment of oropharyngeal candidiasis with a topical agent, such as clotrimazole troches, is appropriate first-line therapy. Fluconazole should be reserved for patients with severe disease or denture stomatitis that can be particularly vexing to treat *(14)*.

Vaginal candidiasis is easily treated with topical antifungal agents, such as miconazole or clotrimazole creams. However, fluconazole, 150 mg orally as a single dose, is an attractive alternative, especially for those patients who have underlying illnesses that make topical therapy difficult to use *(3)*.

Candiduria often disappears with removal of the predisposing factors, especially indwelling urethral catheters and antimicrobial agents *(4)*. When candiduria is persistent and thought to be causing symptoms, the most appropriate treatment is fluconazole, 200 mg daily for 5–7 d *(15)*. Amphotericin B bladder irrigation is useful only for bladder involvement and requires the placement of a urethral catheter.

Amphotericin B has been the mainstay of treatment for serious *Candida* infections but has significant toxicity *(16)*. Nephrotoxicity occurs in most patients receiving amphotericin B but is especially difficult in elderly individuals with pre-existing renal insufficiency. Nephrotoxicity can be minimized by salt and water loading prior to infusion, but this may not be feasible in elderly individuals with heart disease. Immediate reactions that accompany amphotericin B infusion—fever, chills, hypotension, and nausea—can usually be decreased with pre-infusion medications, allowing continued use of the agent.

Recent studies have shown that candidemia can be treated equally well with either amphotericin B (0.5–0.7 mg/kg/d intravenously) or fluconazole (400 mg/d), an agent that is much less toxic *(17)*. All intravascular lines should be removed or replaced, and treatment should be continued for 2 wk beyond the time of the last positive blood culture.

2.4.2. Cryptococcosis

The most appropriate therapy for cryptococcal meningitis in older adults has not been established by randomized treatment trials, but studies in AIDS patients with cryptococcal meningitis have shown that the best results are obtained when induction therapy is carried out with the combination of amphotericin B (0.7 mg/kg/d) and flucytosine (100 mg/kg/d) for at least 2 wk, followed by consolidation therapy with fluconazole, 400 mg/d for a minimum of 10 wk *(18)*. Initial therapy with fluconazole alone is not adequate for patients with meningitis. In spite of appropriate therapy, symptoms of dementia may not improve in older patients *(7)*.

2.4.3. Aspergillosis

The most appropriate agent for treating invasive aspergillosis is intravenous amphotericin B. In patients with acute infection, amphotericin B should be given at a dosage of 1–1.5 mg/kg/d. Chronic necrotizing pulmonary aspergillosis in patients who are not acutely ill can be treated effectively with itraconazole, 200 mg given twice daily with food. Most patients with sino-orbital aspergillosis should be treated initially with amphotericin B, and then, after the infection has improved, therapy can usually be switched to oral itraconazole.

2.4.4. Mucormycosis

Treatment of mucormycosis involves the correction of the underlying immune defect, aggressive debridement of all necrotic tissue, and antifungal treatment with amphotericin B, 1–1.5 mg/kg/d, to a total amount of at least 2 g. There are no available azole drugs with activity against the *Mucorales*. Even with aggressive surgical debridement and antifungal therapy, mortality is extremely high.

3. ENDEMIC MYCOSES

3.1. Epidemiology and Clinical Relevance

As the population of the United States ages, and as older adults remain in better health for a longer period of time, they travel more extensively and indulge in a variety of different outdoor avocations that are associated with increased risk of infection from endemic mycoses *(19)*. Endemic mycoses are found in soil or vegetation; each has its own ecological niche from which it is aerosolized and subsequently inhaled (*see* Table 2). Older persons may become infected while traveling in an area endemic for a certain fungus, but symptoms may appear only after they return home. Thus, a patient who consults a physician in Minnesota with symptoms related to coccidioidomycosis that was acquired in southern California may be the first patient with this infection ever seen by that physician, and the correct diagnosis may not be made.

Several of the endemic mycoses have the propensity to reactivate as immunity wanes because of increasing age or an intercurrent immunosuppressive condition. This reactivation event might occur in a person who retired to an area of the country outside of the endemic area for a particular fungal infection. Thus, although physicians in the southwestern United States are very familiar with coccidioidomycosis, histoplasmosis or blastomycosis might be overlooked in a patient from Kentucky who has retired to Arizona.

Table 2
Endemic Mycoses in Older Adults

Fungal infection	Geographic distribution	Common clinical syndromes
Histoplasmosis	Ohio and Mississippi river valleys	Acute pneumonia, chronic cavitary pulmonary infection, acute disseminated infection, chronic progressive infection
Blastomycosis	Southeastern, south central, and north central states	Pneumonia, mass-like or cavitary pulmonary lesions, verrucous skin lesions, prostatitis
Coccidioidomycosis	Arizona, southern California, New Mexico, western Texas	Acute pneumonia, cavitary pulmonary lesions, ulcerated skin lesions, lytic bone lesions, meningitis

3.1.1. Histoplasmosis

Histoplasma capsulatum is endemic in the Mississippi and Ohio River valleys. It is estimated that hundreds of thousands of people are infected each year with *H. capsulatum*, but usually the illness is benign with minimal flulike symptoms. Histoplasmosis is the only endemic mycosis in which certain manifestations of the disease, specifically chronic cavitary pulmonary infection and progressive disseminated histoplasmosis, occur predominantly in older individuals *(19)*.

3.1.2. Blastomycosis

Blastomyces dermatitidis, the causative agent of blastomycosis, is found most frequently in the southeastern, south central, and north central United States. Although outbreaks have occurred in groups involved in outdoor activities, most often individual cases occur in patients for whom a specific point source of infection cannot be found. There is no evidence that older individuals are at more risk for developing blastomycosis than are younger persons. However, adult respiratory distress syndrome has been described more often in older individuals than in younger patients with blastomycosis *(7)*.

3.1.3. Coccidioidomycosis

As the exodus of retirees to the southwestern United States continues, first-time exposure to *Coccidioides immitis* has increased in older adults. This organism proliferates in the deserts of Arizona and California that comprise the Lower Sonoran Life Zone, typified by flora, such as the saguaro cactus. The conidia are widely dispersed during windstorms, and thus *C. immitis* is highly contagious.

In the mid-1990s, a major epidemic of coccidioidomycosis occurred in Arizona and southern California. In addition to an increase of cases in the usual endemic areas, the epidemic extended as far west as Los Angeles and other coastal areas of southern California. In the last decade, there has been a shift in the age of patients with symptomatic coccidioidomycosis; the annual incidence rate for coccidioidomycosis is now highest in those ≥65 yr old *(20)*. There also is evidence that older individuals are more likely to develop disseminated coccidioidomycosis, and there is an association with dissemina-

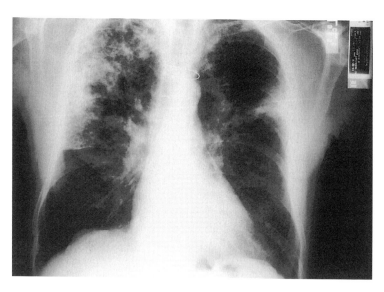

Fig. 5. Chronic cavitary pulmonary histoplasmosis in an elderly man with severe emphysema.

tion and diabetes mellitus, which is more common in older adults. Dark-skinned races are more likely to experience disseminated infection than whites for reasons that are not clear.

3.2. Clinical Manifestations

3.2.1. Histoplasmosis

Two forms of histoplasmosis are seen most often in older adults (*see* Table 2). Chronic cavitary pulmonary histoplasmosis affects mostly middle-aged and elderly men who have emphysema *(19)*. Patients with this form of histoplasmosis have constitutional symptoms of fatigue, weakness, fever, night sweats, and weight loss. Pulmonary symptoms include dyspnea, cough, sputum production, and hemoptysis. The disease is subacute to chronic in its course. Upper lobe cavitary disease is the usual chest radiographic finding (*see* Fig. 5). Progressive scarring, pulmonary insufficiency, and death occur unless treatment is given.

Another form of histoplasmosis that occurs mostly in middle-aged to elderly men is progressive disseminated disease. In this form of histoplasmosis, the host is unable to eradicate the organism from parasitized macrophages, and the disease is fatal if untreated. The clinical manifestations of progressive disseminated histoplasmosis include fever, fatigue, anorexia, and weight loss. Dyspnea and cough are often present, hepatosplenomegaly is usual, and lesions on the buccal mucosa, tongue, palate, or oropharynx are common. The patient may also present with symptoms of Addison's disease because of adrenal destruction. Pancytopenia and increased alkaline phosphatase are frequent, and diffuse pulmonary infiltrates are often present on chest radiograph.

3.2.2. Blastomycosis

Pulmonary blastomycosis in older patients tends to mimic tuberculosis (*see* Table 2). Symptoms include dyspnea, cough, and sputum production, as well as fever, weight

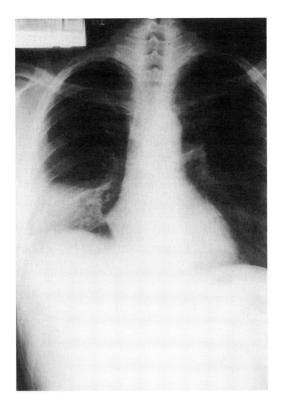

Fig. 6. Pulmonary blastomycosis initially thought to be lung cancer. Bronchoscopy with biopsy showed granulomas and thick-walled budding yeasts typical of *B. dermatitidis*.

loss, and fatigue. When the pulmonary lesions are predominantly nodular or mass-like, the initial diagnosis is often carcinoma of the lung (*see* Fig. 6).

Although blastomycosis begins in the lungs, subsequent dissemination to other organs is common; frequently, the only clinical symptom is the development of one or multiple skin lesions that are usually slowly enlarging, verrucous, and crusting with discrete areas of purulence (*see* Fig. 7). Spread to bone or to the GU tract gives rise to manifestations reflecting involvement of those organs.

3.2.3. Coccidioidomycosis

Coccidioidomycosis may present in many different ways (*see* Table 2). Patients experiencing primary disease usually have a flu-like illness consisting of fever, cough, headache, and fatigue. Chronic pulmonary coccidioidomycosis may give nodular or cavitary lesions, progressive pneumonia, or diffuse miliary infiltrates on chest radiograph (*see* Fig. 8).

The most frequently involved organs with disseminated coccidioidomycosis are skin, bone, GU tract, and meninges. Meningitis, the most feared complication, presents with chronic headache months after the initial infection.

3.3. Diagnostic Methods

Diagnosis of the endemic mycoses can be made using several different diagnostic methods: cultures obtained from the infected tissue; histopathologic or cytologic examination of tissue, body fluids, or purulent material; and serologic assays for antibodies.

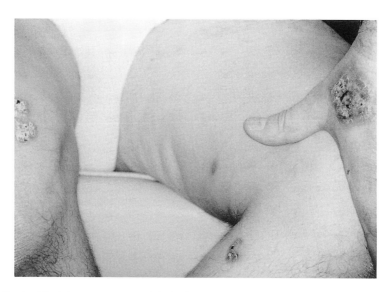

Fig. 7. Typical indolent verrucous skin lesions of blastomycosis on the hands and legs of an elderly gentleman (photo courtesy of Dr. Gunner Deery).

The most definitive method of diagnosis is growth of the organism, but for histo-plasmosis and blastomycosis, culture requires special media and growth may take 4–6 wk. *C. immitis* grows on fungal or regular media within several days usually. Because *C. immitis* is highly contagious in the laboratory setting, clinicians must inform the laboratory that coccidioidomycosis is a possibility so that precautions can be taken.

Histopathologic or cytologic demonstration of the organism in tissues or body fluids is extremely helpful for diagnosis, especially for those patients who are acutely ill. The typical thick-walled yeasts of *B. dermatitidis*, showing single broad-based buds, are readily identified in cytological or potassium hydroxide preparations of sputum or syn-ovial fluid and histopathological examination of tissue biopsies. The tiny intracellular yeast forms of *H. capsulatum* are best visualized in tissues using methenamine silver stains and in bone marrow and other tissue aspirates using Giemsa stain. *C. immitis* is quite distinctive in tissues. The large spherules (80–100 μm) can be seen in tissue sections and in purulent drainage.

Serology plays an important role in the diagnosis of histoplasmosis and coccidioido-mycosis. A positive test prompts the clinician to consider more invasive procedures, such as bronchoscopy or bone marrow and liver biopsies, to establish a diagnosis. There are occasions when the only evidence for infection is the presence of antibodies; this is especially true of meningitis, in which the fungus is exceedingly difficult to grow but CSF serology is positive. For blastomycosis, specific and sensitive serologic assays are not commercially available.

3.4. Treatment

The azole antifungal agents have revolutionized the treatment of the endemic mycoses *(21)*; they are much less toxic than amphotericin B, and oral administration is obviously a benefit in treating chronic diseases. However, there are several adverse effects of azoles that impact on treatment in older adults *(22)*. Ketoconazole suppresses

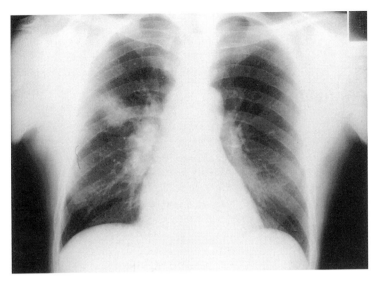

Fig. 8. Right upper lobe pneumonia due to *C. immitis* in a marine sent to southern California for training.

both androgenic and corticosteroid hormones, causing decreased libido and gyneco-mastia and, rarely, Addison's disease. Itraconazole does not have these effects when given at recommended doses but does cause edema, hypokalemia, and hypertension in a small percentage of patients. All of the azole agents have been noted to cause hepati-tis in a small number of patients.

Absorption of ketoconazole and itraconazole is dependent on gastric acidity. Because older adults are more likely to be achlorhydric, absorption may be decreased. Histamine (H2) receptor antagonists, proton pump inhibitors, and antacids should not be used when itraconazole or ketoconazole are prescribed. Itraconazole also requires administration with food to enhance absorption. Fluconazole requires neither gastric acidity nor food for absorption.

Drug interactions, many of which have serious implications for older adults, are frequently encountered with the azole antifungal drugs. Interactions with warfarin, phenytoin, and carbamazepine occur in varying degrees with all of the azole drugs in current use. Itraconazole can increase serum digoxin levels with subsequent toxicity, and ketoconazole and fluconazole can increase the effect of oral hypoglycemics. The antihistamine astemizole and the motility drug cisapride should never be used concur-rently with azoles because of QT prolongation and ventricular arrhythmias.

In spite of these issues, the azoles are exceedingly useful in older adults with endemic mycoses. Most therapy is now given in the outpatient setting. Itraconazole is the preferred agent because of its greater intrinsic activity against the endemic mycoses when compared with fluconazole and better tolerability when compared with ketoconazole. The usual dosage is 200 mg once or twice a day given with food to enhance absorption. Depending on the fungal infection, therapy is given for 6–12 mo and sometimes longer. For those patients who develop coccidioidal meningitis, fluconazole is preferred because of its superior CSF penetration. The dosage is 800 mg daily with normal renal function, and therapy must be given for life, as the organism is rarely eradicated from the central nervous system *(23)*. Overall, results with therapy for the endemic mycoses are excellent, although older patients with advanced emphysema and cavitary histoplasmosis rarely return to their prior functional state and those with coccidioidal meningitis often have a protracted course with a poor outcome.

REFERENCES

1. Narhi, T. O., Ainamo, A., and Meurman, J. H. (1993) Salivary yeasts, saliva, and oral mucosa in the elderly. *J. Dent. Res.* **72,** 1009–1014.
2. Budtz-Jorgensen, E. (1981) Oral mucosal lesions associated with the wearing of removeable dentures. *J. Oral Pathol.* **10,** 65–80.
3. Sobel, J. D. (1994) *Candida* vaginitis. *Infect. Dis. Clin. Pract.* **3,** 334–339.
4. Kauffman C. A., Vazquez, J. A., Sobel J. D., et al. (2000) A prospective multicenter surveillance study of funguria in hospitalized patients. *Clin. Infect. Dis.* **30,** 14–18.
5. Nguyen, M. H., Peacock, J. E. Jr., Tanner, D. C., et al. (1995) Therapeutic approaches in patients with candidemia. *Arch. Intern. Med.* **155,** 2429–2435.
6. Harvey, R. L. and Myers, J. P. (1987) Nosocomial fungemia in a large community teaching hospital. *Arch. Intern. Med.* **147,** 2117–2120.
7. Kauffman, C. A. (1992) Fungal infections. *Clin. Geriat. Med.* **8,** 777–791.
8. Jahrsdoerfer, R.A., Ejercito, V.S., Johns, M.M.E., et al. (1979) Aspergillosis of the nose and paranasal sinuses. *Am. J. Otolaryngol.* **1,** 6–14.
9. Binder, R. E., Faling, J., Pugatch, R. D., et al. (1982) Chronic necrotizing pulmonary aspergillosis: A discrete clinical entity. *Medicine (Balt.)* **61,** 109–124.
10. Parfrey, N. A. (1986) Improved diagnosis and prognosis of mucormycosis. *Medicine (Balt.)* **65,** 113–123.
11. Daly, A. L., Velazquez, L. A., Bradley, S. F., et. al. (1989) Mucormycosis: associated with deferoxamine therapy. *Am. J. Med.* **87,** 468–471.
12. Feigin, D. S. (1983) Pulmonary cryptococcosis: radiologic-pathologic correlates of its three forms. *Am. J. Roentgenol.* **141,** 1262–1272.
13. Washburn, R. G., Kennedy, D. W., Begley M. G., et al. (1988) Chronic fungal sinusitis in apparently normal hosts. *Medicine (Balt.).* **67,** 231–247.
14. Budtz-Jorgensen, E., Holmstrup, P., and Krogh, P. (1988) Fluconazole in the treatment of Candida-associated denture somatitis. *Antimicrob. Agents Chemother.* **32,** 1859–1863.
15. Jacobs, L. G. (1996) Fungal urinary tract infections in the elderly. Treatment guidelines. *Drugs & Aging* **8,** 89–96.
16. Kauffman, C. A. (1997) Amphotericin B, in *Invasive Fungal Infections* (Lynch, J. P., ed.) *Sem. Resp. Crit. Care Med.* **18,** 281–287.
17. Rex, J. H., Bennett, J. E., Sugar A. M., et al. (1994) A randomized trial comparing fluconazole with amphotericin B for the treatment of candidemia in patients without neutropenia. *N. Engl. J. Med.* **331,** 1325–1330.
18. Van der Horst, C. M., Saag, M. S., Cloud, G. A., et al. (1997) Treatment of cryptococcal meningitis associated with the acquired immunodeficiency syndrome. *N. Engl. J. Med.* **337,** 15–21.
19. Kauffman, C. A. (1995) Endemic mycoses in older adults. *Infect. Dis. Clin. Pract.* **4,** 41–45.
20. Mosley, D., Komatsu, K., Vaz, V., et al. (1996) Coccidioidomycosis—Arizona, 1990–1995. *M.M.W.R.* **45,** 1069–1073.
21. Kauffman, C. A. (1994) Newer developments in therapy for endemic mycoses. *Clin. Infect. Dis.* **19(1 Suppl),** S28–S32.
22. Kauffman, C. A. (1993) Antifungal agents, in *Antimicrobial therapy in the Elderly Patient* (Yoshikawa, T. T. and Norman, D. C., eds.), Marcel Dekker, New York, pp. 441–456.
23. Dewsnup, D. H., Galgiani, J. N., Graybill, J. R., et al. (1996) Is it even safe to stop azole therapy for *Coccidioides immitis* meningitis? *Ann. Intern. Med.,* **124,** 305–310.

19

Viral Infections

Ann R. Falsey

1. RESPIRATORY VIRUSES

1.1. Influenza

Of the viral infections that cause disease in older adults, influenza is recognized as one of the greatest causes of morbidity and mortality. Pneumonia and influenza together comprise the fifth leading causes of death in persons aged 65 yr and older. Influenza viruses are enveloped ribonucleic acid (RNA) viruses that are classified as A, B, or C, based on stable internal proteins (1). The virus contains two major surface proteins, hemagglutinin (H) and neuraminidase (N), which can undergo minor antigenic changes leading to yearly epidemics or major changes resulting in influenza pandemics. Currently, there are two circulating influenza A viruses, H1N1 and H3N2, in addition to influenza B, present in the United States. H1N1 viruses do not appear to cause serious problems in older persons, possibly due to previous immunity (2).

1.1.1. Epidemiology and Clinical Relevance

Peak influenza activity typically lasts 6–8 wk in a community with attack rates highest in preschool and school-aged children and lowest in older persons. During non-pandemic influenza, attack rates are approx 10% in the elderly (3). Despite lower attack rates, hospitalization rates and complications are highest in this age group (4). Mortality from influenza rises dramatically with age and the presence of underlying medical conditions contribute significantly to influenza-related mortality (5). The presence of one high-risk medical condition (cardiovascular, pulmonary, renal, metabolic, neurologic, or malignant disease) increases the risk of death from influenza 39-fold. The devastating impact of influenza is most dramatically seen in long-term care facilities where explosive epidemics may occur. During outbreaks, rates of pneumonia and hospitalization are as high as 52% and 29%, respectively, with case fatality rates of 30% (6). In addition to the suffering caused by influenza, the economic burden is enormous, resulting in more than one billion dollars spent by Medicare in 1989–1990 alone for excess hospitalizations (7).

From: *Infectious Disease in the Aging*
Edited by: Thomas T. Yoshikawa and Dean C. Norman
© Humana Press Inc., Totowa, NJ

Table 1
Respiratory Viral Infections

	Peak season	Incubation (d)	Clinical clues	Antiviral therapy
Influenza A	Winter	1–3	High fever, headache,	Amantadine
			myalgias	Zanamivir, Oseltamivir
				Rimantadine
				Zanamivir, Oseltamivir
Influenza B	Winter	1–3	High fever, headache,	Zanamivir, Oseltamivir
			myalgias	
RSV	Winter	3–5	Rhinorrhea, wheezing	Ribavirin
Parainfluenza	Fall-spring	1–2	Pharyngitis, hoarseness	None
Rhinovirus	All	1–2	Rhinorrhea	None
Coronavirus	Winter-spring	1–2	Non-specific	None

RSV, respiratory syncytial virus.

1.1.2. Clinical Manifestations

The classic presentation of influenza is that of the abrupt onset of fever, chills, head-ache, and myalgias (*see* Table 1). Dry cough, sore throat, and ocular pain are also common *(1)*. Although nasal congestion and discharge occur with influenza, rhinor-rhea is usually not as profuse as with other respiratory viruses. Fever remains a common finding in the elderly, although the height of the fever may be lower compared with young persons. Although many elderly adults have classic influenza symptoms, a substantial number may have more subtle presentations such as fever and confusion or worsening of chronic cardiopulmonary disease. Thus, it is important to consider the possibility of influenza in the ill elderly adult during the winter months.

Lower respiratory tract involvement increases steadily with advancing age with the rates of pneumonia 4–8% in persons aged 5–50 yr and rising to 73% in persons over age 70 *(1)*. Secondary bacterial pneumonia following acute influenza also occurs more frequently in older persons. In addition to the immediate complications of influenza, residents of nursing homes who survive influenza experience a significant functional decline in activities of daily living *(8)*.

1.1.3. Diagnostic Tests

The diagnosis of influenza can be made in a variety of ways including viral culture, rapid antigen testing, and serology. Although many physicians use clinical features to make a diagnosis of "the flu," laboratory confirmation is best if therapeutic decisions are needed, as influenza may be difficult to distinguish from other respiratory viruses. Virus can be detected in nasopharyngeal secretions or sputum. Older persons typically shed less virus than young persons but will have culturable virus for 3–4 d into the illness *(9)*. Rapid antigen testing may be done directly on nasopharyngeal specimens using an enzyme immunoassay (EIA) *(10)*. Although not as sensitive as viral culture, rapid tests offer several hour turnaround times and may be useful for infection control and treatment decisions *(11)*. Influenza infection can also be confirmed retrospectively by demonstrating a greater than fourfold rise in antibody by hemagglutination inhibition assay or enzyme immunoassay (EIA). A single acute titer is not useful for diagnosis of influenza, as all persons have preexisting antibodies.

1.1.4. Treatment

At the present time, four antiviral agents, amantadine, rimantadine, zanamivir, and oseltamavir are approved for the treatment of influenza A. These agents are 70–90% effective as prophylactic agents and also reduce illness severity, duration of symptoms, and viral shedding when given within 48 h of symptom onset *(12)*. Central nervous symptoms are a problem in older persons given amantadine. Rimantadine is more costly but appears to be better tolerated. Although resistance develops rapidly on therapy with either agent, a net therapeutic benefit is preserved *(13)*. The appropriate dose of amantadine or rimantadine for most elderly persons is 100 mg/day taken orally with further dose adjustments necessary for amantadine based on renal function. Zanamivir and oseltamavir are new agents that inhibit the action of viral neuraminidase and show promise for prophylaxis and treatment of influenza A or B *(14–16)*. Resistance and central nervous system side effects do not appear to be a problem.

1.1.5. Prevention

The cornerstone of infection control in long-term care facilities is yearly vaccination of residents and staff. (*See* also Chapter 23.) In addition, the Centers for Disease Control and Prevention (CDC) recommends that antiviral prophylaxis be given to all residents once influenza A has been documented in the institution *(17)*. Chemoprophylaxis is given regardless of vaccination status and is continued until 1 wk after the onset of the last influenza case. Because some authorities remain concerned about adverse side effects of amantadine, more conservative approaches have been put forward that recommend antivirals to those ill less than 48 h and to their roommates and reserve institutionwide prophylaxis only when more than 10% of residents are ill *(18)*.

Influenza vaccination has been clearly shown to be efficacious and cost effective in older persons and is recommended for all persons aged 65 and older *(17,19)*. Although serologic response is diminished in residents of nursing homes, vaccination reduces the severity of disease and prevents hospitalization and death *(17)*. The current vaccine contains antigens from two type A and one type B viruses. Mild acute local reactions occur in approx one third of vaccinees and systemic reactions, such as fever and myalgias are uncommon in older persons. Influenza vaccine may be safely given simultaneously with pneumococcal vaccine, and the only contraindication to vaccination is anaphylactic hypersensitivity to eggs or other components of the vaccine *(17)*.

1.2. Respiratory Syncytial Virus

1.2.1. Epidemiology and Clinical Relevance

RSV is an enveloped RNA virus that belongs to the paramyxovirus family and consists of two antigenically distinct groups, designated A and B. RSV has long been recognized as the leading cause of lower respiratory tract disease in children; however, recently, it has been increasingly implicated as a cause of serious disease in elderly persons *(20)*. Although the magnitude of the problem of RSV in the elderly has not been completely defined, it appears to rank second to influenza as a major viral respiratory pathogen in this group *(21,22)*.

RSV was initially recognized as a pathogen in older persons when several outbreaks were described in long-term care facilities *(23,24)*. Since 1977, there have been
20 studies published that have identified RSV infections in nursing homes *(25–29)*.
Attack rates are variable and may be as high as 90% during outbreaks, but are more
commonly range from 1–7% when residents are followed prospectively *(28,30)*. Rates
of pneumonia range from 0–53% and death from 0–55% in published reports
(28,31,32). The variable severity may be in part due to case selection bias in some
studies, but also may reflect differences in strain virulence. In addition to long-term
care facilities, RSV has also been found to be a frequent problem in senior daycare
centers *(33)*.

Although less data are available, RSV appears to cause serious disease in community-dwelling older persons as well *(21,22)*. Similar to influenza, when peaks of RSV
activity occurred among children in the United Kingdom, a peak in excess acute respiratory infection and mortality occurred in persons aged 65 and older *(22)*. In a 3-yr
study examining persons aged 65 and older admitted to the hospital with acute cardiopulmonary conditions, RSV accounted for 10% of cases compared with 13% due to influenza A or B *(21)*. The impact of RSV illness was significant; 18% required intensive
care, 10% needed ventilatory support, and 10% died. Finally, a large study of community-acquired pneumonia in adults found RSV to be the third most commonly identified pathogen at 4.4% compared to 6.2% due to *Streptococcus pneumoniae* and 5.4%
due to influenza *(34)*. A recent analysis of the economic burden of RSV in adults concluded that 0.04–0.2% of the population 65 yr of age and older are hospitalized yearly
with RSV pneumonia with estimated annual health-care costs of $150–680 million *(35)*.

1.2.2. Clinical Manifestations

Manifestations of RSV infection can be difficult to distinguish from other viral respiratory infections, particularly influenza. Most individuals with RSV have nasal discharge, cough, sputum production, and constitutional symptoms *(21,34)*. In addition,
wheezing is a frequent complaint *(30)*. Fever is present in approx half of the cases but
is usually lower than in influenza infection. Although overlap exists, there are some
helpful clues to differentiate RSV from influenza. High fever, sore throat, myalgias,
and gastrointestinal complaints are more characteristic of influenza, whereas rhinor-
rhea and wheezing are more frequently associated with RSV infection *(21,27,34)*.

1.2.3. Diagnostic Tests

The diagnosis of RSV infection can be accomplished by viral culture, rapid antigen
tests, or serology. Unfortunately, because of the labile nature of the virus and low titers of
virus in nasal secretions in adults, diagnosis of acute RSV infection is very difficult.
Under ideal circumstances, viral culture is only 50% sensitive when compared with serology using EIA *(30)*. Both commercial rapid antigen tests and indirect immunofluorescence have poor sensitivity in adults *(36)*. New molecular tests, such as polymerase
chain reaction (PCR), may offer a significant advantage for the diagnosis of acute RSV
in this population and need further development. Infection can also be demonstrated
retrospectively by a ≥fourfold rise in RSV-specific IgG, either by complement fixation
or EIA. Because RSV in adults always represents reinfection, a single elevated titer is
not useful for acute diagnosis. RSV-specific IgM has been detected in 11–81% of older
subjects with acute RSV, but its clinical utility has yet to be defined *(26,37)*.

1.2.4. Treatment

The treatment of RSV infection in adults is largely supportive. Supplemental oxygen and bronchodilators may be useful and antibiotics should be considered if bacterial super-infection is suspected. Ribavirin is a nucleoside analogue which has broad antiviral activity, including RSV *(38)*. Although inhaled ribavirin is approved in young children with RSV, no controlled data exist in adults. Anecdotal experience suggests it may be beneficial in selected cases; however, general recommendations on its use cannot be made due to lack of data *(39)*. Although relatively nontoxic, the major problems with ribavirin are its high cost and difficulty with administration. The recommended 12–18 h/d of aerosol at 20 mg/mL concentrations may be quite difficult for the elderly adult to tolerate. Recent data indicate that higher concentrations (60 mg/mL) given three times a day may also be effective.

1.2.5. Prevention

Although research is ongoing, an effective RSV vaccine has yet to be developed. Thus, prevention of RSV is limited to good basic infection control policies. RSV is spread primarily by large droplet inoculation and fomites. Therefore, close person-to-person contact or contact with contaminated environmental surfaces is required for transmission to occur. Handwashing is the single most important measure in the control of RSV. Because compliance with hand washing is frequently poor, some authorities advocate the use of gowns and gloves when caring for RSV-infected patients *(40)*.

1.3. Parainfluenza Viruses

1.3.1. Epidemiology and Clinical Relevance

The parainfluenza viruses (PIV) are most commonly thought of as the etiologic agents of croup, bronchiolitis, and pneumonia in young children. Although comprehensive studies are lacking, these common respiratory viruses also affect older adults. The parainfluenza viruses are members of paramyxovirus family with four serotypes and two subgroups recognized (1, 2, 3, 4a, and 4b); PIV-3 is endemic throughout the year, whereas PIV-1 and PIV-2 tend to occur during the fall. Most reinfections in young adults result in mild upper respiratory infections; however, occasional outbreaks of pneumonia have been described *(41)*. Although PIV infections are not commonly documented in older adults, several studies of community-acquired pneumonia implicate PIV as a cause in 2–11% of cases *(42,43)*. The PIV-1 and 3 serotypes account for the majority of isolates in older persons, with PIV-2 being relatively uncommon *(44)*.

1.3.2. Clinical Manifestations

Similar to RSV, outbreaks of PIV infections in nursing homes have been described *(44–46)*. High attack rates and significant morbidity and mortality have been reported. Clinical characteristics of PIV infection are not distinctive and include rhinorrhea, sore throat, hoarseness, and cough with high rates of pneumonia ranging from 20–30%. In a recent institutional outbreak of PIV-3, the attack rates among residents and nursing staff were 31% and 11%, respectively. The epidemic pattern, with a steady number of new cases over a 1-mo period, suggested person-to-person transmission *(46)*.

1.3.3. Diagnostic Tests and Treatment

Diagnosis of PIV infection can be made by viral culture or by demonstrating a rise in serum antibody by EIA or complement fixation. Both PIV-1 and 3 infections result in cross-reactive antibody responses and, thus, cannot be distinguished serologically. At present, a rapid antigen test for PIV is not commercially available and no antiviral agents have been approved for the treatment of PIV infection. Therefore, treatment is supportive

1.4. Rhinoviruses

1.4.1. Epidemiology and Clinical Relevance

Rhinoviruses are the most commonly identified cause of the "common cold," accounting for approx 25–50% of upper respiratory infections *(47)*. These ubiquitous viruses are members of the picornavirus family with over 100 antigenic types. Rhinoviruses circulate at all times of the year, but peak activity tends to be during the spring and fall. Infections with rhinoviruses are common throughout life and, although a major cause of school and work absenteeism, illnesses are generally mild in young persons *(48)*. Pneumonia due to rhinovirus is very uncommon, even in immunocompromised persons and is likely because the virus does not replicate well at the lower airway temperature of 37°C *(49)*.

There are little data on the incidence of rhinovirus infections in independent elderly persons living in the community. However, a recent prospective study from the United Kingdom indicates that rhinoviruses are an important cause of debility and lower respiratory disease in elderly people in the community *(50)*. Rhinoviruses accounted for 121 of 497 (24%) respiratory illnesses that occurred in a cohort of 533 persons over a 2-yr period. Seminested reverse transcriptase (RT)-PCR was used to identify rhinovirus infection and the increased sensitivity of this technique was likely responsible for the high infection rates. Although death and hospitalization rates were low, the mean length of illness was 16 d and 6% were unable to perform their normal household activities. Fifty-six percent had evidence of lower respiratory tract involvement such as productive cough or wheezing. The presence of chronic medical conditions and smoking increased the likelihood of lower respiratory tract complications. Because of the frequency of rhinovirus infection, the overall burden of disease in the elderly may approach influenza *(50)*.

1.4.2. Clinical Manifestations

Rhinovirus infections are also common in senior daycare settings and long-term care facilities *(30,51,52)*. In frail elderly persons, nasal congestion (79–89%), cough (71–94%), constitutional symptoms (43–91%) and sore throat (21–51%) characterize illnesses. Similar to independent seniors, illnesses were prolonged, lasting approx 2 wk and approx 50% had lower respiratory involvement.

1.4.3. Diagnostic Tests and Treatment

The diagnosis of rhinovirus is usually made by viral culture of nasopharyngeal secretions. Although the use of RT-PCR greatly increases detection rates, this technique is currently only available in research settings *(50)*. Treatment is supportive and care should be exercised when prescribing "cold" medications to elderly persons as many contain combinations of sympathomimetics and antihistamines. At the present time, specific antiviral therapy of rhinoviruses is not available. Recently, a new compound, tremacamra, which blocks the cellular receptor for rhinovirus, intercellular adhesion molecule 1 (ICAM), shows promise for the treatment of rhinovirus infections *(53)*.

1.5. Coronaviruses

Coronaviruses are RNA viruses of which two major serotypes, 229E and OC43, cause respiratory disease in humans *(54)*. Peak viral activity occurs in the winter and spring *(55)*. Reinfections with coronaviruses are common throughout life, and similar to rhinoviruses; illnesses are generally mild upper respiratory infections in healthy adults. Symptoms include malaise, headache, sore throat, and nasal congestion *(54)*. Exacerbations of chronic obstructive pulmonary disease have been linked to coronavirus infections in several studies *(56)*.

Coronavirus infections have been evaluated in the community-dwelling elderly in one prospective study from the U.K. and accounted for 9.5% of the respiratory illnesses *(57)*. They were associated with lower respiratory tract symptoms in more than 40% of cases. Coronavirus infections have been documented in long-term care facilities and in frail elderly people attending daycare centers *(52,58)*. The most common symptoms were cough (94%), constitutional symptoms (88%), and nasal congestion (84%). Significantly, 66% had a productive cough, 34% experienced shortness of breath, and 22% developed wheezing. Illnesses lasted approx 2 wk and almost half of the patients required antibiotics. Although many of the subjects were very frail, all recovered without sequelae. Unfortunately, diagnosis of coronavirus infections is not generally available outside of research facilities due to the fastidious nature of the virus and the lack of commercial reagents for serologic diagnosis. No antiviral agents are available and treatment is supportive.

2. VIRAL HEPATITIS

2.1. Hepatitis A

Hepatitis A (HAV) is an RNA virus in the picornavirus family *(see* Table 2). The virus is easily transmitted by the fecal-oral route. In countries where the virus is endemic and sanitation is poor, most people become infected in early childhood when the disease is mild and life-long immunity results *(59)*. Recently, a shift in the prevalence of cases from childhood to adulthood has occurred, presumably due to improved living conditions. In the United States and other industrialized nations, the prevalence of anti-HAV antibodies increases with advancing age *(60)*. Seroprevalence in an ambulatory geriatric population (mean age 75) in New York was 94%. In a 1994 serologic study from Colorado, the prevalence of anti-HAV antibodies at ages 60, 70, and 80 was 40%, 60%, and 80%, respectively *(59)*. The steady increase in seroprevalence with age is seen in men and women and in all races and ethnic groups.

The clinical manifestations of acute hepatitis A become more severe and are associated with prolonged cholestasis with advancing age *(61,62)*. In the United States, the overall case fatality rate for HAV infection is 1/1000; however, it rises to 27/1000 in persons 50 yr or older *(61)*. Approx 100 HAV-related deaths occur in the U.S. each year of which 70% are in persons over age 49 *(63)*. The increased death rates in the older population is attributable to higher rates of fulminant hepatitis since chronic infection does not occur *(59)*.

Table 2
Viral Hepatitis

Virus	Transmission	Incubation range in days (average)	Clinical characteristics in older persons	Chronic infection
A	Fecal-oral	14–50 (28)	Prolonged cholestasis Increased mortality	No
B	Parenteral Sexual	45–160 (120)	Milder acute infection, but chronic infection more common. Sequelae: cancer and cirrhosis	Yes
C	Parenteral Other ?	15–150 (42)	Same as hepatitis B virus (HBV)	Yes
D	Parenteral Sexual	45–130	May worsen existing cirrhosis from HBV	Yes
E	Fecal-oral	14–60	No data	No
G	Parenteral	Limited data	Clinical significance unknown	Yes

An inactivated hepatitis A vaccine has been available since 1993, and clinical studies have shown the vaccine to be safe, very well tolerated, and highly immunogenic in all age groups *(64)*. Similar to young adults, seroconversion rates are 100% in older adults (40–61 yr) *(65)*. Immunogenicity in frail elderly persons, such as residents of long-term care, has not been reported. Although disease may be more severe in older adults current vaccination policies do not specifically target the elderly. However, vaccination is recommended for older travelers who plan to visit countries endemic for HAV.

2.2. Hepatitis B

Hepatitis B (HBV) is a complex deoxyribonucleic acid (DNA) virus composed of double-stranded DNA, core antigen (HBcAg), surface antigen (HBSAg), and soluble nucleocapsid antigen (HBeAg). Hepatitis B surface antigen is detectable during acute illness and disappears when antibody to HBSAg develops. Transmission of HBV is by percutaneous and mucous membrane exposure to infectious body fluids. Serum, saliva, and semen have been shown to contain HBSAg. Hepatitis D (HDV), also known as Delta agent, is a small single-stranded, circular RNA particle that is coated with HBSAg. Infection with HDV requires either simultaneous infection with HBV or chronic HBV infection. The co-infection may result in fulminant hepatitis *(60)*.

Infection with HBV accounts for approx 20% of cases of acute viral hepatitis in older adults *(60,66)*. Because the primary risk group in the U.S. and Europe is intravenous drug abusers, a group not highly represented in the elderly population, acute infection is not common in this age group. Transfusion-related HBV infection from contaminated blood in the window period of detection is a now an uncommon event with risk estimated to be 1 in 63,000 transfusions *(67)*. Long-term care facilities were at one time considered a risk area for HBV when several outbreaks occurred during the 1970s–1980s *(60)*. However, recent surveys of geriatric hospitals indicate the prevalence of HBSAg is similar to the general geriatric population (<1%) *(60,68)*.

Acute HBV in older adults is usually mild and many cases are subclinical or present with a cholestatic picture *(66)*. In addition to the typical symptoms of jaundice, anorexia, and fatigue, diarrhea is a common complaint in elderly persons *(66)*. Complaints reflecting immune complex disease such as myalgias and arthalgias are rare in older adults. Although acute HBV is generally not a severe disease in older adults, the mortality from fulminant HBV increases with age *(60)*. In a multivariant analysis of prognostic factors in 115 patients with HBV, age was an independent predictor of survival. Chronic carriage rates also increase when individuals are infected at older ages. Compared with a 10% carriage rate in young adults, approx 60% of older persons become chronic carriers *(60)*. However, most elderly HBV chronic carriers were infected early in life and have carried the virus for a prolonged period and, although HBSAg is detected, there is little evidence of active viral replication as determined by the presence of HBeAg or viral DNA in the serum *(60)*.

In addition to cirrhosis from chronic active hepatitis, one of the major complications of HBV infection is hepatocellular carcinoma. The length of time infected is an important factor in the development of cancer and, thus, elderly persons who have been infected for many years are at greatest risk *(69)*. The rate of hepatocellular carcinoma rises from 197/100,000 in 30- to 39-yr olds to 927/100,000 in 60- to 69-yr-old chronic HBV carriers *(62)*.

The treatment of elderly persons with chronic HBV is largely supportive. Although α-interferon shows evidence of suppressing viral replication and may decrease the risk of progression to cirrhosis or cancer, side effects of therapy increase with advancing age *(60)*. Therapy should be reserved for patients in overall good health except for their liver disease and who have evidence of active viral replication. Lamivudine, a nucleoside analogue, holds promise as a new anti-HBV agent.

The currently licensed hepatitis B vaccine is a genetic recombinant vaccine consisting of highly purified HBSAg particles expressed in yeast. The vaccine is very well tolerated and highly immunogenic with excellent protective efficacy in children and young adults. However, response rates to HBV vaccine diminish significantly with increased age. Ninety percent of persons under age 40 achieve an adequate seroresponse compared with only 50% in persons over age 60.

2.3. Hepatitis C

Hepatitis C (HCV) is an RNA virus in the flavivirus family and accounts for the majority of cases of acute viral hepatitis in the older adults. The virus is transmitted parenterally and accounts for approx 90% of new cases of posttransfusion hepatitis. Other exposures to contaminated blood, either via occupation or intravenous drug abuse, may also transmit HCV. Although 40–50% of community-acquired HCV cases do not report a parenteral exposure, nonparenteral transmission of HCV is not well understood. Sexual transmission, if it occurs, is not efficient *(61)*. The major risk factor for HCV in older persons is transfusion and most became infected with HCV prior to 1990 when routine screening of the blood supply began *(60)*. The current risk of acquiring HCV from transfusion is approx 1 in 103,000 *(67)*. The seroprevalence of HCV increases with advancing age from 0.6% among 18- to 25-yr olds to 2.5% of persons over age 60. The increased prevalence in older persons is likely due to a greater chance of transfusion *(60)*. The seroprevalence in long-term care facilities is approx that of the general elderly population. In a Canadian and an Italian chronic care facility, the prevalences of anti-HCV antibodies were 1.4% and 2.2%, respectively, both reflecting rates similar to the community at large *(68,70)*.

The clinical manifestations of acute HCV are generally mild and nonspecific. In a series of 20 older people with acute non-A non-B hepatitis, approx 30–40% had fever, abdominal pain, and jaundice *(60)*. Fulminant hepatitis is rare with HCV, but development of chronic liver disease is very common *(61,66,71)*. Virtually all persons become chronically infected and a significant number develop chronic liver disease. Chronic active hepatitis or cirrhosis develops in 29–76%, on average 20 yr after initial infection *(71)*. In older patients with chronic HCV, the HCV–RNA titer is significantly higher than in younger patients, and there is evidence that disease progression is more rapid *(60)*. Hepatocellular carcinoma is clearly associated with chronic HCV infection, and the relative risk of cancer from HCV may be even greater than that from HBV (52 vs. 15) *(69)*. In a study of 25 older persons with HCV in the U.K., 36% developed hepatocellular carcinoma *(71)*.

Alpha interferon is administered to patients with chronic HCV infection as an attempt to prevent progression to cirrhosis and possibly liver cancer. Persons with high viral load and viral genotype 1 have a low response rate to α-interferon, and many patients who do have an initial response relapse when therapy is discontinued *(60)*. Most studies of interferon treatment of HCV have not included older participants. In one study from Japan, interferon was administered to 19 patients aged 65 and older with HCV, and the response rate was 26% compared with 33% in younger persons. Of note, the older subjects had higher HCV–RNA titers and more severe fibrosis on liver biopsy compared with young subjects. Response rates in elderly persons correlated with lower HCV–RNA titers *(72)*. Because older persons have more side effects and a lower response rate to interferon, therapy should be reserved for those persons with a low RNA titer, viral genotypes other than 1, and minimal fibrosis on biopsy *(60)*.

2.4. Hepatitis E

Hepatitis E virus (HEV) is an enterically transmitted virus found in Africa, Asia, and Mexico. Attack rates of HEV are highest in persons ages 15–40, and mortality is high in pregnant women. Seroprevalence increases with age, reaching 70% in persons over age 60 living in endemic areas *(60)*. No cases of HEV have been reported in the United States.

2.5. Hepatitis G

Hepatitis G virus (HGV) is a recently discovered novel agent belonging to the flavivirus family and is distantly related to HCV. The epidemiology and clinical significance of this HGV is still being defined, but it is felt to be a possible cause of the transfusion-associated hepatitis *(73)*. The pattern of HGV seroprevalence is similar to HCV and increases with age, peaking in the sixties *(60)*. In 105 elderly Italian persons with a mean age of 73, anti-HGV antibodies were found in 24%, and 3% were viremic. No subject had clinical evidence of hepatitis *(73)*.

3. GASTROENTERITIS VIRUSES

Recent studies from the CDC have described increased morbidity and mortality associated with gastroenteritis in the elderly. Although deaths related to diarrhea have traditionally been thought to be a problem of young children in developing countries, 51% of the 28,538 diarrhea-related deaths in the United States from 1979–1987 occurred in adults over age 74 compared with 11% in children <5 yr old *(74)*. The odds ratio of dying during a hospitalization involving gastroenteritis was 52.6 for adults over age 70 compared with children less than age 5. Residents of nursing facilities are at particular risk for infectious diarrhea illness because of the outbreaks which can occur in closed populations. The majority of nursing facility outbreaks of gastroenteritis are probably viral in origin since bacterial causes are not usually identified. These include rotavirus, enteric adenoviruses, calicivirus, Norwalk-like agent, Snow Mountain agent, and small round structured viruses (SRSV) *(74–76)*.

Rotaviruses are small RNA viruses in the retrovirus family and are the most important cause of gastroenteritis in infants and young children worldwide. The mode of transmission is assumed to be fecal-oral, and the virus is relatively resistant to common disinfectants and thus facilitating nosocomial dissemination. Several outbreaks of rotavirus infection in elderly residents of long-term care facilities have been reported *(77–79)*. Attack rates have ranged from 36–66% with mortality rates of 1–10%. The typical illness included voluminous vomiting and watery diarrhea with low-grade fever. Blood in stool was not seen, and diarrhea typically lasts 2–3 d. Death resulted from dehydration progressing to oliguria and acidosis *(77,79)*. Rotavirus serum antibody titers offer some protection against severe disease and tend to diminish with increasing age *(79)*.

In 1998, a live attenuated rotavirus vaccine was approved for use in infants. The vaccine provides 88% protection from severe diarrhea and 75% from dehydration, and produced a 70% reduction in hospital admissions *(80)*. No data on safety or immunogenicity in the elderly exists; however, given the mortality rates in this age group, further study would be reasonable.

4. HUMAN IMMUNODEFICIENCY VIRUS

Human immunodeficiency virus (HIV) is the cause of a worldwide pandemic with estimates that 50–100 million individuals will be infected by the year 2000. (*See* also Chapter 25.) Although acquired immunodeficiency syndrome (AIDS) is primarily a disease of young persons, elderly persons are also affected and diagnosis is frequently unrecognized *(81–83)*. As of June 1996, 10% of the AIDS cases in the United States were in persons older than age 50 *(81)*. Of these, 28% were over age 60 and 13% were 65 yr and older. Until recently, the primary source of HIV in the elderly was blood transfusion during the period between 1978 and 1985. Currently, the most common risk factor among AIDS patients over age 50 is homosexuality. It is estimated that in the United States, one million homosexuals persons are aged 65 and older *(82)*. Intravenous drug use ranks second and a history of blood transfusion now ranks third as the most common HIV risk factors in older persons *(82)*. In addition, older adults have a greater probability of having no identifiable risk factors that may reflect heterosexual transmission from at-risk partners *(81,82)*. Finally, older at-risk Americans are much less likely to have adopted AIDS-preventing strategies than persons in their twenties *(84)*. Persons over age 50 are one-sixth as likely to use condoms during sex and one-fifth as likely to have ever been HIV tested.

HIV infection appears to progress more rapidly in older persons. Age over 40 yr is an independent risk factor for poor survival among patients with transfusion-related AIDS *(85)*. Older AIDS patients who develop an AIDS-defining opportunistic infection are also more likely to progress quickly and die. Approx 37% of persons over age 80 die within the same month as they have AIDS diagnosed compared with 12% in young adults *(82)*. The decreased survival time is likely due to a combination of comorbid disease, immunosenescence, and most importantly, delayed diagnosis *(81,83)*. In general, the most frequent illness in older persons with HIV infection is bacterial pneumonia, although opportunistic infections do occur and are similar to those in younger AIDS patients. A significant problem in the elderly is AIDS dementia, as it may be mistaken for Alzheimer's disease or Parkinson's disease. If unrecognized, the opportunity for a trial of antiretroviral medication is lost. Regardless of age, all patients with clinical syndromes compatible with AIDS should be evaluated for HIV infection.

5. HERPES VIRUS INFECTIONS

5.1. Varicella Zoster

Varicella-zoster virus (VZV) is a DNA virus and a member of the herpes virus family. It causes two distinct clinical syndromes: primary disseminated infection, which is manifested as chickenpox, and reactivation of latent virus in the dorsal root ganglia, leading to herpes zoster or "shingles." Herpes zoster is a painful, vesicular exanthem which erupts in one to two dermatomes after a prodrome of days to weeks and may take up to a month to heal *(86)*. Most patients report a deep aching or burning sensation, altered sensation to touch with paresthesias, dysesthesia, or hyperesthesia. Herpes zoster is a common condition with a cumulative lifetime incidence of 10–20% with most of the risk concentrated in older age *(87)*. The overall incidence is 215 per 100,000 person-years, but rates rise sharply with increasing age to 1425/100,000 for persons older than 75 yr.

Postherpetic neuralgia (PHN) is the presence of pain more than 1 mo after onset of the eruption *(86)*. PHN afflicts the elderly much more frequently than the young, occurring in 27–68% of persons age 60 and older, compared with 3–10% of persons under age 50 *(88)*. In addition to age, severity of acute pain, rash severity, prodromal symptoms, and the degree of sensory impairment are predictors of PHN *(89)*. Approx 20% of persons with PHN who are over age 60 will have pain for more than 1 yr. The pathological changes seen in PHN include fibrosis and loss of neurons in the dorsal ganglion and axon and myelin loss in the affected side *(86)*. Once PHN develops, treatment of pain is often ineffectual. The great variety of treatments that are available for PHN is an indication that none are very effective. Topical formulations of aspirin and anesthetics, such as lidocaine and prilocaine, may provide some short-term benefit *(86)*. Capsaicin cream, which depletes the neurotransmitter, substance P, is the only drug approved for the treatment of PHN by the Food and Drug Administration. Neuropathic pain is generally not very responsive to narcotics, although some patients derive benefit. The most beneficial systemic agents available for PHN are the tricyclic antide-

Table 3
Therapy for Acute Herpes Zoster Within 72 Hours of Rash

Antiviral	Dose	Duration
Valacyclovir	1 g, three times a day	7 d
Famciclovir	750 mg, three times a day	7 d
Acyclovir	800 mg, five times a day	7–10 d

Consider in persons with no contraindications[a] to corticosteroids: antiviral + prednisone 60 mg/d, tapered over 21 d.

[a]Contraindications include: diabetes, hypertension, and glaucoma.

pressant drugs. Randomized clinical trials of amitriptyline and desipramine showed that 45–65% of elderly PHN patients achieved some pain relief *(88)*. Anticonvulsants, such as phenytoin, carbamazepine, and gabapentin, may be helpful to reduce the lacinating component of neuropathic pain *(86)*. Other treatments, such as transcutaneous electrical nerve stimulation (TENS), biofeedback, relaxation therapy, and regional neuron blockade have all been used with variable success.

Because PHN is often refractory to treatment, efforts have been directed toward prevention using antivirals and corticosteroids. Five controlled trials have evaluated the use of corticosteroids to prevent PHN. Two studies showed a benefit, but the other two did not *(86)*. The fifth study was done in 208 persons over age 50 with localized zoster of less than 72 h duration. Treatments included acyclovir, 800 mg, five times a day for 21 d, and prednisone, starting at 60 mg/d, with a taper over 21 d. Four treatment arms include acyclovir and prednisone, acyclovir alone, prednisone alone, and placebo. The acyclovir-plus-prednisone group showed accelerated time to cessation of acute pain, time to uninterrupted sleep and time to return to daily activities *(90)*. Of note, no effect on chronic pain at 6 mo was observed. The new antivirals, famciclovir and valacyclovir, also show significant reduction in the duration of zoster pain in placebo-controlled trials *(88,91)*. However, 20% of patients in both studies developed chronic pain despite early treatment with antiviral drugs.

In summary, if begun within 72 h of the rash, acyclovir, famciclovir, and valacyclovir all reduce acute pain in immunocompetent adults with zoster and, thus, are worthwhile, regardless of their effect on PHN. Corticosteroids also do not alter the course of PHN but may improve the quality of life after zoster, and their use, in combination with an antiviral, is reasonable in persons over 50 yr of age with no contraindication to corticosteroids *(see* Table 3) *(86)*.

The optimal way to prevent PHN may be to prevent zoster itself. Trials to evaluate the live OKA-strain varicella vaccine in older adults to prevent herpes zoster are ongoing. Immunization of adults who are immune to varicella-zoster results in increases in humoral and cellular immune responses. However, it will take many years to know if these encouraging results translate into decreased rates of herpes zoster *(86)*.

5.2. Epstein-Barr Virus

The Epstein–Barr Virus (EBV) is a double-stranded DNA virus in the herpes virus family. Infection with EBV establishes lifelong infection. Primary infection may occur in childhood when infection is asymptomatic or during adolescence when the symptoms of classic mononucleosis are most often observed *(92)*. Although primary infection is uncommon in old age, the manifestations may be different than in youth, making diagnosis challenging.

Seroepidemiologic studies indicate that 3–10% of older adults are at risk for primary infection as indicated by the absence of EBV antibodies *(92)*. Because primary EBV infection is uncommon in older age, the diagnosis is often not considered. Diagnosis is also often delayed because symptoms may be misleading. Lymphadenopathy, pharyngitis, and splenomegaly are significantly less common and jaundice is more common in older persons as compared with the young *(93)*. The neurologic manifestations of EBV infection are protean, and acute EBV encephalitis has been documented in an elderly woman *(94)*. To add to the difficulty in making a correct diagnosis, development of atypical lymphocytosis may be absent or delayed in the elderly. Diagnosis of primary EBV is made by the presence of heterophile antibodies or EBV-specific IgM. Although acyclovir has in vitro activity against EBV, no benefit has been demonstrated in the treatment of acute EBV infection. Therefore treatment is supportive.

REFERENCES

1. Betts, R. (1995) Influenza, in *Principles and Practices of Infectious Diseases* (Mandell, G. L., Bennett, J. F., and Dolin, R., eds.), Churchill Livingston, New York , pp. 1546–1567.
2. Cate, T. R. (1987) Clinical manifestations and consequences of influenza. *Am. J. Med.* **82,** 15–19.
3. Glezen, W. P. and Couch, R. B. (1978) Interpandemic influenza in the Houston area, 1974–1976. *N. Engl. J. Med.* **298,** 587–592.
4. Perrotta, D. M., Decker, M., and Glezen, W. P. (1985) Acute respiratory disease hospitalizations as a measure of impact of epidemic influenza. *Am. J. Epidemiol.* **122,** 468–476.
5. Barker, W. H. and Mullooly, J. P. (1980) Impact of epidemic A influenza in a defined adult population. *Am. J. Epidemiol.* **112,** 798–811.
6. Goodman, R. A., Orenstein, W. A., Munro, T. F., et al. (1982) Impact of influenza A in a nursing home. *JAMA* **247,** 1451–1453.
7. McBean, A. M., Babish, J. D., and Warren, J. L. (1993) The impact and cost of influenza in the elderly. *Arch. Intern. Med.* **153,** 2105–2111.
8. Barker, W. H., Borisute, H., and Cox, C. (1998) A study of the impact of influenza on the functional status of frail older people. *Arch. Intern. Med.* **158,** 645–650.
9. Schirm, J., Luijt, D. S., Pastoor, G. W., et al. (1992) Rapid detection of respiratory viruses using mixtures of monoclonal antibodies on shell viral cultures. *J. Med. Virol.* **38,** 147–151.
10. Waner, J. L., Todd, S. J., Shalaby, H., et al. (1991) Comparison of Directigen FLU-A with viral isolation and direct immunofluorescence for the rapid detection and identification of influenza A virus. *J. Clin. Microbiol.* **29,** 479–482.
11. Leonardi, G. P., Leib, H., Birkhead, G. S., et al. (1994) Comparison of rapid detection methods for influenza A virus and their value in health care management of institutionalized geriatric patients. *J. Clin. Microbiol.* **32,** 70–74.
12. Douglas, R. G. (1990) Prophylaxis and treatment of influenza. *N. Engl. J. Med.* **322,** 443–450.
13. Hayden, F. G., Sperber, S. J., Belshe, R. B., et al. (1991) Recovery of drug-resistant influenza A virus during therapeutic use of rimantadine. *Antimicrob. Agent Chemother.* **35,** 1741–1747.
14. Center for Disease Control and Prevention (1999) Neuraminadase inhibitors for the treatment of influenza A and B infection. *M.M.W.R.* **48** (No. RR-14), 1–9.
15. Schilling, M., Povinelli, L., Krause, P., et al. (1998) Efficacy of zanamivir for chemoprophylaxis of nursing home influenza outbreaks. *Vaccine* **16,** 1771–1774.

16. Hayden, F. G., Osterhaus, A. D., Treanor, J. J., et al. (1997) Efficacy and safety of the neuraminidase inhibitor zanamivir in the treatment of influenza virus infections. *J. Med.* **337,** 874–880.

17. Anonymous (1996) Prevention and control of influenza - recommendations of the Advisory Committee on Immunization Practices. *M.M.W.R.* **45 RR-5,** 1–24.

18. Gravenstein, S., Miller, B. A., and Drinka, P. (1992) Prevention and control of influenza A outbreaks in long term care facilities. *Infect. Control Hosp. Epidemiol.* **13,** 49–54.

19. Nichol, K. L., Margolis, K. L., Wuorenma, J., et al. (1994) The efficacy and cost effectiveness of vaccination against influenza among elderly persons living in the community. *N. Eng. J. Med.* **331,** 778–784.

20. Nicholson, K. G. (1996) Impact of influenza and respiratory syncytial virus on mortality in England and Wales from January 1975 to December 1990. *Epidemiol. Infect.* **116,** 51–63.

21. Falsey, A. R., Cunningham, C. K., Barker, W. H., et al. (1995) Respiratory syncytial virus and influenza A infections in the hospitalized elderly. *J. Infect. Dis.* **172,** 389–394.

22. Fleming, D. M. and Cross, K. W. (1993) Respiratory syncytial virus or influenza? *Lancet* **342,** 1507–1510.

23. Mathur, U., Bentley, D. W., and Hall, C. B. (1980) Concurrent respiratory syncytial virus and Influenza A infections in the institutionalized elderly and chronically ill. *Ann. Intern. Med.* **93,** 49–52.

24. Centers for Disease Control (1977) Epidemiologic notes and reports: respiratory syncytial virus -Missouri. *M.M.W.R.* **26,** 351.

25. Falsey, A. R. (1991) Noninfluenza respiratory virus infection in long-term care facilities. *Infect. Control Hosp. Epidemiol.* **12,** 602–608.

26. Agius, G., Dindinaud, G., Biggar, R. J., et al. (1990) An epidemic of respiratory syncytial virus in elderly people: clinical and serological findings. *J. Med. Virol.* **30,** 117–127.

27. Wald, T. G., Miller, B. A., Shult, P., et al (1995) Can respiratory syncytial virus and influenza A be distinguished clinically in institutionalized older persons? *J. Am. Geriatr. Soc.* **43,** 170–174.

28. Osterweil, D. and Norman, D. (1990) An outbreak of an influenza-like illness in a nursing home. *J. Am. Geriatr. Soc.* **38,** 659–662.

29. Public Health Laboratory Service Communicable Diseases Surveillance Centre. (1983) Respiratory syncytial virus infection in the elderly 1976–1982. *Br. Med. J.* **287,** 1618–1619.

30. Falsey, A. R., Treanor, J. J., Betts, R. F., et al. (1992) Viral respiratory infections in the institutionalized elderly: clinical and epidemiologic findings. *J. Am. Geriatr. Soc.* **40,** 115–119.

31. Sorvillo, F. J., Huie, S. F., Strassburg, M. A., et al. (1984) An outbreak of respiratory syncytial virus pneumonia in a nursing home for the elderly. *J. Infect.* **9,** 252–256.

32. Garvie, D. G. and Gray, J. (1980) Outbreak of respiratory syncytial virus infection in the elderly. *Br. Med. J.* **281,** 1253–1254.

33. Falsey, A. R., McCann, R. M., Hall, W. J., et al. (1995) Acute respiratory tract infection in daycare centers for older persons. *J. Am. Geriatr. Soc.* **43,** 30–36.

34. Dowell, S. F., Anderson, L. J., Gary, H. E. J., et al. (1996) Respiratory syncytial virus is an important cause of community acquired pneumonia among hospitalized adults. *J. Infect. Dis.* **174,** 456–462.

35. Han, L. L., Alexander, J. P., and Anderson, L. J. (1999) Respiratory syncytial virus pneumonia among the elderly: an assessment of disease burden. *J. Infect. Dis.* **179,** 25–30.

36. Falsey, A. R., McCann, R. M., Hall, W. J., et al. (1996) Evaluation of four methods for the diagnosis of respiratory syncytial virus infection in older adults. *J. Am. Geriatr. Soc.* **44,** 71–73.

37. Vikerfors, T., Grandien, M., Johansson, M., et al. 1988) Detection of an immunoglobulin M response in the elderly for early diagnosis of respiratory syncytial virus infection. *J. Clin. Microbiol.* **26,** 808–811.

38. Falsey, A. R. (1996) Viral respiratory infections, tract infections in elderly persons. *Infect. Dis. Clin. Pract*. **5,** 53–58.

39. Aylward, B. R. and Burdge, D. R. (1991) Ribavirin therapy of adult respiratory syncytial virus pneumonitis. *Arch. Intern. Med.* 2303,2304.

40. Graman, P. S. and Hall, C. B. (1989) Epidemiology and control of nosocomial viral infections. *Infect. Dis. Clin. North Am.* **3,** 815–841.

41. Wenzel, R. P., McCormick, D. P., and Beam, W. E. J. (1972) Parainfluenza pneumonia in adults. *JAMA* **221,** 294,295.

42. Fransen, H., Heigl, Z., Wolontis, S., et al. (1969) Infections with viruses in patients hospitalized with acute respiratory illness, Stockholm 1963–1967. *Scand J. Infect. Dis.* **1,** 127–136.

43. Monto, A. S. and Sullivan, K. M. (1993) Acute respiratory illnesses in the community: frequency of illness and the agents involved. *Epidemiol. Infect.* **110,** 145–160.

44. Public Health Laboratory Service Communicable Disease Surveillance Centre (1983) Parainfluenza infections in the elderly 1976–82. *Br. Med. J.* **287,** 1619.

45. Epidemiologic Notes and Reports. (1978) Parainfluenza outbreaks in extended care facilities—United States. *M.M.W.R.* **27,** 475–476.

46. Glasgow, K. W., Tamblyn, S. E., and Blair, G. (1995) A respiratory outbreak due to parainfluenza virus type 3 in a home for the aged. *Ontario Can. Comm. Dis. Rep.* **21,** 57–61.

47. Gwaltney, J. M., Hendley, J. O., Simon, G., et al. (1966) Rhinovirus infections in an industrial population—I. the occurrence of illness. *N. Engl. J. Med.* **275,** 1261–1268.

48. Monto, A., Bryan, E. R., and Ohmit, S. (1987) Rhinovirus infections in Tecumseh, Michigan: frequency of illness and number of serotypes. *J. Infect. Dis.* **156,** 43–49.

49. Gwaltney, J. M. (1995) Rhinoviruses, in *Principles and Practices of Infectious Diseases* (Mandell, G. L., Bennett, J. E., and Dolin, R., eds.), Churchill Livingstone, New York, pp. 1656–1662.

50. Nicholson, K. G., Kent, J., Hammersley, V., et al. (1996) Risk factors for lower respiratory complications of rhinovirus infections in elderly people living in the community: prospective cohort study. *Br. Med. J.* **313,** 1119–1123.

51. Wald, T. G., Shult, P., Krause, P., Miller, et al. (1995) A rhinovirus outbreak among residents of a long-term care facility. *Ann. Intern. Med.* **123,** 588–593.

52. Falsey, A. R., McCann, R. M., Hall, W. J., et al. (1997) The common cold in frail older persons: impact of rhinovirus and coronavirus in a senior daycare center. *J. Am. Geriatr. Soc.* **45,** 706–711.

53. Turner, R. B., Wecker, M. T., Pohl, G., et al. (1999) Efficacy of tremacamra, a soluble intercellular adhesion molecule 1, for experimental rhinovirus infection. *JAMA* **281,** 1797–1804.

54. Larson, H. E., Reed, S. E.,and Tyrrell, D. A. J. (1980) Isolation of rhinoviruses and coronaviruses from 38 colds in adults. *J. Med. Virol.* **5,** 221–229.

55. McIntosh, K., Kapikian, A. Z., Turner, H. C., et al. (1970) Seroepidemiologic studies of coronavirus infection in adults and children. *Am. J. Epidemiol.* **91,** 585–592.

56. Wiselka, M. J., Kent, J., Cookson, J. B., et al. (1993) Impact of respiratory virus infection in patients with chronic chest disease. *Epidemiol. Infect.* **111,** 337–346.

57. Nicholson, K. G., Kent, J., Hammersley, V., et al. (1997) Acute viral infections of upper respiratory tract in elderly people living in the community; comparative, prospective, population based study of disease burden. *Br. Med. J.* **315,** 1060–1064.

58. Nicholson, K. G., Baker, D. J., Farquhar, A., et al. (1990) Acute upper respiratory tract viral illness and influenza immunization in homes for the elderly. *Epidemiol. Infect.***105,** 609–618.

59. Melnick, J. L. (1995) History and epidemiology of hepatitis A virus. *J. Infect. Dis.* **171,** S2–S8.

60. Marcus, E. and Tur-Kaspa, R. (1997) Viral hepatitis in older adults. *J. Am. Geriatr. Soc.* **45,** 755–763.

61. Alter, M. J. and Mast, E. E. (1994) The epidemiology of viral hepatitis in the United States. *Gastroenterol. Clin. North Am.* **23,** 437–455.
62. MacMahon, M. and James, O. F. W. (1994) Liver disease in the elderly. *J. Clin. Gastroenterol.* **18,** 330–334.
63. Bader, T. F. (1996) Hepatitis A vaccine. *Am. J. Gastroenterol.* **91,** 217–222.
64. Clemens, R., Safary, A., Hepburn, A., et al. (1995) Clinical experience with an inactivated hepatitis A vaccine. *J. Infect. Dis.* **171,** S44–S49.
65. Scheifele, D. W. and Bjornson, G. J. (1993) Evaluation of inactivated hepatitis A vaccine in Canadians 40 years of age or more. *Can. Med. Assoc. J.* **148,** 551–555.
66. Goodson, J. D., Taylor, P. A., Campion, E. W., et al. (1982) The clinical course of acute hepatitis in the elderly patient. *Arch. Intern. Med.* **142,** 1485–1488.
67. Schreiber, G. B., Busch, M. P., Kleinman, S. H., et al. (1996) The risk of transfusion-transmitted viral infections. The Retrovirus Epidemiology Donor Study. *N. Engl. J. Med.* **334,** 1685–1690.
68. Simor, A. E., Gordon, M., and Bishai, F. R. (1992) Prevalence of hepatitis B surface antigen, hepatitis C antibody, and HIV-1 antibody among residents of a long-term-care facility. *J. Am. Geriatr. Soc.* **40,** 218–220.
69. Sallie, R. and DiBisceglie, A. M. (1994) Viral hepatitis and hepatocellular carcinoma. *Gastroenterol. Clin. North Am.* **23,** 567–579.
70. Floreani, A., Bertin, T., Soffiati, G., et al. (1992) Anti-hepatitis C virus in the elderly: a seroepidemiological study in a home for the aged. *Gerontology* **38,** 214–216.
71. Brind, A. M., Watson, J. P., James, O. F. W., et al. (1996) Hepatitis C virus infection in the elderly. *Q. J. Med.* **89,** 291–296.
72. Horiike, N., Masumoto, T., Nakanishi, K., et al. (1995) Interferon therapy for patients more than 60 years of age with chronic hepatitis C. *J. Gastroenterol. Hepatol.* **10,** 246–249.
73. Sampietro, M., Caputo, L., Corbetta, N., et al. (1998) Hepatitis G virus infection in the elderly. *Ital. J. Gastroenterol. Hepatol.* **30,** 524–527.
74. Bennett, R. and Greenough, W.B. (1993) Approach to acute diarrhea in the elderly. *Gastroenterol. Clin. North Am.* **22,** 517–533.
75. Humphrey, T. J., Cruickshank, J. G., and Cubitt, W. D. (1984) An outbreak of calicivirus associated gastroenteritis in an elderly persons home. A possible zoonosis? *J. Hygiene* **93,** 293–299.
76. Jiang, X., Turf, E., Hu, J., et al. (1996) Outbreaks of gastroenteritis in elderly nursing homes and retirement facilities associated with human calciviruses. *J. Med. Virol.* **50,** 335–341.
77. Marrie, T., Lee, S., Faulkner, R., et al. (1982) Rotavirus infection in a geriatric population. *Arch. Intern. Med.* **142,** 313–316.
78. Cubitt, W. D. and Holzel, H. (1980) An outbreak of rotavirus infection in a long-stay ward of a geriatric hospital. *J. Clin. Pathol.* **33,** 306–308.
79. Halvorsrud, J. and Orstavik, I. (1980) An epidemic of rotavirus-associated gastroenteritis in a nursing home for the elderly. *Scand. J. Infect. Dis.* **12,** 161–164.
80. Perez-Schael, I., Guntinas, M. J., Perez, et al. (1997) Efficacy of the rhesus rotavirus-based quadrivalent vaccine in infants and young children in Venezuela. *N. Engl. J. Med.* **337,** 1181–1187.
81. El-Sadr, W. and Gettler, J. (1995) Unrecognized human immunodeficiency virus infection in the elderly. *Arch. Intern. Med.* **155,** 184–186.
82. Gaeta, T. J., LaPolla, C., and Melendez, E. (1996) AIDS in the elderly: New York City vital statistics. *J. Emerg. Med.* **14,** 19–23.
83. Newcomer, V. D. (1997) Human immunodeficiency virus infection and acquired immunodeficiency syndrome in the elderly. *Arch. Dermatol.* **133,** 1311,1312.
84. Stall, R. and Catania, J. (1994) AIDS risk behaviors among late middle-aged and elderly Americans. *Arch. Intern. Med.* **154,** 57–63.

85. Sutin, D. G., Rose, D. N., Mulvihill, M., et al. (1993) Survival of elderly patients with transfusion-related acquired immunodeficiency syndrome. *J. Am. Geriatr. Soc.* **41,** 214–216.

86. Kost, R. and Straus, S. (1996) Postherpetic neuralgia—pathogenesis, treatment, and prevention. *N. Engl. Med.* **335,** 32–42.

87. Donahue, J., Choo, P., Manson, J., et al. (1995) The incidence of herpes zoster. *Arch. Intern. Med.* **155,** 1605–1609.

88. Schmader, K. (1998) Postherpetic neuralgia in immunocompetent elderly people. *Vaccine* **16,** 1768–1770.

89. Whitley, R. J., Shukla, S., and Crooks, R. J. (1998) The identification of risk factors associated with persistent pain following herpes zoster. *J. Infect. Dis.* **178,** S71–S75.

90. Whitley, R., Weiss, H., Gnann, J., et al. (1996) Acyclovir with and without prednisone for the treatment of herpes zoster. *Ann. Intern. Med.* **125,** 376–383.

91. Dworkin, R. H., Boon, R. J., Griffin, D. R. G., et al. (1998) Postherpetic neuralgia: impact of famciclovir, age, rash severity, and acute pain in herpes zoster patients. *J. Infect. Dis.* **178,** S76–S80.

92. Schmader, K., van der Horst, C. M., and Klotman, M.E. (1989) Epstein-Barr virus and the elderly host. *Rev. Infect. Dis.* **11,** 64–73.

93. Horwitz, C. A., Henle, W., Henle, G., et al. (1976) Clinical and laboratory evaluation of elderly patients with heterophil-antibody positive infectious mononucleosis. *Am. J. Med.* **61,** 333–339.

94. Edelstein, H. and Knight, R. T. (1989) Epstein-Barr virus causing encephalitis in an elderly woman. *South. Med. J.* **82,** 1192–1193.

III
Special Infectious Disease Problems

20

Infections and Infection Control in the Long-Term Care Setting

Suzanne F. Bradley

1. EPIDEMIOLOGY OF INFECTION IN LONG-TERM CARE

In the United States, long-term care residents continue to outnumber the number of patients in the acute care setting. Infections in long-term care facilities occur at rates similar to those found in acute care hospitals ranging in incidence from 1.8–9.4 1000 patient-care days *(1–4)*. Urinary tract infections (UTI) occur most often followed by infections of the respiratory tract, gastrointestinal tract, or soft-tissue infection. It has been estimated that 10–30% of nursing facility residents die each year, but how often infection contributes to mortality rates is not known *(1)*. Pneumonia has been reported to result in death in 6–23% of cases, whereas bacteremia has been associated with death in 10–25% of cases *(1,4)*. This chapter discusses the prevention and control of common infectious problems in the long-term care setting. The reader should refer to related chapters in this book for in-depth discussion of the diagnosis and treatment of specific clinical syndromes and pathogens.

2. RISK FACTORS FOR INFECTION IN LONG-TERM CARE RESIDENTS

Infections occur commonly in residents of nursing facilities (nursing homes) as a consequence of different factors. The majority of persons residing in nursing facilities are 65 yr of age or older. Comorbid illnesses, such as obstructive uropathy, that increase with age can predispose the patient to UTI. Chronic obstructive pulmonary disease and congestive heart failure contribute to development of respiratory tract infections. Vascular insufficiency and neuropathy, frequent complications of diabetes mellitus, are associated with increased risk of skin infection.

Alterations in a patient's functional status, such as impaired feeding, bathing, toileting, and mobility, can also lead to infection. Use of enteral devices to assist in feeding can promote aspiration and lead to pneumonia, whereas urethral catheters to prevent incontinence can contribute to the development of UTI. Decreased mobility and incontinence are significant risk factors for the development of pressure ulcers and potential secondary infection. The increased need for nursing assistance in the performance of activities of daily living can facilitate transmission of pathogens between nursing facility residents.

Medications used to treat comorbid illnesses can inadvertently impair important host defenses. Medications that are sedating can impair the cough reflex and increase the risk for pneumonia or reduce mobility and increase the risk for skin infection. Medications may also reduce oropharyngeal secretions and facilitate colonization of the

From: *Infectious Disease in the Aging*
Edited by: Thomas T. Yoshikawa and Dean C. Norman
© Humana Press Inc., Totowa, NJ

oropharynx with pathogens. Drugs can also contribute to decreased urinary outflow, stasis, and the development of bacteriuria *(1,2,4)*.

3. ESSENTIAL ELEMENTS OF AN INFECTION CONTROL PROGRAM

Each nursing facility should have an infection control program in accordance with state or national regulations and guidelines. Infection control programs in the long-term care setting are required by the Omnibus Budget Reconciliation Act of 1987 (OBRA) for skilled-care facilities, the Health Care Financing Administration (HCFA) for Medicare or Medicaid patients, the Occupational Safety and Health Administration (OSHA) for blood-borne pathogens and tuberculosis exposures, and the Joint Commission on Accreditation of Healthcare Organizations' (JCAHO) Long-term Care Standards *(4)*. National organizations such as the Society for Healthcare Epidemiology of America (SHEA), The Association for Professionals in Infection Control and Epidemiology (APIC), and The Centers for Disease Control and Prevention (CDC) also provide infection control guideline information specific for the long-term care setting.

An organizational structure that defines responsibilities for implementation and coordination of a written infection control policy should be established. An actual infection control committee that meets formally on a regular basis may not be required or necessary depending on the size of the nursing facility. However, a small group composed of a representative from administration, the physician staff (medical director), nursing staff, and a infection control practitioner should meet as necessary to oversee infection control activities. This committee or oversight group is responsible for establishing and updating policies, reviewing the infection prevalence reports, and monitoring adherence to policies and procedures. Specific policies should be developed in advance to meet regulatory guidelines as well as the needs of the individual facility (*see* Table 1). Meetings should occur as often as are necessary to identify problems, recommend solutions, and assess the efficacy of those actions. Regardless of the organizational structure chosen, written minutes should be maintained *(1,2,4)*.

The infection control practitioner is responsible for infection surveillance, analysis of surveillance to date, and preparation of reports back to the organizational body. The infection control practitioner is also responsible for implementation of infection control policy, education, and notification of public health authorities when appropriate. Depending on the size of the facility, many nursing facility infection control practitioners are hired on a part-time basis to perform infection surveillance in addition to other duties. It has been suggested that facilities with 250–300 beds may require a full-time infection control practitioner. The level of formal training in infection control among practitioners in the long-term care setting appears to be increasing. It is important that the institution define the amount of time to be spent on infection surveillance in the infection control practitioner's job description and assure protection of time to carry out those duties *(1,2,4)*.

4. SURVEILLANCE FOR INFECTION IN THE LONG-TERM CARE SETTING

Surveillance for infection can be carried out by identifying rates of infection by clinical syndrome, pathogen, or pattern of resistance to an antibiotic or class of antibiotics. Location in the facility and date of onset should be recorded. Review of physician notes, nursing records, or hospital discharge summaries; laboratory and radiology reports; and medication or treatment records, as well as conducting formal rounds or informal discussions with staff can be useful in detecting potential infection control problems.

Table 1
Essential Infection Control Policies in the Long-Term Care Setting

Routine infection control, detection, and surveillance

    Establish routine infection control procedures
        Hand disinfection
        Precautions to be used in the care of all patients
        Employee education
        Organism-specific precautions (*see below*)

    Establish infection case definitions to assist in detection and surveillance
        Identify cases of infection
        Determine normal rates of infection by institution
        Establish threshold for investigation for possible outbreaks

Identification, investigation, and control of outbreaks
Organism-specific infection control policies and procedures
    Influenza
    Tuberculosis
    Group A streptococci
    Scabies, lice
    Blood-borne pathogens
        Hepatitis B, hepatitis C, HIV
    Gastroenteritis
        Food-borne
        Other
    Multiple drug-resistant bacteria, including MRSA, and VRE

Review of antimicrobial use

Monitoring of patient care practice guidelines
    Aspiration precautions
    Pressure ulcer prevention
    Use of invasive devices
    Feeding tubes, urinary catheters, intravenous devices

Facility management issues
    Environmental cleaning and disinfection
    Collection, cleaning, and disposal of laundry
    Collection, containment, and disposal of infectious waste
    Food preparation, transport, and holding

Pre-admission and resident health program
    Tuberculosis
        Two-step PPD
        Baseline CXR —repeat if PPD converts or patient is symptomatic
    Vaccination status
        Influenza, pneumococcal? tetanus-diphtheria (Td)

Pre-employment and employee health program
    Tuberculosis
        Annual screening PPD skin test
        Baseline CXR — repeat if PPD converts or patient is symptomatic
    Vaccination/immune status
        Influenza, hepatitis B, ? tetanus-diphtheria, varicella-zoster, hepatitis A
    Occupational exposure program
        Blood-borne pathogens— HIV, hepatitis B, hepatitis C
        Tuberculosis
        Scabies

HIV, human immunodeficiency virus; MRSA, methicillin-resistant *S. aureus;* VRE, vancomycin-resistant enterococci; PPD, purified protein derivatives; CXR, chest X-ray.

Identification of infection by clinical syndrome can be difficult in the long-term care setting as CDC hospital-based definitions are often not met. CDC definitions of infection rely heavily on laboratory or other diagnostic studies *(5)*. In the nursing facility setting, clinical presentation of infection in the elderly may be atypical, vital signs are taken infrequently, documentation is scant, and use of laboratory tests and radiology studies is infrequent *(1,4)*. Case definitions for UTI and other clinical syndromes have been suggested for the long-term care setting, but these criteria have not been validated *(6,7)*. Each nursing facility should establish a case-definition for the most common clinical syndromes—UTI, respiratory-tract infection, gastroenteritis, and soft-tissue infection that will be used for the purposes of infection surveillance (*see* Table 2).

Routine surveillance of cultures obtained for clinical purposes can assist the infection control practitioner to determine if infections due to a specific pathogen or if resistance to certain kind of antibiotics is increasing in the facility. It is important to differentiate whether the infection was present at the time the resident was admitted (hospital or community-acquired infection) or after >72 h of admission (nursing-facility acquired infection). Correlation between the presence of a potential pathogen and the presence of appropriate symptoms or signs must be made, when available, to determine if the isolate is truly causing infection, is just asymptomatically colonizing the patient, or is a culture contaminant. Obtaining cultures specifically for surveillance purposes in asymptomatic individuals when an outbreak of infection has not been documented is not recommended.

The infection control practitioner should routinely determine the number of new nursing-facility acquired infections by clinical syndrome, pathogen, and antibiotic-resistance pattern. Generally, this information is obtained weekly and reported on a monthly basis and expressed as (the number of new infections/ number of residents × number days in the month) × 1000 or the number infections per 1000 resident days. Knowledge of infection rates over time allows the practitioner to establish what is normal for a given nursing facility and to set a threshold above which an investigation for a possible outbreak might ensue *(4)*.

5. ROUTING PREVENTION OF INFECTION

Infections are generally spread from patient to patient by small airborne respiratory droplets, by exposure to large droplets, by direct skin-to-skin contact, or by contact with the environment or inanimate fomites. Infection control procedures to prevent infection in hospitals are based on the most likely mechanism of transmission for a given pathogen (*see* Table 3). Most of these measures are applicable to the long-term care setting with some exceptions, which are discussed as follows.

5.1. Standard Precautions

Standard precautions emphasize hand washing before and after care of patients and the use of gowns and gloves when soiling of clothes with potentially infectious body fluids is likely *(8)*. Protective eyewear or face shields are recommended when spattering of body fluids is likely. Sharp implements should be disposed of in puncture-resistant containers. Equipment soiled with body fluids should be cleaned after use with each patient. Environmental surfaces should be cleaned between patient use. Soiled linens should be handled and transported in a manner to minimize exposure to staff and other patients. These routine simple procedures are used in the care of all patients, regardless of infection status, and have been shown to be effective in preventing the transmission of blood-borne pathogens to healthcare workers and the spread of pathogens to patients. These simple measures are inexpensive and well within the limited resources of long-term care facilities. The infection control procedures listed below are performed in addition to standard precautions when indicated.

5.2. Airborne Precautions

Suspension of tiny airborne droplets, i.e., <5 millimicrons in the air for prolonged periods of time with potential dispersion by air currents is the major mode of transmission of tuberculosis. To prevent this spread, *airborne precautions* (negative pressure rooms, the use of appropriate N95 respirators, and strict confinement of patients to their rooms with the door closed) are required *(8)*. Negative pressure rooms are generally not available in long-term care facilities. Care of patients with tuberculosis may be particularly hazardous in closed facilities that care for debilitated elderly residents. Therefore, transfer of nursing facility residents with diseases transmitted by the airborne route to hospital is generally warranted. These patients may be transferred back to the nursing facility when they are no longer considered contagious.

5.3. Droplet Precautions

Droplet precautions prevent the transmission of infection by large respiratory particles (>5 millimicrons) in size that are transmitted by coughing, sneezing, or talking *(8)*. Typical droplet-related infections in the long-term care setting include *Mycoplasma pneumoniae*, influenza, and adenovirus. Patients are placed in a private room or cohorted together. Surgical masks are worn within 3 ft of the patient. Patients may be removed from isolation when they are no longer considered contagious. Because the duration of these infections and the need for isolation is limited, the care needs of residents with droplet infections can be met by nursing facilities with limited infection control resources.

5.4. Contact Precautions

The greatest controversy exists regarding the use of hospital-derived *contact precautions* in the long-term care setting. Contact precautions prevents transmission of infectious agents from patient to patient by the hands of personnel or by contact with the patient's environment. In the acute care hospital, patients are confined to private rooms or cohorted together for the duration of the infectious episode or until discharge. Patient transport outside of the room is limited. Routine use of gowns, gloves, and antimicrobial soap or waterless disinfection with all patient contact is recommended *(5)*. In the long-term care setting, strict adherences to contact precautions as applied in hospitals can be problematic unless the need for isolation is of limited duration. Prolonged isolation is detrimental to resident rehabilitation, and use of private rooms or cohorting can be costly for the facility. Therefore, some modifications in contact precautions for long-term care facilities have been recommended, particularly with regard to policies for multidrug-resistant bacteria.

Table 2
A Comparison of Case Definitions for Clinical Infectious Syndromes Used in the Long-Term Care Setting[a]

Clinical syndrome	McGeer criteria	CDC criteria
Principles of case definition	**New or acutely worse symptoms** Exclude non-infectious causes by laboratory evidence supportive of diagnosis *if compatible symptoms/signs are present*	Based on physician diagnosis Based on pathogen isolation, laboratory/radiologic evidence
Respiratory tract infection		
URI/pharyngitis	*Two or more symptoms:* Runny nose or sneezing Stuffy nose/congestion Sore throat/hoarseness/difficulty swallowing Dry cough Tender cervical lymphadenopathy	Two symptoms *and:* cause identified from site, blood serology, or physician diagnosis
Tracheobronchitis	*Three of the following:* Change in cough, sputum Fever ≥ 38°C (100.4°F) Pleuritic chest pain New physical finding (rales, rhonchi, or wheezing) Change in breathing status (new or worsened) shortness breath/RR ≥ 25 min *or change in mental status*	No radiologic evidence of pneumonia *and* at least two symptoms *and* isolation of pathogen by culture or rapid test
Pneumonia	*Two signs or symptoms of tracheobronchitis and chest radiograph with pneumonia, possible pneumonia, or new infiltrate present*	Rales or dullness to percussion *and* purulent sputum *or* pathogen identified by BAL[b]/biopsy *or isolated from blood or* New or progressive infiltrate, cavity, or pleural effusion *and* new purulent or change in sputum or identification of pathogen in blood, BAL/ biopsy, or serology
Urinary tract infection	Bacteriuria must be symptomatic *Three* of the following *without* catheter: Fever ≥38°C or chills Dysuria, frequency, urgency	Bacteriuria can be asymptomatic *One* symptom/sign *and* ≥10⁵ cfu/mL urine of one pathogen *or* *Two* symptoms/signs *and* pyuria *or*

Infection	Criteria	
	Flank or suprapubic pain Character of urine Change in mental or functional status from baseline *Two* the following with catheter: Fever >38°C or chills Flank or suprapubic pain Character of urine Change in mental or functional status from baseline	repeated in isolation same pathogen *or* physician diagnosis/treatment No symptoms, catheter with 7d and bacterium ≥10^5 cfu
Conjunctivitis	*One* of the following ≥24 h: Purulence from one or both eyes Redness conjunctivae	Pathogens isolated *or* Symptoms *and* Gram stain, ELISA, biopsy, or serologic evidence
Cellulitis/soft tissue infection	Four of the following symptoms or signs: Fever ≥38°C Change in functional capacity Redness Pain Tenderness or serous drainage at affected site *or* *One* symptom/sign *and* purulent wound or lesion	Presence of pustules, boils, or purulent drainage *or* Two symptoms *and*: pathogen isolated from aspirate, drainage or blood or antigen detection, biopsy, or serology positive
Gastroenteritis	*One* of the following: Two or more watery stools beyond the patient norm *or* Two or more episodes of vomiting in 24 h *or* Culture or toxin assay positive with at least one symptom (nausea, vomiting, pain, tenderness, diarrhea)	Liquid stool ≥ 12 h *or* Two symptoms *and* pathogen isolated or detected by microscopy, toxin-assay, antigen detection, serology
Primary Bloodstream Infection	*Two* or more blood cultures positive for same organism *or* *One* blood culture positive *with* *one* of the following: Fever ≥ 38°C (100.4°F), hypothermia <34.5°C (94.1°F), Decrease systolic blood pressure ≥ 30 Hg from baseline, Change mental or functional status	Recognized pathogen *and* not related to infection at another site *or* *One* symptom *and* possible contaminants grown ≥ two cultures on separate occasions *or* *One* positive culture associated with intravascular catheter and treated

[a]Adapted from refs. 5 and 6.
[b]BAL, bronchoalveolar lavage; RR, respiratory rate; cfu, colony forming units; ELISA, enzyme-linked immunosorbent assay; URI, upper respiratory infection.

Table 3
Isolation Precautions for Infections Known to Cause Outbreaks in Long-Term Care Facilities[a]

Precaution type	Clinical setting	Essential elements
Standard	All patients	Handwashing before, after, and between patient contacts
		Use plain (nonantimicrobial) soap unless outbreak identified
		Gowns/gloves when contact with patient's moist secretions likely
		Use faceshields if splattering or spray with possible mucocutaneous exposure of face likely
		Reusable equipment contaminated with secretions should be cleaned between uses
		Clean and disinfect environmental surfaces and equipment between patient use
		Minimize staff exposure to soiled linens
		Appropriate sharps disposal
		Resuscitation devices
Airborne	*Mycobacterium tuberculosis*	Negative pressure[b]
	Disseminated herpes zoster	Private room
		N95 respirator
		Limit transport, patient masked

252

Droplet	*Mycoplasma pneumoniae* Influenza Adenovirus Pertussis Diphtheria	Private room or cohorting Mask within 3 ft of patient Limit transport, patient masked

Contact	Contagious skin infections/persist on dry skin
	  Scabies
	  Pediculosis
	  Impetigo
	  Major (noncontained) abscesses, cellulitis,
	    pressure ulcers
	  Herpes zoster
	  Herpes simplex (mucocutaneous)
	  Viral/hemorrhagic conjunctivitis
	Enteric infections (low infectious dose/ long
	  environmental survival)
	  C. difficile
	  Diapered/incontinent patients with:
	    Shigella, rotavirus, hepatitis A,
	    enterohemorrhagic *E. coli*
	Multidrug-resistant bacteria — see text
		Private room or cohort
		Emphasize standard precautions
		Utilize antimicrobial soap/waterless
		Limit patient transport
		Dedicated equipment disinfection

[a]Adapted from ref. 8.
[b]Beyond the resources of most long-term care facilities. Transfer to acute care.

Viral conjunctivitis and skin infections due to herpes simplex, localized herpes
zoster, scabies, lice, staphylococci, and streptococci are spread by direct contact. Respiratory syncytial virus, parainfluenza virus, and enteroviruses can also be spread in
this manner. Direct contact is important in the spread of enteric infections due to
Escherichia coli 0157:H7, rotavirus, hepatitis A, and *Shigella* in incontinent or dia-
pered patients. Many of these infections are of limited duration, the need for isolation is of short duration, and patients can be removed from isolation when they are no
longer contagious.

Direct contact is the major means of spread for multi-drug resistant bacteria, such as
methicillin-resistant *Staphylococcus aureus* (MRSA) or vancomycin-resistant enterococci (VRE). (See also chapter, "Multi-Drug Resistant Organisms in Long-term Care
Facilities"). Direct contact is also a major means of spread of *Clostridum difficile*.
Asymptomatic colonization with MRSA,VRE, and *C. difficile* is common in residents
in many long-term care facilities. Colonization with these bacteria is often prolonged,
for months or even years, in the long-term care resident *(9)*. Confinement of the nursing facility resident to a private room or even cohorting is obviously impractical *(9,10)*.
It has been recommended that nursing facilities monitor rates of infection, not colonization, with these pathogens. In the absence of unacceptably high rates of infection or
an outbreak, residents do not need to be confined to their rooms if they are capable of
practicing good hygiene (hand washing). Contaminated wounds must be covered by a
bandage. If the patient is continent they need not be isolated, and contaminated urine
must be contained by a urinary device or diaper and feces by a diaper in incontinent
patients. Patients with MRSA-contaminated sputum need not be isolated if they can
cover their mouths or tracheostomy when they cough. Incontinent patients with
uncontained contaminated excretions, patients with large contaminated wounds not
contained by a bandage, and colonized residents who cannot cover their mouths when
coughing or use good handwashing should be isolated *(9)*.

6. DETECTION AND CONTROL OF EPIDEMICS

Epidemics of infection due to a variety of pathogens have been noted in the long-
term care setting *(11–25)* (*see* Table 4). An epidemic should be suspected if there is an
increase in the rate of infection due to a single pathogen or clinical syndrome. Cases of
infections with a specific pathogen should be reviewed to see if all the isolates seem to
be the same (similar antimicrobial susceptibility pattern) and if there is evidence of
transmission between patients, e.g., the infections occurred at a similar time, in the
same location, or patients shared the same staff. If there appears to be evidence that
transmission is occurring, knowledge of how that pathogen is spread will allow the
practitioner to hypothesize how the outbreak occurred and how to prevent further
spread. Infected residents should be placed in appropriate isolation and employees
should be re-educated about infection control principles. Monitoring should be ongoing for new cases of infection. If new cases of infection continue to develop despite
institution of appropriate isolation procedures and education, then alternative hypoth-
eses may need consideration. For some organisms, e.g., *S. aureus*, group A streptococci, multidrug-resistant *Streptococcus pneumoniae*, and *C. difficile*, an asymptomatic
carrier state, may exist among nursing facility residents or staff that perpetuate an out-

**Table 4
Causes of Epidemic Infection and Associated Clinical Syndromes
in the Long-Term Care Setting**

Clinical syndrome	Bacterial	Viral	Parasitic
Respiratory tract	*Chlamydia pneumoniae*	Influenza	
	M. pneumoniae	Respiratory syncytial virus	
	Group A streptococci	Parainfluenza	
	Haemophilus influenzae	Adenovirus	
	M. tuberculosis	Rhinovirus	
	C. psittaci		
	S. pneumoniae		
Soft-tissue infections			
Conjunctivitis	*S. aureus*	Adenovirus	
	Group A streptococci		
Cellulitis/fasciitis	*S. aureus*		
	Group A streptococci		
Rash			Scabies
Gastroenteritis			
Invasive	*Salmonella*		*Entamoeba histolytica*
	Shigella		
	Campylobacter		
Noninvasive	Rotavirus		*Giardia lamblia*
	Norwalk agent		
Toxin-mediated			
Food-borne	*E. coli* 0157:H7		
	S. aureus		
	C. perfringens		
	Bacillus cereus		
Non-food-borne	*C. difficile*		

break. In the event of increased rates of infection, it may be appropriate to identify asymptomatic carriers and isolate them in an attempt to disrupt the chain of transmission. For some infections (MRSA, multidrug-resistant *S. pneumoniae*, group A streptococci) decolonization with systemic or topical antimicrobial agents has been attempted to disrupt transmission and stop an outbreak. Consultation with an expert in epidemiology should be considered if reasonable measures are not effective. Failure to detect new cases indicates that the epidemic has abated and a return to routine infection control procedures can be considered.

REFERENCES

1. Nicolle, L. E. and Garibaldi, R. A. (1995) Infection control in long-term-care facilities. *Infect. Control Hosp. Epidemiol.* **16,** 348–353.
2. Nicolle, L. E., Strausbaugh, L. J., and Garibaldi, R. A. (1996) Infections and antibiotic resistance in nursing facilities. *Clin. Microbiol. Rev.* **9,** 1–17.
3. Jackson, M. M. and Fierer, J. (1984) Infections and infection risk in residents of long-term care facilities: a review of the literature, 1970–1984. *Am. J. Infect. Control* **13,** 63–77.

4. Smith, P. W. and Rusnak, P. G. (1997) Infection prevention and control in the long-term-care facility. *Infect. Control Hosp. Epidemiol.* **18,** 831–849.

5. Garner, J. S., Jarvis, W. R., Emori, T. G., et al. (1988) CDC definitions for nosomial infections. *Am. J. Infect. Control* **16,** 128–140.

6. McGeer, A., Campbell, B., Emori, T. G., et al. (1991) Definitions of infection for surveillance in long-term care facilities. *Am. J. Infect. Control* **19,** 1–7.

7. Smith, P. W. and The Consensus Conference Participants. (1987) Consensus conference on nosocomial infections in long-term care facilities. *Am. J. Infect. Control* **15,** 97–100.

8. Garner J. S. and The Hospital Infection Control Practices Advisory Committee. (1996) Guideline for isolation precautions in hospitals. *Infect. Control Hosp. Epidemiol.* **17,** 53–80.

9. Bradley S. F. (1999) Issues in the management of resistant bacteria in long-term-care facilities. *Infect. Control Hosp. Epidemiol.* **20,** 362–366.

10. Strausbaugh, L. J., Crossley, K. B., Nurse, B. A., et al. (1996) Antimicrobial resistance in long-term care facilities. *Infect. Control Hosp. Epidemiol.* **17,** 129–140.

11. Bennett, R. G. (1998) Gastrointestinal infections among the elderly, in *Bailliere's Clinical Infectious Diseases,* vol. 5, (Bula, C. J. and Kauffman, C. A., eds.), Bailliere Tindall, London, pp. 83–103.

12. Boyce, J. M., Jackson, M. M., Pugliese, G., et al. (1994) Methicillin-resistant *Staphylococcus aureus* (MRSA): a briefing for acute care hospitals and nursing facilities. *Infect. Control Hosp. Epidemiol.* **15,** 105–115.

13. Bradley, S. F. and the Society for Healthcare Epidemiology of America Committee on Long-Term Care. (1999) Prevention of influenza in chronic care facilities: a position statement. *Infect. Control. Hosp. Epidemiol.* **20,** 629–637.

14. Cantrell, M. and Norman, D. C. (1998) Skin and soft-tissue infections in the elderly, in *Bailliere's Clinical Infectious Diseases,* vol. 5, (Bula, C. J. and Kauffman, C. A., eds.), Bailliere Tindall, London, pp. 71–81.

15. Crossley, K. and The Long-Term-Care Committee of the Society for Healthcare Epidemiology of America. (1998) Vancomycin-resistant enterococci in long-term care facilities. *Infect. Control Hosp. Epidemiol.* **19,** 521–525.

16. Degelau, J. (1992) Scabies in long-term care facilities. *Infect. Control Hosp. Epidemiol.* **13,** 421–425.

17. Falsey, A. R. (1991) Noninfluenza respiratory virus infection in long-term care facilities. *Infect. Control Hosp. Epidemiol.* **12,** 602–608.

18. Levine, W. C., Smart, J. F., Archer, D. L., et al. (1991) Foodborne disease outbreaks in nursing facilities, 1975 through 1987. *JAMA* **266,** 2105–2109.

19. Marcus, E. L. and Tur-Kaspa, R. (1997) Viral hepatitis in older adults. *J. Am. Geriatr. Soc.* **45,** 755–763.

20. Marrie, T. J. (1998) Pneumonia, in *Balliere's Clinical Infectious Diseases*, vol. 5, (Bula, C. J. and Kauffman , C. A., eds.), Bailliere Tindall, London, pp. 35–51.

21. Muder, R. R. (1998) Pneumonia in residents of long-term care facilities: epidemiology, etiology, management, and prevention. *Am. J. Med.* **105,** 319–330.

22. Rajagopalan, S. (1997) Infectious diarrheas in older adults. *Infect. Dis. Clin. Pract.* **6,** 313–316.

23. Rajagopalan, S. and Yoshikawa, T. T. (1998) Tuberculosis in the elderly, in *Bailliere's Clinical Infectious Diseases*, vol. 5, (Bula C. J. and Kauffman, C. A., eds.), Bailliere Tindall, London, pp. 105–118.

24. Schwartz, B. and Ussery, X. T. (1992) Group A streptococcal outbreaks in nursing facilities. *Infect. Control Hosp. Epidemiol.* **13,** 742–747.

25. Yoshikawa, T. T. (1994) The challenge and unique aspects of tuberculosis in older patients. *Infect. Dis. Clin. Pract.* **3,** 62–66.

21

Multi-Drug Resistant Organisms in Long-Term Care Facilities

Robert A. Bonomo and Louis B. Rice

1. CLINICAL RELEVANCE

Infections in long-term care facilities (LTCFs) represent a major cause of morbidity and mortality in the elderly *(1–3)*. Because of this increased infection rate, antimicrobials are among the most frequently prescribed medications *(4)*. Studies have shown that antibiotics account for nearly 40% of all systemic drugs used in LTCFs *(5)*. In this unique environment, the most challenging questions facing the geriatrician are not which antibiotics are available that can treat the suspected infection, but which are the most appropriate to use.

Although antibiotics are necessary to treat infections in the elderly, their use may be excessive *(6)*. In a study performed by Zimmer and colleagues *(7)*, in 37.6% of cases, the evidence to start an antibiotic was considered inadequate. Of all antibiotic classes, cephalosporins were the most frequently overused *(8)*. As a result of frequent antibiotic use in LTCFs, we are now challenged with the problem of increasing antimicrobial resistance *(9)*. Nearly 10 years ago, it was articulated that LTCFs would become the reservoir for the evolution of antibiotic resistant genes *(10)*. At that time, attention centered on methicillin resistance in staphylococci and third-generation cephalosporin resistance in enteric bacilli. Trimethoprim/sulfamethoxazole (TMP/SMX) resistance and aminoglycoside resistance in Gram-negative bacteria were recognized as significant problems for nearly 20 years *(11,12)*. Geriatricians are now facing the fear of treating multiresistant organisms in a population that is relatively immunocompromised *(13–16)*. In many ways, the activities and practices in LTCFs are ideal for the emergence of resistant bacteria.

Bacteria possessing antibiotic resistance determinants arise in LTCFs by one of two ways. The transfer of infected or colonized patients from hospital to LTCF is believed to be the primary way resistant bacteria are introduced into nursing facilities (nursing homes). A contemporary example of this is the spread of methicillin-resistant *Staphylococcus aureus* (MRSA) to LTCFs from tertiary care centers *(17)*. In this study, a single asymptomatic carrier passed MRSA to 24 veterans in a skilled care unit. Second, the excessive and inappropriate use of antibiotics can select for mutations in bacterial gene(s) that confer a selective advantage. Examples of this are (1) the selection of mutations in β-lactamase genes that confer resistance to third-generation cephalospor-

From: *Infectious Disease in the Aging*
Edited by: Thomas T. Yoshikawa and Dean C. Norman
© Humana Press Inc., Totowa, NJ

ins *(18,19)*, (2) the selection of quinolone-resistant bacteria with mutations in *gyrA* and *gyrB* or *parC (20,21)*, and (3) mutations in *dhfr*, which confer resistance to TMP/SMX *(22)*. Once endemic to an LTCF, the antibiotic resistance genes can be transferred from one patient to another and from one species or genus to another *(23)*.

2. RESISTANCE IN GRAM-POSITIVE BACTERIA

2.1. β-Lactam-Resistant Staphylococci

Penicillin resistance in staphylococci dates back to the 1950s *(24)*. Hence, it is now rare to find staphylococci susceptible to penicillin. Despite its prevalence, the ubiquitous nature of penicillin resistance in staphylococci should not be accepted with complacency. The staphylococcal penicillinase (PC1) is an inducible β-lactamase exo-enzyme. Four variants (A–D) exist. The staphylococcal penicillinase genes are carried on plasmids and transposons and can be readily spread to other strains of staphylococci and possibly even to enterococci *(25)*. The semisynthetic penicillins (nafcillin, oxacillin, methicillin, cloxacillin, and dicloxacillin) are resistant to the action of staphylococcal penicillinases. The β-lactamase inhibitors (clavulanate, sulbactam, and tazobactam) are also effective inhibitors of PC1 β-lactamase. The medicinal chemist has exploited the use of a β-lactam with a β-lactamase inhibitor to create a potent combination *(26)*. Hence, the penicillinase-resistant penicillins and the β-lactam β-lactamase inhibitors (amoxicillin/clavulanate, ampicillin/sulbactam, piperacillin/tazobactam, and ticarcillin/clavulanate) have become the treatment option for susceptible staphylococcal infections in the elderly. From a clinical standpoint, the oral penicillinase-resistant penicillins can be problematic to administer in the elderly. They often require frequent dosing (four times a day) and can have significant gastrointestinal side effects. On the other hand, the dosing of dicloxacillin, nafcillin, and oxacillin do not need to be adjusted for patients with renal insufficiency. The β-lactam β-lactamase inhibitors are also associated with gastrointestinal side effects (diarrhea can occur in up to 18% of patients receiving amoxicillin/clavulanate). The dose of amoxicillin/clavulanate needs to be reduced in patients with renal insufficiency.

2.2. Methicillin-Resistant S. aureus

In the past decade, colonization and infection with methicillin-resistant *S. aureus* (MRSA) has proven to be one of the most difficult issues facing geriatricians in LTCFs *(27)*. In the United States, approximately 40% of staphylococci are resistant to methicillin. This highly resistant and virulent pathogen is the etiologic agent in epidemics of conjunctivitis, skin and soft-tissue infections, pneumonia, infected pressure ulcers, catheter-associated urinary tract infections, and osteomyelitis. The term "methicillin resistance" is actually a misnomer. In reality, these strains of staphylococci are resistant to all β-lactams and penicillinase-resistant penicillins (cefazolin, cefadroxil, nafcillin, oxacillin, dicloxacillin, and the like). The most commonly accepted criteria for MRSA are a minimum inhibitory concentration (MIC) of ≥ 4 μg/dL to oxacillin and ≥ 8 μg/mL to methicillin. Some investigations use ≥ 8 μg/mL and > 16 μg/mL for oxacillin and methicillin, respectively, as criteria for MRSA. Not only is MRSA resistant to penicillins and cephalosporins, it has also acquired resistance determinants to multiple antimicrobial agents (quinolones, aminoglycosides, rifampin, sulfamethoxazole, trimethoprim, erythromycin, and clindamycin). Hence, it is probably more accurate to refer to this organism as "multiresistant *S. aureus*." The presence of MRSA in an LTCF leads to fewer treatment options when infections do occur.

MRSA is a frequent colonizer of debilitated patients. In a study performed by Bradley and co-workers, MRSA colonization rate was around 25% *(27)*. In contrast, infection rates are only 3%. Risk factors for MRSA colonization include (1) residence on a medical ward or medical intensive care unit, or prolonged hospitalization (>3 wk), (2) age, and (3) history of invasive procedures *(28)*. Colonization by MRSA is often a hallmark of significant short-term disability. In a study by Nicales and co-workers, the relative risk of dying within 6 mo in MRSA carriers compared with noncarriers was 2.29 (95% CI = 1.04–5.04) *(29)*. This relative risk remained stable (1.57–2.40) even after adjustment for covariables. After 1 yr, the relative risk was reduced to 1.30 (95% CI = 0.65–2.58). Univariate survival analysis confirmed a difference in survival between carriers and noncarriers after 6 mo, but no difference after 1 yr. There was no relationship found between carriage and the likelihood of hospitalization or indicators of functional status. These results suggest a possible relationship between 6 mo mortality and MRSA carriage in nursing-home patients.

Differences in the epidemiology and significance of MRSA colonization between veterans and nonveteran patients in LTCFs have also been examined *(30)*. The prevalence of MRSA nares colonization, the patterns of MRSA acquisition, and the risk for subsequent MRSA infection between a hospital-based, Department of Veterans Affairs (VA) LTCF and community-based nursing facilities were compared. It was found that the prevalence of MRSA colonization was significantly higher in the VA LTCFs than in the community nursing facilities. A trend toward an increased rate of infection was seen in colonized individuals residing in the community nursing facilities versus those in the VA LTCF . In contrast to residents of the VA LTCFs, MRSA colonization in the community facilities was a marker for high mortality.

Common sites of colonization by MRSA are the nares and wounds. Colonization rates of these two sites range from 8–53%, and 30–82%, respectively *(31)*. The routine use of surveillance cultures and antibacterials in an attempt to permanently eradicate MRSA colonization from nursing facility residents has not been successful, and resistance has quickly emerged. Systemic antibiotics to eradicate colonization should be avoided in LTCFs. Topical antibiotics, such as the nasal administration of mupirocin, should be reserved for use in outbreaks *(32)*. Clinicians underestimate the ability of MRSA to spread rapidly among debilitated patients. In a well-studied outbreak, an epidemic MRSA strain spread from a patient in India who was subsequently hospitalized in British Columbia. This patient was transferred to a hospital in Vancouver. A subsequent patient who was colonized in Vancouver passed the organism to a patient in Winnipeg, Manitoba. This all occurred in 6 wk and was all due to the same strain as determined by pulsed-field gel electrophoresis (PFGE) *(33)*.

It is estimated that residents of LTCFs who are colonized with MRSA have a four- to six-fold increase in infection rate *(31)*. In a study by Muder and colleagues *(34)*, 25% of MRSA carriers had an episode of staphylococcal infection compared with only 4% of carriers with methicillin-susceptible staphylococci. These authors concluded that MRSA colonization may predict the development of staphylococcal infection in LTCFs. Unfortunately, once residents acquire MRSA, they remain persistently colonized. The different MRSA strains that circulate in LTCFs often mirror the strains found in local referring hospitals. Infection control practices that disrupt transmission by direct contact (hand washing) should be implemented, thus preventing the potential spread of MRSA. Hand washing, gloves, and gowns are generally effective in limiting the spread of MRSA. In contrast, surveillance of the MRSA colonization status is not necessary when these universal barrier precautions are applied to the care of all patients. If an increase in the rate of MRSA infections is documented, more intensive infection control measures should be implemented. Clinicians should be aware that health care workers (HCWs) are also a source of MRSA. The need to instruct HCWs regarding hand washing has been a serious, perennial problem.

Molecular fingerprinting techniques (e.g., PFGE) are rapidly becoming indispensable tools for tracing and analyzing MRSA colonization and infection *(35)*. The utility of PFGE was recently demonstrated in a study performed in New York City. In this recent cooperative report, 270 MRSA isolates from 12 hospitals in the New York metropolitan area were collected and analyzed. The same PFGE pattern was found in 42% of the isolates and was the predominant clones in 9 hospitals. Based on this study and a previous pilot analysis *(36)*, the authors concluded that epidemiological and surveillance studies can be done that would provide a surveillance network to assist hospitals, clinics, and LTCFs in controlling the spread of multidrug-resistant pathogens, particularly MRSA.

The molecular basis for resistance to methicillin is the introduction of the *mecA* element into *S. aureus*. In brief, *mecA* gene is a complex 30–50 kilobase (kb) element that encodes production of an alternative penicillin-binding protein (PBP), named PBP2' (or PBP2a) that assumes the function of PBP2. The presence of the *mecA* gene can be demonstrated by using a specific probe or PCR amplification reaction. The level of methicillin resistance also depends on *fem* and *aux* determinants; *fem* (factors essential for methicillin resistance) and any *aux* (auxiliary) genes are usually located at distant sites on the staphylococcal chromosome and are outside of the *mec* element. These genes are involved in the synthesis of peptidoglycan and influence the level of resistance to methicillin *(37)*.

2.3. Vancomycin-Intermediate S. aureus

Vancomycin resistance in *S. aureus* (defined by a minimum inhibitory concentration [MIC] of vancomycin of 8 to 16 µg/mL) has been recently described in the United States *(38–40)*. These strains of *S. aureus* with elevated MICs against vancomycin or glycopeptides have been called vancomycin intermediate *S. aureus* (VISA or GISA). In May 1996, the world's first documented clinical infection of VISA was reported from Japan *(39)*. So far, VISA has been recovered from three patients in the United States (Michigan, New York, and New Jersey). All of these patients carry disease burdens similar to those cared for by geriatricians in LTCFs. Data regarding the molecular biology of VISA showed that the glycopeptide-resistant strains have increased extracellular material (thicker extracellular matrix) associated with their cell walls. The glycopeptide-intermediate *S. aureus* isolates also differed by two bands on PFGE. Whether these genetic differences are related to the expression of glycopeptide resistance is unclear. There is some small comfort with knowing that this resistance determinant is not transferable on a plasmid. No transmission was documented among contacts of the two patients. Guidelines for the control of VISA have been proposed *(41)*. If the same high-level vancomycin resistance that is described in vancomycin-resistant enterococci (VRE) were found in methicillin-resistant *S. aureus*, it would result in a "virulent pathogen for which effective antimicrobial therapy would not be available *(41)*." Given that the spread of VISA may mimic MRSA, containment of a virulent strain of VISA would be difficult in an LTCF.

2.4. Penicillin-Resistant Pneumococci

Pneumonia due to *Streptococcus pneumoniae* is one of the most frequent causes of lower respiratory tract infection in the United States. In the past, clinicians resorted to penicillin to treat this infection. The pneumococci were exquisitely susceptible (MIC <0.1 µg/mL). Pneumococci that are intermediate resistant, resistant, and highly resistant have MICs to penicillin of 0.1–1.0 µg/mL, >1.0–1.9 µg/mL, and ≥ 2.0 µg/mL, respectively. Penicillin-resistant pneumococci (PRP) have now emerged as a significant threat in the therapy of the pneumonia in the elderly. This threat stems from the fear of outbreaks of pneumococcal infection in institutionalized settings. Studies by Millar and colleagues *(42)* and Denton and co-workers *(43)*, were among the first to describe PRP infection in the elderly institutionalized, debilitated patients.

The threat of penicillin resistance has been emerging for nearly 40 yr. Penicillin resistance was first noted in the 1967 *(44)*. By the late 1970s, Jacobs and colleagues reported isolates with decreased susceptibility to penicillin *(45)*. By the 1980s, PRPs were described in Hungary, Spain, the United States, and Korea *(46)*. Currently, the Centers for Disease Control report that in some areas of the United States nearly 40% of pneumococcal isolates of blood or spinal fluid of persons >65 yr have reduced susceptibility to penicillin *(47)*. A worrisome characteristic of PRP is the concomitant finding of resistance to erythromycin, tetracycline, quinolones, clindamycin, sulfa, and other antibiotics *(48)*. In this most recent survey, 55% of PRP were resistant to erythromycin and 35% to clindamycin. This pattern mimics the same concerns addressed with MRSA.

A significant outbreak of PRP in an LTCF in rural Oklahoma was recently reported *(49,50)*. In this outbreak the predominant strain was serotype 23F, a serotype included in the vaccine. Pneumonia developed in 13% of the residents in this nursing facility. The mortality rate in this outbreak was 23%. Resistant isolates were recovered in 64% of residents with pneumonia (type 23F) and from 23% of noninfected (colonized) residents. Antibiotic use was associated with both colonization and disease. It is surprising to note that the pneumococcal vaccination rate was less than 25% in this LTCF. Low rates of vaccination have been reported in other nursing facilities *(51)*. (*See also* Chapter 23.)

Resistance to penicillin and other β-lactam antibiotics in the pneumococcus involves alterations or remodeling of the penicillin binding proteins (PBPs) *(52,53)*. PBPs are bacterial enzymes that are responsible for cell wall synthesis. It is speculated that DNA from the PBP genes of relatively penicillin-resistant streptococci that colonize the oropharynx (e.g., *S. oralis* or other viridans streptococci) has been incorporated into the pneumococcal PBP genes, presumably by natural transformation and homologous recombination. It is interesting to note that even though these altered PBPs have decreased affinity for penicillins, the carbapenems and certain third-generation cephalosporins are still active.

Penicillin resistance has occurred mainly in serotypes 6B, 9V, 14, 19A, 19F, and 23F *(53)*. Partial protection against invasive infection by the strains that are penicillin resistant can be achieved by immunizing with the pneumococcal polysaccharide vaccine *(54)*. Hence, immunization of the elderly and other high-risk individuals in LTCFs assumes high priority. Despite substantial educational efforts, this practice has not gained universal acceptance. In addition to questions concerning efficacy, the difficulty in ascertaining correct immunization history has dampened enthusiasm for this practice *(55)*. Hence, reimmunization with pneumococcal polysaccharide vaccine after 4–6 yr remains an ideal, but elusive, goal. Pneumococcal revaccination is relatively safe and has proven extremely beneficial *(56)*. (*See also* Chapter 23.)

Penicillin resistance is most worrisome in patients suspected to be afflicted with pneumococcal meningitis *(57)*. The poor penetration of penicillin through the meninges makes it difficult to achieve sufficient levels in the cerebrospinal fluid; hence the use of ceftriaxone, cefotaxime and vancomycin is advocated. Meropenem, a carbapenem antibiotic that possesses the potency of imipenem/cilastatin but not the neurotoxicity, may prove eventually to be the treatment of choice for pneumococcal meningitis *(58,59)*.

Retrospective studies have shown that penicillin is effective therapy for intermediate resistant (MIC ≤ 1 µg/mL) pneumococcal pneumonia *(60)*. Nevertheless, many clinicians are concerned about the efficacy of penicillin in the treatment of non-meningeal infections by strains of pneumococci expressing high-level resistance (i.e., MICs ≥ 2 µg/mL) *(61)*. The concern raised by many regarding the increasing prevalence of high-level penicillin and ceftriaxone resistance has focused attention to the use of the newer fluoroquinolone agents (e.g., levofloxacin and sparfloxacin) in the treatment of pneumonia *(62)*. These agents offer enhanced activity against the pneumococcus when compared with ciprofloxacin. As a group, the newer fluoroquinolones have MICs against pneumoccoci between 0.25 µg/mL and 1.0 µg/mL *(61)*. Whether these agents are absolutely necessary for the empiric treatment of community-acquired pneumonia is debated *(63)*. How excessive use of these agents will impact on the colonizing flora of nursing facility residents also remains to be seen.

2.5. Vancomycin-Resistant Enterococci

According to recent national nosocomial infections surveillance studies, enterococci have emerged as the second most common organism in nosocomial infections *(64)*. This "success" may be due to their intrinsic resistance to virtually all antibiotics. Enterococci have also acquired resistance to cephalosporins, penicillins, aminoglycosides (gentamicin and streptomycin), macrolides, and quinolones. They are inherently resistant to the folate antagonists (TMP/SMX) and clindamycin. The most worrisome resistance traits in the enterococci are resistance to ampicillin, vancomycin, and aminoglycosides. Ampicillin and gentamicin resistance abrogate the possibility of using synergistic therapy in the treatment of serious enterococcal infections. Vancomycin resistance has created the feared scenario—a microbial infection in which no therapy is effective.

The problems of ampicillin and aminoglycoside resistance are most notable when geriatricians are faced with treating enterococcal endocarditis in the elderly. Enterococcal endocarditis is the third most common cause of endocarditis and the incidence of this disease is likely to grow as the population ages and as more elderly undergo valve replacement *(65,66)*. Ampicillin (or penicillin) resistance in the enterococcus is a critical phenomenon. Vancomycin resistance is restricted only to glycopeptide antibiotics (teicoplanin, ramoplanin and vancomycin). Ampicillin resistance affects all β-lactams. Alteration in the prokaryotic cell wall synthesizing mechanisms mediated by changes in the structure and regulation of PBPs is the major factor responsible for ampicillin resistance *(67)*. High-level aminoglycoside resistance in the enterococcus is mediated by the acquisition of aminoglycoside-modifying enzymes *(68)*.

Resistance to vancomycin was first noted in enterococci in 1986, almost 30 yr after the release of the drug *(69,70* and references therein). Vancomycin-resistant enterococci (VRE) have now become one of the most important pathogens in the world *(71)*. A review of the mechanism of resistance to vancomycin is as follows.

Vancomycin inhibits cell wall synthesis in Gram-positive bacteria by forming direct hydrogen bonds with cell wall precursors that terminate in D-alanyl- D-alanine, which prevents formation of important cross bridges *(69)*. Vancomycin resistance is known to be a result of the presence of mobile genetic elements encoding operons with nine unique genes. In the VanA operon, *vanR* and *vanS* are responsible for sensing the presence of vancomycin in the bacterial environment. *VanH* and *vanA* genes are responsible for the synthesis of D-ala-D-lactate (D-ala-D-lactate is attached to the growing pentapeptide essential for cross-linking of bacterial cell wall). *VanX* controls a dipeptidase that cleaves D-ala-D-ala, thereby decreasing the cellular pool of normal dipeptide precursors. With D-ala-D-lactate incorporated in the cell wall, vancomycin binds with a significantly decreased affinity. Two subsequent genes on the transposon contribute in minor ways to glycopeptide resistance (*vanY* and *Z*). Only *vanH*, *vanA*, and *vanX* are required for expression of resistance.

Five phenotypes of VRE have been described (*see* Table 1) *(70,71)*. The VanA phenotype is characterized by high-level resistance to vancomycin and teicoplanin (MICs >64 µg/mL). VanB strains show variable resistance to vancomycin, with MICs from 4–1000 µg/mL, but are susceptible in vitro to teicoplanin. Resistance conferred by the VanB phenotype is mediated by the VanB operon, which is very similar in organization to VanA and is also transferable. The VanC phenotype is an intrinsic characteristic of certain enterococcal species of minimal pathogenic potential (*Enterococcus gallinarium* and *E. casseliflavus*). This phenotype is characterized by only moderate levels of resistance to vancomycin (MICs between 8 and 16 µg/mL), and susceptibility to teicoplanin and is not transferable. Both *vanA* and *vanB* are inducible in the presence of vancomycin. VanA and VanB phenotypes are also transferable; hence they can be disseminated easily on plasmids and transposons. The clinical significance of the VanD and VanE phenotypes is as yet unknown.

Identified risk factors for the emergence of VRE are (1) the use of oral vancomycin and metronidazole to treat antibiotic-induced colitis, (2) excessive cephalosporin use, (3) previous antibiotic use, and (4) increased disease burden *(72)*. Enterococci acquire resistance characteristics through exchange of genes carried on conjugative transposons and broad host range plasmids.

Numerous studies are published suggest there is facile transfer of VRE between institutions *(73)*. From these studies it appears that VRE can spread by direct patient-to-patient contact, indirectly via transient carriage on hands of personnel, contami-

Table 1
Vancomycin Resistance in Enterococci

Type	MIC	Expression	Transfer
	(Vancomycin)		
	µg/mL		
Van A	64–1000	I	+ (P)
Van B	4–1000	I	+ (?)
Van C	2–32	C	–(Ch)
Van D	16–64	?	–(Ch)
Van E	16	C	–(Ch)

MIC, minimum inhibitory concentration; I, inducible; C, constitutive; P, plasmid; Ch, chromosomal. Adapted from ref. *(71)*.

nated environmental surfaces, and patient care equipment. The prevalence rate of VRE colonization in patients admitted to acute care hospitals from LTCFs may be as high as 47% of patients *(74)*.

VRE has become a serious challenge for geriatricians. Given that enterococci are one of the major causes of urine, wound, and bloodstream infection in the debilitated elderly, it is easy to understand why geriatricians are facing the problem of VRE infection and colonization in the nursing facility. Urinary tract infections (UTIs) and infected pressure ulcers are among the most common VRE infections found in LTCFs. Many of these patients with pressure ulcers and UTIs are administered multiple courses of antibiotics and are frequently hospitalized. Their translocation from tertiary care institutions to LTCFs and back can easily spread flora from the hospital to the nursing facility. In a study done by Edmond and colleagues, the attributable mortality due to VRE bacteremia was 37%, and patients with VRE bacteremia were twice as likely to die than closely matched controls *(75)*. In this study, 27 patients with VRE bacteremia were studied and septic shock occurred in 37% of cases. It is tempting to speculate that the lack of effective therapy is related to increased mortality.

As an example of the difficulty VRE colonization presents to geriatricians, the epidemiology of colonization with VRE in a 400-bed veterans LTCF was reviewed *(74)*. Twenty-four of 36 patients were colonized with VRE when they were transferred from an acute care hospital to the VA LTCF. VRE persisted for 67 d and was associated with antibiotic administration. Interestingly, only three patients acquired colonization, suggesting that in this high-risk, disabled population, person-to-person transmission is infrequent.

The recommendations for containment of VRE in hospitals have proven to be impractical in nursing homes. The financial, social, and psychological burdens associated with implementation of these guidelines are significant. The use of barrier precautions and isolation practice can be implemented in the hospital but are not feasible in the long-term care setting. The Society for Healthcare Epidemiology of America (SHEA) recommends that patients colonized with VRE be isolated in private rooms until this organism is "cleared"—usually two to three negative stool cultures 1 wk apart.

Modified contact isolation (gloves, gown, and private room if available) is also strongly encouraged *(76,77)*.

A variety of methods have been tried to eradicate VRE colonization; unfortunately, none have proved effective *(78)*. Treatment of infections caused by VRE is also unsatisfactory. The oxazolidinones, a novel class of antibiotics highly effective against Gram-positive bacteria, may prove effective against VRE, but the large number of drug–drug interactions (interaction with antidepressants, anticonvulsants, and the like) may preclude widespread use in the elderly *(79,80)*. Preliminary experience with this novel class of drugs indicates that these agents will probably be used successfully against VRE, multiresistant pneumococci, and staphylococci *(79)*. These new agents' mode of action is by inhibiting the formation of an initiation complex in bacterial translation systems by preventing formation of the N-formylmethionyl-tRNA-ribosome-mRNA ternary complex *(81)*. Although it is anticipated that resistance will eventually emerge, these agents may prove to be an effective antimicrobial against resistant Gram-positive organisms (VRE, MRSA, and PRP) *(82,83)*.

2.6. Erythromycin-Resistant Pneumococci

Erythromycin, as a representative of the macrolide antibiotic class, has long been regarded as the most favorable alternative to penicillin in penicillin-allergic patients for the treatment of pneumococcal and group A streptococcal infections. Macrolides had also enjoyed a unique role as the treatment of choice for community-acquired pneumonia. Erythromycin's mode of action is binding to the 50S subunit of the prokaryotic ribosome. Resistance to erythromycin has been described in *S. pneumoniae* and other Gram-positive pathogens. Up to 65% of PRPs are also erythromycin resistant *(84)*. Three mechanisms are responsible for erythromycin resistance: one mechanism is the presence of erythromycin methylases, a second is the presence of the alteration of the 50S ribosome that prevent the binding of erythromycin to that subunit, and the third is the expression of macrolide efflux (MEF) proteins. Erythromycin resistance is emerging as a potential problem in the treatment of pneumococcal upper respiratory infections (URI) and lower respiratory tract infection (LRTI) in LTCFs. To date, there have not been any studies examining the carriage of erythromycin-resistant pneumococci in elderly populations confined to LTCFs.

3. RESISTANCE IN GRAM-NEGATIVE ORGANISMS

3.1. Aminoglycoside-Resistant Gram-Negative Bacteria

Aminoglycosides (gentamicin, tobramycin, netilimicin, and streptomycin) are intravenous and intramuscular bactericidal antibiotics that are particularly potent against Gram-negative bacteria. As a class these antibiotics bind to the 16S ribosome RNA and interfere with protein synthesis in prokaryotes. The exact mechanism by which aminoglycoside antibiotics kill Gram-negative bacteria is unknown *(85)*. Aminoglycoside resistance can arise by three distinct mechanisms. The most important mechanism of resistance is by aminoglycoside-modifying enzymes (acetyltransferases, adenyltransferase, and phosphotransferases). Alterations in the L6 and S12 ribosomal subunit are also associated with reduced affinity for aminoglycoside binding. Mutations in terminal cytochrome oxidases and quinones have also been described. In a recent survey of resistant bacteria in LTCFs, up to 90% of resistant enterobacteriaceae were resistant to gentamicin *(86)*.

3.2. Trimethoprim/Sulfamethoxazole-Resistant Gram-Negative Bacteria

Trimethoprim combined with sulfamethoxazole (TMP/SMX) is an effective oral antibiotic combination, primarly against enteric Gram-negative bacilli, *Haemophilus influenzae*, and many strains of streptococci. The major clinical uses of this combination had been in the treatment of urinary tract infections (UTIs), upper respiratory infections (URIs) (bronchitis, sinusitis, otitis media), and gastrointestinal infections (dysentery). However, the widespread use of TMP/SMX has resulted in the emergence of resistance. In geriatric units this was described by Gruneberg and Bendall in 1979 *(87)*. Major organisms resistant to TMP/SMX now are *S. pneumoniae*, *H. influenzae*, and many enteric Gram-negative bacilli (*Escherichia coli, Klebsiella* spp.). The target of sulfamethoxazole is the enzyme dihydropteroate synthetase. Sulfamethoxazole competitively inhibits this enzyme and prevents the formation of pteridines and nucleic acids. Alterations in dihydropteroate synthetase reduce the ability of sulfamethoxazole to inhibit this pathway. Trimethoprim, the partner antibiotic, binds to dihydrofolate reductase (DHFR). Alterations in DHFR, as with dihydropteroate synthetase, result in diminished binding of trimethoprim. Altered *dhfr* genes are found in the bacterial chromosome and on plasmids. Walker and co-workers *(88)* have shown that cephalosporins and TMP/SMX are significant risk factors for the asymptomatic carriage of *Clostridium difficile* in LTCFs.

3.3. Extended-Spectrum β-Lactamases

β-Lactamase enzymes are the major mechanisms by which bacteria inactivate β-lactam antibiotics. Numerous cephalosporin and penicillin antibiotics have been developed to combat these enzymes. Although the third-generation cephalosporins promised to be the safest and most effective drugs against this problem, in the past 10 yr there have been described more than 75 extended-spectrum β-lactamases (ESBLs) able to inactivate many currently available penicillins and advanced generation cephalosporins *(89)*. Many of these β-lactam-inactivating enzymes are derived from the plasmid-borne TEM-1 and SHV-1 β-lactamases, the most common β-lactamase found in enteric bacilli.

The prevalence of ESBLs in LTCFs can be alarming. In a study of an LTCF in Chicago, 31 of 35 patients from eight nursing facilities harbored an ESBL. Not only were these strains resistant to ceftazidime, but they were also resistant to gentamicin, tobramycin, TMP/SMX, and ciprofloxacin *(90)*. In this analysis, risk factors associated with colonization by ESBLs include (1) poor functional status, (2) gastrostomy tube or pressure ulcer, and (3) ciprofloxacin and/or TMP/SMX use.

Horizontal transfer of β-lactam resistance on plasmids in *E. coli* and *Klebsiella* spp. has resulted in the dissemination of multiple antibiotic resistance traits, as these mobile genetic elements often carry resistance determinants against many antibiotics (e.g., aminoglycosides) *(91)*.

Point mutations in the plasmid-determined β-lactamase genes are the major mechanism by which resistance to third-generation cephalosporin antibiotics develops in these ESBLs *(92)*. These point mutations permit the enzymes to inactivate β-lactams before they reach the PBPs. The altered amino acids change the conformation of the active site such that third-generation cephalosporins can be hydrolyzed. More recently, plasmid-encoded β-lactamases resistant to inactivation by β-lactamase inhibitors have also been described *(93,94)*. The appearance of these newer enzymes is of significant concern. By MIC testing, most ESBLs are highly susceptible to inactivation by β-lactamase inhibitors (clavulanate, sulbactam, or tazobactam). The clinical formulations—ampicillin/sulbactam, amoxicillin/clavulanate, piperacillin/tazobactam, and ticarcillin/clavulanate—can be used to treat infections by ESBL-producing enterics. Unfortunately, this may not be true in each case. To date, only one plasmid-determined β-lactamase resistant to inactivation by β-lactamase inhibitors and able to efficiently hydrolyze third-generation cephalosporins has been described in the clinic (TEM-50) *(94)*. This unique β-lactamase enzyme has incorporated in its gene sequence the necessary mutations to confer resistance to β-lactamase inhibitors and extend the substrate spectrum to include hydrolysis of third-generation cephalosporins. Fortunately, it has not become widespread.

Resistance to both third-generation cephalosporins and β-lactam/β-lactamase inhibitor combinations in clinical isolates has also been attributed to the production of more than one β-lactamase enzyme, hyperproduction of an ESBL, and the production of a plasmid-mediated AmpC β-lactamase *(95)*. The production of chromosomally mediated AmpC type β-lactamase confers β-lactam resistance to several clinically important Gram-negative bacilli (*Enterobacter, Citrobacter, Serratia, Pseudomonas*). Elevated production of this β-lactamase can result from induction by exposure to cefoxitin, clavulanic acid, or imipenem *(96)*. Mutations in the regulatory mechanism controlling expression of these AmpC β-lactamase enzymes are also well described *(97)*. Important characteristics of these AmpC cephalosporinases are that they are able to inactivate all cephalosporins including cefoxitin (with the possible exception of cefepime) and that they are generally resistant to inhibition by currently available β-lactamase inhibitors.

The importance of induction of β-lactamases and recycling of cell wall materials has also been recently elucidated *(98)*. It has been shown that AmpC β-lactamase induction in *Enterobacteriaceae* requires a balance between a variety of genes that control β-lactamase production and the transport of cell wall products into the bacterial cytoplasm. This work is important because it highlights the "bidirectional communication" between cell wall synthesis and bacterial transcription. The clinical consequence of the induction of these chromosomal β-lactamases in *Enterobacter* has been examined by Chow and colleagues *(99)*. In this prospective multicenter study, ceftazidime-resistant *Enterobacter* spp. isolates were associated with a higher mortality rate. This increased mortality rate as a reflection of increased antibiotic resistance somehow suggests that virulence and resistance are linked. A frightening new development is the increasing number of AmpC β-lactamases found on plasmids. On mobile genetic elements these β-lactamases can be spread among enteric bacilli.

Outbreaks of bacteria resistant to third-generation cephalosporins have been reported in VA chronic care facilities as well *(100)*. Frequent use of third-generation cephalosporins has been blamed for the emergence of this problem *(101)*. In the VA outbreak reported by Rice and co-workers *(100)* ceftazidime use was implicated. The switch to piperacillin/tazobactam decreased the percentage of ceftazidime-resistant isolates. Suc-

cessful treatment of these types of infections will require the use of a carbapenem antibiotic or the combination of β-lactam/β-lactamase inhibitor (ampicillin/sulbactam,
amoxicillin/clavulanate, piperacillin/tazobactam, ticarcillin/clavulanate). Experimental animal models are being actively studied to evaluate the most effective therapy
(102). To date, of the β-lactam-type agents, the carbapenems (meropenem and
imipenem) offer the most promise against ESBL and AmpC type-producing enterics.

3.4. Multiresistant Gram-Negative Bacilli
3.4.1. Quinolone Resistance

The target of quinolone action in Gram-negative bacteria is the A subunit of DNA
gyrase *(103,104)*. DNA gyrase is a bacterial type II topoisomerase and is made up of a
tetramer of two parts, A2 and B2. This protein converts relaxed DNA into supercoiled
DNA. The A subunit is responsible for breakage and resealing of chromosomal DNA.
The B subunit is responsible for energy transduction from ATP hydrolysis. Quinolones
interrupt the resealing of double-stranded DNA by forming a quinolone–gyrase–DNA
ternary complex. This inhibition is associated with rapid bacterial killing. Additional
antibacterial activity is expressed through inhibition of topoisomerase IV. This enzyme
is responsible for the separation of daughter DNA strands during bacterial cell division
in Gram-positive bacteria. Topoisomerase IV is likely to be the primary target for
quinolone action in Gram-positive bacteria. In addition to DNA gyrase and topoisomerase IV, quinolones are bactericidal by other mechanisms *(104,105)*. Three mechanisms, A, B, and C, have been proposed. Mechanism A requires RNA and protein
synthesis as well as cell division for bactericidal action. Mechanism B is the ability to
kill nondividing cells without concomitant protein or RNA synthesis. Mechanism C is
the bactericidal activity that occurs in the absence of multiplication, yet in the presence
of protein and RNA synthesis. Utilization of these mechanisms is organism specific.

Resistance to quinolone antibiotics is generally mediated by alterations in the chromosomal DNA of bacteria. In the main, most bacteria accumulate several mutations
that affect both DNA gyrase and permeability. Mutations in the regulatory genes that
govern permeability porins or efflux pumps are commonly found in quinolone-resistant bacteria. Point mutations in residues 67–106 of the A subunit of DNA gyrase, the
quinolone-resistance determining region, result in resistance. Mutations in this region
are associated with increased resistance to all quinolones.

Resistance to quinolone agents can emerge rapidly during therapy. Ciprofloxacin-
resistant *P. aeruginosa*, *S. aureus*, and *S. epidermidis* have been well described *(106)*.
Once organisms develop resistance, therapeutic options are severely limited.
Clinafloxacin, a newer generation quinalone, offers enhanced activity against
ciprofloxacin-resistant organisms *(107)*, but this drug is not in our current pharmacopeia.

Quinolone resistance in LTCFs and debilitated patients is becoming a serious concern *(108,109)*. In cancer patients, exposure to quinolones as prophylactic agents can
alter the colonizing flora. In one study, ciprofloxacin resistance developed in 32% of
patients receiving fluoroquinolones; persistence of colonization lasted in approximately
7% of these patients. The clinical consequences of colonization by quinolone-resistant
bacteria are unknown.

3.4.2. Multidrug Efflux Pumps

Multidrug efflux pumps have proved to be important mechanisms for the expression
of resistance to a variety of antibiotic classes, including β–lactams, tetracyclines, and,

most prominently in recent years, fluoroquinolones. The species for which these pumps have proved to be of greatest importance is *P. aeruginosa*, in which three distinct pumps have been described. The antibiotic classes expelled by these pumps varies somewhat but in all cases prominently includes fluoroquinolone antibiotics. An efflux pump (designated NorA) has also proved to be of importance in the expression of resistance to fluoroquinolones in *S. aureus*.

4. INFECTION CONTROL AND ANTIBIOTIC USE

The Society for Health Care Epidemiology has drafted recommendations to help control antibiotic resistance in LTCFs and cross-infection include antibiotic restriction practices, surveillance, nontreatment of asymptomatic bacteruria, minimizing topical antibiotics, hand washing, and barrier precautions for wound care *(108)*. We propose that, for LTCFs, the following additional items be specifically stressed (1) education, (2) surveillance, (3) antibiotic control, and (4) immunization.

Continuing medical education concerning the imprudent use of antibiotics needs to be the first step. Alerting staff to the dangers of excess antibiotic use and epidemiology of current outbreaks will help with enforcing infection control guidelines in the community. Education of nursing staff is also needed to determine if infection is really present. As a guide we encourage the use of the definitions of infection in LTCFs developed by McGeer and colleagues *(110)*. Nursing personnel who are instructed in the use of these guidelines can assist physicians with treatment decisions. Infection control surveillance also helps to identify the presence and spread of resistance. It is our belief that identifying patients coming from hospitals where PRP, VRE, and ESBLs are endemic should be a nursing facility physician and infection control priority. Identifying nursing facility residents who have been treated with multiple courses of antibiotics in hospital will also alert health care workers to this potential problem. Although not proven in prospective studies, screening high-risk patients for colonization by antibiotic-resistant bacteria, particularly ESBLs, may help contain a potential outbreak *(111)*. Screening for VRE should also be a consideration in high-risk LTCFs.

Clinicians should be "ecologically responsible" in their prescribing of antibiotics. The unnecessary use of broad-spectrum antibiotics to treat susceptible organisms should be strongly discouraged. There should be clear guidelines in place for using vancomycin in the nursing facility (e.g., MRSA, β-lactam allergy, metronidazole failures in treatment of *C. difficile* colitis, or surgical prophylaxis in β-lactam-allergic patients). Limits to the length of antibiotic administration should also be enforced. Using third-generation cephalosporins and quinolones in LTCFs only when they are absolutely necessary in the treatment of UTIs or URI/LRTIs may limit the emergence of multiresistant Gram-negative bacilli and VRE. Restricting antibiotic formularies for LTCFs has been suggested as a potential means to this end. Alerting physicians to the number of treatment courses of quinolones or advanced generation cephalosporins used can stem overprescribing. Treatment algorithms are not yet a common practice in the nursing home and should be developed.

Immunization of the elderly with pneumococcal polysaccharide vaccine should also be a clinical and administrative priority. The vaccine should be strongly encouraged in everyone 65 yr and older admitted to an LTCF. It can be given at the time of influenza vaccine and should be part of a nursing facility admission medical care regimen. Careful review of patient records should be undertaken to ensure immunization when the patient's or family's recollection is not reliable. Once administered, the information can be entered in a patient log book that serves as a reminder for the next immunization. Pneumococcal polysaccharide vaccination is extremely safe and can and should be repeated every 6 yr for select high-risk groups of elderly persons. (*See* Chapter 23.)

REFERENCES

1. Irvine P. W., Van Buren N., and Krossley, K. (1984) Causes for hospitalization of nursing home residents: the role of infection. *J. Am. Geriatr. Soc.* **32,** 103–107.
2. Alvarez, S., Shell, C. G., Wooley, T. W., et al. (1988) Nosocomial infections in long-term care facilities. *J. Gerontol. (Med. Sci.)* **43,** M9–17.
3. Norman, D. C., Castle, S. C., and Cantrell, M. (1987) Infections in the nursing home. *J. Am. Geriatr. Soc.* **35,** 796–805.
4. Crossley, K., Henry, K., Irvine, P., et al. (1987) Antibiotic use in nursing homes: prevalence, cost, and utilization. *Bull. N. Y. Acad. Med.* **63,** 510–518.
5. Warren, J. W., Palumbo, F. B., Fisherman, L. et al. (1991) Incidence and characteristics of antibiotic use in aged nursing home patients. *J. Am. Geriatr. Soc.* **39,** 963–972.
6. Nicolle, L. E., Bentley, D., Garibaldi, R., et al. (1996) Antimicrobial use in long-term-care facilities. *Infect. Control Hosp. Epidemiol.* **17,** 119–128.
7. Zimmer, J. G., Bentley, D. W., Valenti, W. M., et al. (1986) Systemic antibiotic use in nursing homes. A quality assessment. *J. Am. Geriatr. Soc.* **34,** 703–710.
8. Jones, S. R., Parker, D. F., Liebow, E. S., et al. (1987) Appropriateness of antibiotic therapy in long-term care facilities. *Am. J. Med.* **83,** 499–502.
9. Yoshikawa, T. T. (1998) VRE, MRSA, PRP, and DRGNB in LTCF: lessons to be learned from this alphabet. *J. Am. Geriatr. Soc.* **46,** 241–243.
10. John, Jr. J. F. and Ribner, B. S. (1991) Antibiotic resistance in long term care facilities: *Infect. Control Hosp. Epidemiol.* **12,** 245–250.
11. Gaynes, R. P., Weinstein, R. A., Chamberlin, W., et al. (1985) Antibiotic-resistant flora in nursing home patients admitted to the hospital. *Arch. Intern. Med.* **145,** 1804–1807.
12. Gaynes, R. P., Cooksey, R., Thornsberry, C., et al. (1987) Mechanism of aminoglycoside resistance among beta-lactam resistant Escherichia coli in the United States. *Diagn. Microbiol. Infect. Dis.* **7,** 45–50.
13. Nicolle, L. E., Strausbaugh, L. J., and Garibaldi, R. A. (1996) Infections and antibiotic resistance in nursing homes. *Clin. Microbiol. Rev.* **9,** 1–17.
14. McCue, J. D. (1997) Antibiotic resistance: why is it increasing in nursing homes? *Geriatrics* **52,** 39–43.
15. Strausbaugh, L. J., Crossley, K. B., Nurse, B. A. et al. (1996) Antimicrobial resistance in long-term-care facilities. *Infect. Control Hosp. Epidemiol.* **17,** 129–140.
16. Bradley, S. F. (1999) Issues in the management of resistant bacteria in long-term-care facilities. *Infect. Control Hosp. Epidemiol.* **20,** 362–366.
17. Strausbaugh, L. J., Jacobson, C., Swell, D. L., et al. (1992) Methicillin resistant *Staphylococcus aureus* in extended care facilities: experiences in a Veteran's Affairs nursing home and a review of the literature. *Infect. Control Hosp. Epidemiol.* **13,** 711–718.
18. Rice, L. B., Willey, S. H., Papanicolaou, G. A., et al. (1990) Outbreak of ceftazidime resistance caused by extended-spectrum β-lactamases at a Massachusetts chronic care facility. *Antimicrob. Agents Chemother.* **34,** 2193–2199.
19. Bradford, P. A., Urban, C., Jaiswal, A., et al. (1995) SHV-7, a novel cefotaxime-hydrolyzing β-lactamase, identified in *Escherichia coli* from hospitalized nursing home patients. *Antimicrob. Agents Chemother.* **39,** 899–905.

20. Deguchi, T., Fukuoka, A., Yasuda, M., et al. (1997) Alterations in the GyrA subunit of DNA gyrase and the ParC subunit of topoisomerase IV in quinolone-resistant clinical isolates of Klebsiella pneumoniae. *Antimicrob. Agents Chemother.* **41,** 699–701.

21. Hooper, D. C. (1995) Bacterial resistance to fluoroquinolones: mechanisms and patterns. *Adv. Exp. Med. Biol.* **390,** 49–57.

22. Huovinen, P., Sundstrom, L., Swedberg, G., et al. (1995) Trimethoprim and sulfonamide resistance. *Antimicrob. Agents Chemother.* **39,** 279–289.

23. Shales, D. M., Lehman, M. H., Currie-McCumber, C. A., et al. (1986) Prevalence of colonization with antibiotic resistant gram-negative bacilli in a nursing home care unit: The importance of cross-colonization as documented by plasmid analysis. *Infect. Control* **7,** 538–547.

24. Lowy, F. D. (1998) *Staphylococcus aureus* infections. *N. Engl. J. Med.* **339,** 520–532.

25. Murray, B. E., Mederski-Samoraj, B., Foster, S. K., et al. (1986). In vitro studies of plasmid mediated penicillinase from *Streptococcus faecalis* suggests a staphylococcal origin. *J. Clin. Invest.* **77,** 289–299.

26. Moellering, R. C., Jr. (1991) Beta-lactamase inhibition: therapeutic implications in infectious diseases—an overview. *Rev. Infect. Dis.* **13(Suppl. 9),** S723–S726.

27. Bradley, S. F., Terpenning, M. S., Ramsey, M. A., et al. (1991) Methicillin-resistant *Staphylococcus aureus*: colonization and infection in a long-term care facility. *Ann. Intern. Med.* **115,** 417–422.

28. Asensio, A., Guerrero, A., Quereda, C., et al. (1996) Colonization and infection with methicillin-resistant *Staphyloccus aureus*: associated factors and eradication. *Infect. Control Hosp. Epidemiol.* **17,** 20–28.

29. Nicales, L., Buntinx, F., Banuro, F., et al. (1999) Consequences of MRSA carriage in nursing home residents. *Epidemiol. Infect.* **122,** 235–239.

30. Mulhausen, P. I., Harrel, L. J., Weinberger, M., et al. (1996) Contrasting methicillin-resistant *Staphylococcus aureus* colonization in Veterans Affairs and community nursing homes. *Am. J. Med.* **100,** 24–31.

31. Bradley, S. F. (1999) Methicillin-resistant *Staphylococcus aureus*: long-term care concerns. *Am. J. Med.* **106(5A),** 2S-10S.

32. Kauffman, C. A., Terpenning, M. S., Zairns, L. T., et al. (1993). Attempts to eradicate methicillin resistant *Staphylococcus aureus* from a long-term care facility with the use of mupirocin ointment. *Am. J. Med.* **94,** 371–378.

33. Roman, R. S., Smith, J., Bryne, S., et al. (1997) Rapid geographic spread of methicillin-resistant *Staphylococcus aureus* strain. *Clin. Infect. Dis.* **25,** 698–705.

34. Muder, R. R., Brennen, C., Wagener, M. M., et al. (1991) Methicillin-resistant staphylococcal colonization and infection in a long-term care facility. *Ann. Intern. Med.* **114,** 107–112.

35. Roberts, R. B., deLencastre, A., Eisner, W., et al. (1998) Molecular epidemiology of methicillin-resistant *Staphylococcus aureus* in 12 New York hospitals. MRSA Collaborative Study Group. *J. Infect. Dis.* **178,** 164–171.

36. deLencastre, H., Severina, E. P., Roberts, R. B., et al. (1996) Testing the efficacy of a molecular surveillance network: methicillin-resistant *Staphylococcus aureus* (MRSA) and vancomycin-resistant *Enterococcus faecium* (VREF) genotypes in six hospitals in the metropolitan New York City area. The BARG Initiative Pilot Study Group. Bacterial Antibiotic Resistance Group. *Microb. Drug Resist.* **2,** 343–351.

37. Chambers, H. F. (1997) Methicillin resistance in staphylococci: molecular and biochemical basis and clinical implications. *Clin. Microbiol. Rev.* **10,** 781–791.

38. Rotun, S. S., McMath, V., Schoomaker, D. J., et al. (1999) *Staphylococcus aureus* with reduced susceptibility to vancomycin isolated from a patient with fatal bacteremia. *Emerg. Infect. Dis.* **5,** 147–149.

39. Smith, T. L., Pearson, M. L., Wilcox, K. R., et al. (1999) Emergence of vancomycin resistance in *Staphylococcus aureus*. Glycopeptide-Intermediate *Staphylococcus aureus* Working Group. *N. Engl. J. Med.* **340,** 493–501.

40. Sieradzki, K., Roberts, R. B, Haber, S. W., et al. (1999) The development of vancomycin resistance in a patient with methicillin-resistant *Staphylococcus aureus* infection. *N. Engl. J. Med.* **340,** 517–523.

41. Edmond, M. B., Wenzel, R. P., and Pasculle, A. W. (1996) Vancomycin resistant *Staphylococcus aureus*: Perspectives on measures for control. *Ann. Intern. Med.* **124,** 329–334.

42. Millar, M. R., Brown, N. M., Tobin, G. W., et al. (1994) Outbreak of infection with penicillin resistant *Streptococcus pneumoniae* in a hospital for the elderly. *J. Hosp. Infect.* **27,** 99–104.

43. Denton, M., Hawkey, P. M., Hoy, C. M., et al. (1993) Co-existent cross-infection with *Streptococcus pneumoniae* and group B streptococci on an adult oncology unit. *J. Hosp. Infect.* **23,** 271–278.

44. Hansman, D. and Bullen, M. M. (1967) A resistant pneumococcus. *Lancet* **1,** 264–265.

45. Jacobs, M. R., Koornhof, H. J., Robins-Browne, R. M., et al. (1978) Emergence of multiply resistant pneumococci. *N. Engl. J. Med.* **299,** 735–740.

46. Klugman, K. P. (1990) Pneumococcal resistance to antibiotics. *Clin. Microbiol. Rev.* **3,** 171–196.

47. Butler, J. C. and Cetron, M. S. (1999) Pneumococcal drug resistance: the new "special enemy of old age". *Clin. Infect. Dis.* **28,** 730–735.

48. Fluit, A. C., Schmitz, F. J., Jones, M. E., et al. (1999) Antimicrobial resistance among community-acquired pneumonia isolates in Europe: first results from the SENTRY antimicrobial surveillance program 1997. *Int. J. Infect. Dis.* **3,** 153–156.

49. Nuorti, J. P., Butler, J. C., Crutcher, J. M., et al. (1998) An outbreak of multidrug-resistant pneumococcal pneumonia and bacteremia among unvaccinated nursing home residents. *N. Engl. J. Med.* **338,** 1861–1868.

50. Musher, D. M. (1998) Pneumococcal outbreaks in nursing homes. *N. Engl. J. Med.* **338,** 1915–1916.

51. Quick, R. E., Hoge, C. W., Hamilton, D. J., et al. (1993). Underutilization of pneumococcal vaccine in nursing home in Washington State: report of a serotype-specific outbreak and a survey. *Am. J. Med.* **94,** 149–152.

52. Spratt, B. G. (1994) Resistance to antibiotics mediated by target alterations. *Science* **264,** 388–393.

53. Tomasz, A. (1997) Antibiotic resistance in *Streptococcus pneumoniae*. *Clin. Infect. Dis.* **24(Suppl. 1),** S85–S88.

54. Munford, R. S., and Murphy, T. V. (1994) Antimicrobial resistance in *Streptococcus pneumoniae*: can immunization prevent its spread? *J. Invest. Med.* **42,** 613–621.

55. Ortqvist, A., Hedlund, J., Burman, L. A., et al. (1998) Randomized trial of 23 valent pneumococcal capsular polysaccharide vaccine in middle aged and elderly people. Swedish pneumococcal vaccination study group. *Lancet* **351,** 399–403.

56. Jackson, L. A., Benson, P., Sneller, V. P., et al. (1999) Safety of revaccination with pneumococcal polysaccharide vaccine. *JAMA* **281,** 243–248.

57. Friedland, I. R. and McCracken, G. H. Jr. (1994) Management of infections caused by antibiotic resistant *Streptococcus pneumoniae*. *N. Engl. J. Med.* **331,** 377–382.

58. Quagliarello, V. J. and Scheld, W. M. (1997) Treatment of bacterial meningitis. *N. Engl. J. Med.* **336,** 708–716.

59. Bradley, J. S. and Scheld, W. M (1997). The challenge of penicillin resistant *Streptococcus pneumoniae meningitis*: current antibiotic therapy in the 1990s. *Clin. Infect. Dis.* **24(Suppl. 2),** S213–S221.

60. Pallares, R., Linares, J., Vadillo, M., et al. (1995) Resistance to penicillin and cepha-losporins and mortality from severe pneumococcal pneumonia in Barcelona, Spain. *N. Engl. J. Med.* **333,** 474–480.

61. Bartlett, J. G., Breiman, R. F., Mandell, L. A., et al. (1998) Community-acquired pneumonia in adults: guidelines for management. The Infectious Diseases Society of America. *Clin. Infect. Dis.* **26,** 811–838

62. Klugman, K. P. and Feldman, C. (1999) Penicillin- and cephalosporin-resistant *Streptococcus pneumoniae*. Emerging treatment for an emerging problem. *Drugs* **58,** 1–4.

63. Jacobs, M. R. (1999) Drug-resistant *Streptococcus pneumoniae*: rational antibiotic choices. *Am. J. Med.* **106(5A),** 19S-25S

64. Huycke, M. M., Sahn, D. F., and Gilmore, M. S. (1998) Multiple-drug resistant Enterococci: the nature of the problem and the agenda for the future. *Emerg. Infectious Dis.* **4,** 239–249.

65. Megran, D. W. (1993) Diagnosis and treatment of enterococcal endocarditis. *Hosp. Pract. (Off Ed)*. **28,** 41–44, 47–50.

66. Rice, L. B., Calderwood, S. B., Eliopoulos, G. M., et al. (1991) Enterococcal endocarditis: a comparison of prosthetic and native valve disease. *Rev. Infect. Dis.* **13,** 1–7.

67. Carias, L., Rudin, S. D., Donskey, C. J., et al. (1990) Genetic linkage and co-transfer of a novel *vanB* encoding transposon (TN5382) and a low affinity penicillin binding protein 5 gene in a clinical vancomycin resistant Enterococcus faecium isolate. *J. Bacteriol.* **180,** 4426–4434.

68. Chow, J. W., Donabedian, S. M., Clewell, D. B., et al. (1998) In vitro susceptibility and molecular analysis of gentamicin-resistant Enterococci. *Diagn. Microbiol. Infect. Dis.* **32,** 141–146.

69. Arthur, M. and Courvalin, P. 1993 Genetics and mechanisms of glycopeptide resis-tance in enterococci. *Antimicrob. Agents Chemother.* **37,** 1563–1571.

70. Leclerq, R. and Courvalin, P. (1997) Resistance to glycopeptides in enterococci *Clin. Infect. Dis.* **24,** 545–554.

71. Fines, M., Perichon, B., Reynolds, P., et al. (1999) VanE, a new type of acquired glycopeptide resistance in *Enterococcus faecalis* BM4405. *Antimicrob. Agents Chemother.* **43,** 2161–2164.

72. Centers for Disease Control and Prevention (1993) Nosocomial enterococci resis-tant to vancomycin—United States, 1989–1993. *M. M. W. R.* **42,** 597–599.

73. Morris, J. G., Jr., Shay, D. K., Hebdon, J. N., et al. (1995) Enterococci resistance to multiple antimicrobial agents, including vancomycin. Establishment of endemicity in a university medical center. *Ann. Intern. Med.* **123,** 250–259.

74. Brennan, C., Wagner, M. M., and Muder, R. R. (1998) Vancomycin resistant *Entero-coccus faecium* in a long term care facility. *J. Am. Geriatr. Soc.* **46,** 157–160.

75. Edmond, M. B., Ober, J. F., Dawson, J. D., et al. (1996) Vancomycin-resistant enterococcal bacteremia: natural history and attributable mortality. *Clin. Infect. Dis.* **23,** 1234–1239.

76. Hospital Infection Control Practices Advisory Committee (1995) Recommendations for preventing the spread of vancomycin resistance. *Infect. Control Hosp. Epidemiol.* **16,** 105–113.

77. Crossley, K. (1998) Vancomycin-resistant enterococci in long-term care facilities. *Infect. Control Hosp. Epidemiol.* **19,** 521–525.

78. Chia, J. K., Nakata, M. M., Park, S. S., et al. (1995) Use of bacitracin therapy for infection due to vancomycin resistant *Enterococcus faecium. Clin. Infect. Dis.* **21,** 1520.

79. Eliopoulos, G. M., Wennersten, C. B., Gold, H. S., et al. (1996) In vitro activities of new oxazolidinone antimicrobial agents against enterococci. *Antimicrob. Agents Chemother.* **40**, 1745–1747.

80. Dresser, L. D. and Ryback, M. J. (1998) The pharmacologic and bacteriologic properties of oxazolidinones, a new class of synthetic antimicrobials. *Pharmacotherapy* **18**, 456–462.

81. Swaney, S. M., Aoki, M. J., and Shinabarger, D. L. (1998) The oxazolidone linezolid inhibits initiation of protein synthesis in bacteria. The pharmacologic and bacteriologic properties of the oxazolidone linezolid inhibits initiation of protein synthesis in bacteria. *Antimicrob. Agents Chemother.* **42**, 3251–3255.

82. Patel, R., Rouse, M. S., Piper, K. E., et al. (1999). In vitro activity of linezolid against vancomycin-resistant enterococci, methicillin-resistant *Staphylococcus aureus* and penicillin-resistant *Streptococcus pneumoniae*. *Diagn. Microbiol. Infect. Dis.* **34**, 119–122.

83. Noskin, G. A., Siddiqui, F., Stosor, V., et al. (1999) In vitro activities of linezolid against important gram-positive bacterial pathogens including vancomycin-resistant enterococci. *Antimicrob. Agents Chemother.* **43**, 2059–2062.

84. Corso, A., Severina, E. P., Petruk, V. F., et al. (1998). Molecular characterization of penicillin-resistant *Streptococcus pneumoniae* isolates causing respiratory disease in the United States. *Microb. Drug Resist.* **4**, 325–337.

85. Macinga, D. R. and Rather, P. N. (1999) The chromosomal 2'-N-acetyltransferase of *Providencia stuartii*: physiological functions and genetic regulation. *Front. Biosci.* **4**, D132–D140.

86. Muder, R. R., Brennen, C., Drenning, S. D., et al. (1997) Multiply antibiotic-resistant gram-negative bacilli in a long-term-care facility: a case-control study of patient risk factors and prior antibiotic use. *Infect. Control Hosp. Epidemiol.* **18**, 809–813.

87. Bendall, M. J. and Gruneberg, R. N. (1979) An outbreak of infection caused by trimethoprim-resistant coliform bacilli in a geriatric unit. *Age Ageing* **8**, 231–236.

88. Walker, K. J., Gilliland, S., Vance-Bryant, K., et al. (1993). *Clostridium difficile* colonization in residents of long-term care facilities: prevalence and risk factors. *J. Am. Geriatr. Soc.* **41**, 940–946.

89. Web site. http://www. lahey. org/studies/web. htm

90. Wiener, J., Quinn, J. P., Bradford, P. A., et al. (1999) Multiple antibiotic-resistant *Klebsiella* and *Escherichia coli* in nursing homes. *JAMA* **281**, 517–523.

91. Jacoby, G. A. (1994) Genetics of extended-spectrum β-lactamases. *Eur. J. Clin. Microbiol. Infect. Dis.* **13(Suppl. 1),** 2–11.

92. Mederios, A. A. (1997) Evolution and dissemination of β-lactamases accelerated by generations of β-lactam antibiotics. *Clin. Infect. Dis.* **24(Suppl 1),** S19–S45.

93. Nicolas-Chanoine, M. H. (1997) Inhibitor-resistant β-lactamases. *J. Antimicrob. Chemother.* **40**, 1–3.

94. Sirot, D., Recule, C., Chaibi, E. B., et al. (1997) A complex mutant of TEM-1 β-lactamase with mutations encountered in both IRT-4 and extended spectrum TEM-1, produced by *Escherichia coli* clinical isolates. *Antimicrob. Agents Chemother.* **41**, 322–1325.

95. Bret, L., Chanal-Claris, C., Sirot, D., et al. (1998) Chromosomally encoded AmpC type β-lactamase in a clinical isolate of *Proteus mirabilis*. *Antimicrob. Agents Chemother.* **48**, 1110–1114.

96. Bradford, P. A., Urban, C., Mariano, N., et al. (1997) Imipenem resistance in *Klebsiella pneumoniae* is associated with the combination of ACT-1, a plasmid

mediated Amp C beta-lactamase and the loss of an outer membrane protein. *Antimicrob. Agents Chemother.* **41,** 563–569.

97. Sanders, W. E. and Sanders, C. C. (1988) Inducible β-lactamases: Clinical and epidemiologic implications for use of newer cephalosporins. *Rev. Infect. Dis.* **10,** 830–838.

98. Jacobs, C., Frere, J.-M., and Normack, S. (1997) Cytosolic intermediates for cell wall biosynthesis and degradation control inducible beta-lactam resistance in Gram-negative bacteria. *Cell* **88,** 823–832.

99. Chow, J. W., Fine, M. J., Shlaes, D. M., et al. (1991) *Enterobacter bacteremia*: clinical features and emergence of antibiotic resistance during therapy. *Ann. Intern. Med.* **115,** 585–590.

100. Rice, L. B., Carias, L. L., Bonomo, R. A., et al. (1995). Molecular genetics of resistance to both ceftriaxone and β-lactam β-lactamase inhibitor combinations in *Klebsiella pneumoniae* and in vivo response to β-lactam therapy. *J. Infect. Dis.* **173,** 151–158.

101. Moellering, R. C., Jr. (1990) Interaction between antimicrobial consumption and selection of resistant bacterial strains. *Antimicrob. Agents Chemother.* **39,** 1211–1233.

102. Rice, L. B., Carias, L. L., and Shlaes, D. M. (1993) Efficacy of ampicillin-sulbactam versus cefoxitin for the treatment of *Escherichia coli* infection in the rat abdominal abscess model. *Antimicrob. Agents Chemother.* **37,** 610–612.

103. Shen, L. L. and Pernet, A. G. (1985) Mechanism of inhibition of DNA gyrase by analogues of nalidixic acid; the target of the drugs is DNA. *Proc. Natl. Acad. Sci. USA* **82,** 307–311.

104. Brightly, K. E. and Gootz, T. D. (1997) The chemistry and biological profile of trovafloxacin. *J. Antimicrob. Chemother.* **39(Suppl. B),** 1–14.

105. Wiedemann, B. and Heisig, P. (1994) Mechanism of quinolone resistance. *Infection* **22(Suppl. 2),** S73–S79.

106. Coronado, V. G., Edwards, J. R., and Culver, D. H. (1995) Ciprofloxacin resistance among nosocomial *Pseudomonas aeruginosa* and *Staphylococcus aureus* in the United States. National Nosocomial Infections Surveillance (NNIS). *Infect. Control Hosp. Epidemiol.* **16,** 71–75.

107. Ednie, L. M., Jacobs, M. R., and Appelbaum, P. C. (1998) Comparative activities of clinafloxacin against gram-positive and gram-negative bacteria. *Antimicrob. Agents Chemother.* **42,** 1269–1273.

108. Shlaes, D. M., Gerding, D. N., John, J. F. Jr., et al. (1997) Society for Healthcare Epidemiology of America and the Infectious Disease Society of America Joint Commission on the Prevention of Antimicrobial Resistance. *Infect. Control Hosp. Epidemiol.* **18,** 275–291.

109. Perea, S., Hildalgo, M., Arcediano, A., et al. (1999). Incidence and clinical impact of fluoroquinolone-resistant *Escherichia coli* in the faecal flora of cancer patients treated with high dose chemotherapy and ciprofloxacin prophylaxis. *J. Antimicrob. Chemother.* **44,** 117–120.

110. McGeer, A., Campbell, B., Eckert, D. G., et al. (1991) Definitions of infection for surveillance in long term care facilities. *Am. J. Infect. Control* **19,** 1–7.

111. Bonten, M. J. and Weinstein, R. A. (1996) The role of colonization in the pathogenesis of nosocomial infection. *Infect. Control Hosp. Epidemiol.* **17,** 193–200.

22

Infections in Diabetics

Francisco L. Sapico

1. CLINICAL RELEVANCE

1.1. Epidemiology

Diabetes mellitus affects at least 6% of the U.S. population, and at least another 6% of diabetics may be undiagnosed *(1)*. However, in persons 65 yr and older, 11% have diabetes with probably another 8% being undiagnosed. Of all diabetics in the U.S., 43% are 65 yr and older. The vast majority of these individuals (90–95%) belong to the type II category and the rest belong to type I. Diabetic complications are more common the longer the duration of the disease has been present. A significant percentage of these complications come in the form of infections. Because these complications are generally related to disease duration, clinical problems are very frequently seen in the elderly population. Moreover, infectious complications in older diabetics have poorer outcomes.

Infections by themselves can destabilize diabetic control. Marked hyperglycemia and/or ketoacidosis can, in turn, make the control of infection more difficult.

Clinicians have generally believed that diabetics are more susceptible to infections and that infections are generally more severe in diabetics than they are in nondiabetics. There has been a scarcity of controlled studies that have conclusively shown that certain infections are more common in diabetics as compared to nondiabetics *(2)*. Urinary tract infection and bacteremia have also been shown to be more frequent in the diabetic *(3,4)*. Review of the literature with regards to certain specific infections, however, strongly suggests that diabetics are clearly overrepresented in these infections *(5,6)*. These infections are discussed in detail in this chapter.

1.2. Predisposing Factors

Hyperglycemia and the generalized metabolic imbalance associated with diabetes mellitus are believed to be largely responsible for the disordered immune function seen in this disease. Significant dysfunction of the polymorphonuclear leukocyte (PMNL) chemotaxis, phagocytosis, and intracellular bactericidal capability have been identified *(7–9)*. A recent study has implicated increased levels of cytosolic calcium secondary to hyperglycemia for the phagocytic defect in the diabetic PMNL *(10)*. Improvement of the metabolic control results in improved function of these cells. Similar defects in monocyte function have also been described *(11)*.

From: *Infectious Disease in the Aging*
Edited by: Thomas T. Yoshikawa and Dean C. Norman
© Humana Press Inc., Totowa, NJ

Other host defense defects that have been reported in diabetics include decreased cutaneous and delayed hypersensitivity and decreased lymphocyte responsiveness to phytohemagglutinin stimulation in vitro *(12)*. Diabetics have also been shown to have deficiency in the fourth component of complement as well as decreased opsonization of microorganisms such as *Candida albicans (13)*.

Besides all these defects in immune function, other diabetic complications that predispose to infections include peripheral and autonomic neuropathy as well as large- and small-vessel disease. These deficiencies can lead to dryness and fissuring of the skin and gangrene of extremities, in turn leading to soft-tissue and bone infections; to neuropathic foot lesions and Charcot osteoarthropathy, which also predispose to injuries and secondary infections; and to urinary bladder dysfunction leading to acute and chronic urinary tract infections.

2. SPECIFIC INFECTIONS (*See* Table 1)

2.1. Respiratory Tract Infections

2.1.1. Pneumonitis

Diabetic patients with gastroparesis, diabetic ketoacidosis, hyperosmolar coma, or hypoglycemic seizures may have an increased risk for aspiration pneumonitis. Aging alone increases the susceptibility for pneumonia (*see* Chapter, 6). Higher morbidity and mortality in diabetics have been described with influenza *(14)*, and there appears to be an increased incidence of pneumonitis secondary to *Staphylococcus aureus* and *Klebsiella pneumoniae*. Pneumococcal vaccination has been recommended for all persons aged 65 yr and older as well as diabetics because of potentially increased morbidity from *Streptococcus pneumoniae* infections.

2.1.2. Tuberculosis

Diabetics are at an increased risk of developing active tuberculosis when their tuberculin skin tests are positive with normal chest X-rays. Therefore, they are candidates for isoniazid chemoprophylaxis regardless of age *(15)*. Tuberculosis has been described to be up to 16 times more common in diabetics as compared to nondiabetics *(2)*.

2.1.3. Rhinocerebral Mucormycosis

More than 75% of the reported cases of the fungal disease rhinocerebral mucor-mycosis occurs in diabetics; generally these diabetics are in states of poor metabolic control and ketoacidosis (*16*; *see also* Chapter 18). Paranasal sinuses and the palate may be initially involved with this infection, with later spread of this disease to the retroorbital area, the cavernous sinus, and intracranial sites, including the frontal lobes. Fungi belong to the order Mucorales, and the genera *Rhizopus, Absidia, Mucor,* and *Rhizomucor* are often responsible. Local spread of the infection may result in osteomy-elitis, proptosis, ophthalmoplegia, blindness, cavernous sinus thrombosis, meningoen-cephalitis, and brain abscesses. Fungal invasion of blood vessels causes thrombosis and often result in tissue infarctions. Diagnosis is generally made by biopsy of the marginal areas of the necrotic black eschars, which are characteristically seen in this disease entity. Potassium hydroxide (KOH) or stained tissue preparations will show thick hyphae that have rare septations and with right-angle branching.

Table 1
Infections Associated with Diabetes Mellitus

Respiratory tract
    Pneumonitis
    Tuberculosis
    Rhinocerebral mucormycosis
    Invasive external otitis

Gastrointestinal
    Candida esophagitis
    Emphysematous cholecystitis

Urinary tract
    Bacteriuria, cystitis, and uncomplicated pyelonephritis
    Emphysematous pyelonephritis
    Emphysematous cystitis
    Perinephric abscess
    Papillary necrosis
    Fungal infections

Skin and soft-tissue infections
    Superficial, nonnecrotizing infections
    Necrotizing infections
        Superficial necrotizing
            Crepitant (anaerobic) cellulitis
            Necrotizing fasciitis
        Deep necrotizing
            Nonclostridial myonecrosis
            Clostridial myonecrosis
        Foot-related infections

Aggressive surgical extirpation of infected bone and soft tissue is required. Repeated debridement is often necessary. Intravenous (IV) amphotericin B at 1.0 mg/kg/d (or liposomal amphotericin B at 5.0 mg/kg/d) may be given up to total doses of 2.0–4.0 g. The available azoles are inactive against this organism. Despite aggressive therapy, 15–50% mortality may still ensue. Survivors may require extensive plastic reconstruction and psychological support.

2.1.4. Invasive External Otitis

In contrast to the more common external otitis often seen in children ("swimmer's ear"), invasive (or necrotizing) external otitis is a much more aggressive infection (*see* also Chapter 15). Approximately 90% of patients with this disease are diabetics, frequently in poor metabolic control. Except for unusual cases caused by other organisms such as *Aspergillus* and *K. pneumoniae*, virtually all cases are associated with *Pseudomonas aeruginosa*; the presence of granulation tissue at the junction of the bony and cartilaginous portions of the external canal is a characteristic clinical finding *(17)*. Local spread along this cleft or junction may result in osteomyelitis of the temporomandibular joint, parotitis, and mastoiditis. Deeper invasion may result in cranial nerve

IX–XII palsies, septic sigmoid sinus thrombophlebitis, and meningoencephalitis. Involvement of cranial nerve VII resulting in facial palsy (due to inflammation of the stylomastoid canal exit site) is fairly common (30–40% of cases) and may not necessarily imply a dire prognosis. Computed tomographic (CT) and magnetic resonance imaging (MRI) scans have dramatically improved the clinician's ability to determine the extent of involvement of bony and intracranial structure in this disease process.

Management includes early and aggressive debridement of the external auditory canal. Bony sites of involvement may also need debridement and administration of appropriate antimicrobial therapy. Since *P. aeruginosa* is almost always the pathogen involved, therapy frequently consists of parenteral, high-dose anti-pseudomonal β-lactam agent, such as piperacillin, ceftazidime, cefepime, or aztreonam, in combination with an aminoglycoside for synergistic antimicrobial activity. Extreme care should be exercised when giving aminoglycosides to elderly persons and to diabetics, especially those with preexistent renal insufficiency. Since the aminoglycosides under these conditions are given primarily for synergy, maximum doses may not be necessary, and the drug may be given once or twice daily to decrease nephrotoxicity. Anecdotal cases suggest that oral (PO) ciprofloxacin may be effective in selective cases *(18)*. Parenteral therapy with β-lactams will generally require a total minimum duration of 4 wk, but longer therapy (i.e., 3 mo) has been suggested for oral ciprofloxacin.

2.2. Gastrointestinal Infections

2.2.1. Candida Esophagitis

Human immunodeficiency virus (HIV) disease is currently the most common predisposing condition leading to esophageal candidiasis, (*see* also Chapters 18 and 19). *Candida* esophagitis, however, has been reported to occur with increased frequency in diabetics *(19)*. Complaints of dysphagia or odynophagia in a diabetic (with or without concomitant or antecedent course of antimicrobial therapy) should alert the clinician to the possibility of candida esophagitis. Unlike HIV disease, diabetics may have esophagitis without necessarily manifesting oral thrush. Diagnosis is easily made by endoscopy and biopsy. Oral therapy with fluconazole (200 mg the first day followed by 100 mg daily thereafter) for a minimum of 3 wk (at least 2 wk after resolution of symptoms) is generally sufficient.

2.2.2. Emphysematous Cholecystitis

Approximately 35% of the reported cases of the highly virulent emphysematous cholecystitis has occurred in diabetics *(20)*. Compared with the usual form of cholecystitis, this entity has shown a preponderance of males (70%), a high incidence of gallbladder wall gangrene (74%) and perforation (21%), and high mortality (15–25%). Absence of concomitant gallstones is seen in one-half of these cases. Infection is frequently polymicrobial, with Gram-negative bacilli such as *Escherichia coli* and *Klebsiella* spp., as well as *Clostridium perfringens* among the most commonly isolated microorganisms. A high index of suspicion followed by prompt and aggressive surgery and appropriate antimicrobial therapy may help decrease the morbidity and mortality of this disease entity.

2.3. Urinary Tract Infections

2.3.1. Bacteriuria, Cystitis, and Uncomplicated Pyelonephritis

The prevalence of bacteriuria and urinary tract infections (UTI) in diabetic females has been shown to be higher than in nondiabetic females *(3)*. Involvement of the upper urinary tract (pyelonephritis) in diabetics with bacteriuria has also been proposed to occur more frequently in diabetics. Moreover, bacteriuria substantially increases in both females and males with aging (*see* Chapter 10). Factors that may predispose diabetics to UTI include the presence of neurogenic bladder (with associated increase in residual volume), recurrent vaginitis, glycosuria, underlying renal disease, and urinary tract instrumentation.

2.3.2. Emphysematous Pyelonephritis

This condition generally presents as a fulminant, life-threatening illness. Seventy percent to 90% of the cases of emphysematous pyelonephritis reported are diabetic, and the infection is almost always unilateral *(21)*, affecting the left kidney more often than the right. There is characteristic mottled gas found in and around the kidney, often detectable with plain upright abdominal radiograph and clearly demonstrated by CT scan. Associated urinary tract obstruction is seen in 40% of diabetic patients and virtually all of the nondiabetic patients. *E. coli* is the culprit pathogen in 70% of the cases. Pathologically, necrotizing pyelonephritis, cortical abscesses, and sometimes papillary necrosis are present. Clinically, the patient presents with fever, chills, flank pain, confusion, and generalized sepsis. Although a few cases have responded to medical therapy alone, higher survival rates have been associated with combined antibiotic therapy plus nephrectomy. Because aging and diabetes (diabetic nephropathy) are associated with renal insufficiency, careful assessment of kidney function is also essential in the management of this and all forms of UTI in elderly diabetics.

2.3.3. Emphysematous Cystitis

E. coli and other members of the Enterobacteriaceae family are generally responsible for this clinical entity, which is generally more benign than emphysematous pyelonephritis. At least 80% of the reported cases occur in diabetics *(23)*. They may present with pneumaturia, and gas in the urinary bladder wall may be seen on plain abdominal X-ray or by abdominal CT scan. The disease is generally responsive to antimicrobial therapy.

2.3.4. Perinephric Abscesses

This entity should be suspected in patients with urinary tract infection and fever of at least 5 d duration that is unresponsive to appropriate antimicrobial therapy *(23)*. Approximately 35% of the cases have associated diabetes, and about half of the patients will present with abdominal or flank mass.

The diagnosis is generally established by ultrasonography or CT or MRI scan. Surgical drainage done by either open surgery or percutaneous catheter placement, in combination with about 4 wk of antimicrobial therapy, are generally effective in the management of this disease. Ureteral obstruction needs to be excluded. *E. coli* is the most common isolate, and ascending infection is the usual route of spread.

2.3.5. Papillary Necrosis

At least 50% of patients with papillary necrosis are diabetic *(24)*. An associated urinary infection may or may not be present. However, other causes of papillary necrosis include sickle cell disease, analgesic abuse, and obstruction. Most cases present with an acute febrile illness, but a few may present with a more subacute course. Acute-onset flank or abdominal pain, chills, and fever are the usual initial symptoms. Renal insufficiency may be a complication and may become more rapidly apparent in older diabetics. Characteristic findings of papillary necrosis may sometimes be seen on ultrasonography, but the "gold standard" of diagnosis for this disease is generally by retrograde pyelography. If the detached papilla is not passed spontaneously, urinary obstruction may need to be relieved surgically. A minimum course of 2 wk of appropriate antimicrobial therapy may be required if there is associated infection.

2.3.6. Fungal Urinary Tract Infections

Twenty percent to 90% of cases of *C. (Torulopsis) glabrata* UTI have been reported to be in diabetics. High incidences of candiduria (as high as 35%) and *Candida* UTI have been reported in glycosuric diabetics *(25)*. Severe infections resulting in sepsis, fungus ball formation, and obstruction may be seen in some cases. Quantitative colony counts of only 10,000 yeasts/mL urine may be sufficient to cause disease. Fluconazole (IV or PO) is excreted in the urine and is generally effective therapy. Intravenous amphotericin B may be an alternative for renal infection, but cystitis may be managed with bladder catheter instillation of amphotericin B. Obstruction needs to be relieved surgically with removal of fungus balls.

2.4. Skin and Soft-Tissue Infections

2.4.1. Superficial Nonnecrotizing Infections

Increased nasal carriage of *S. aureus* has been reported in insulin-injecting diabetics *(26)*. However, increased propensity of diabetics to staphylococcal furunculosis and carbuncles has not been conclusively proven. Erythrasma, a superficial bacterial infection located in the genitocrural area, is caused by *Corynebacterium minutissimum*, and is more commonly found in men and obese persons with diabetes. Postoperative clean-wound infections have been reported to occur with increased frequency in diabetics.

2.4.2. Necrotizing Infections

2.4.2.1. Superficial Necrotizing

These infections do not extend below the deep fascia enveloping muscles. *Crepitant (anaerobic cellulitis)* infections are frequently superimposed on chronic, nonhealing ulcers and are generally characterized by extensive subdermal and subcutaneous gas dissection produced by multiple organisms, particularly anaerobes. Good clinical outcome is generally seen with thorough debridement and appropriate antimicrobial therapy. *Necrotizing fasciitis* is characterized by extensive dissection of the infection along the superficial fascial planes without involvement of the underlying muscles. Although it may sometimes be caused by single organisms (such as *Streptococcus pyogenes*), mixed infections with aerobes and anaerobes are more frequently seen (i.e., *Bacteroides* spp., *Peptostreptococcus* spp., *E. coli*, *P. mirabilis*, *Enterococcus* spp., and so on) *(27)*. Thrombosis of nutrient vessels to the skin may occur, resulting in patchy areas of skin gangrene. Bullae formation under the skin may develop in the later stages, but early disease may show little external changes (tautness of the skin, mild erythema, and tenderness). Patchy areas of skin anesthesia may occur secondary to destruction of small nerve fibers to the skin in the later stages. Management includes thorough debridement and drainage of the necrotic fascia and the associated purulence (the so-called "filleting procedure," where the subcutaneous tissue is left open and subjected to irrigation with normal saline or Ringer's lactate solutions). Appropriate antimicrobial therapy should be directed toward both the aerobic and anaerobic flora when mixed infection is present. *S. pyogenes* infection is frequently associated with toxic shock syndrome. In this situation, addition of clindamycin to high-dose penicillin G has been suggested, primarily to halt the organism's toxin production. Intravenous gamma globulin administration has also been felt to be helpful. Repeated surgical debridement is frequently required.

2.4.2.2. Deep Necrotizing

Nonclostridial myonecrosis (erstwhile known as necrotizing cellulitis) is an extensive infection, and up to 75% of these cases have been reported to be in diabetics. The bacterial flora involved are similar to necrotizing fasciitis, but infection involves the muscles. Therapy is similar, but resection of necrotic muscle is required. *Clostridial myonecrosis* related to injuries do not appear to occur more frequently in association with diabetes. However, there are some suggestions that the spontaneous or hematogenous form of this disease has a predilection to involve diabetics. *C. septicum* (not *perfringens)* is the organism generally involved, and there is a strong association with the presence of colonic malignancy. *Foot-related infections* may involve deep tissues. The major factors contributing to foot-related infections are diabetic neuropathy, vascular disease, and impaired immune resistance. Superficial and milder infections are frequently monomicrobial (usually from Gram-positive cocci such as *S. aureus*), but more severe infections associated with tissue necrosis and/or gangrene is generally polymicrobial (aerobic and anaerobic) in origin (*see* Table 2). These infections may be associated with gas formation, from proliferation of gas-forming organisms such as *Bacteroides, Prevotella, Porphyromonas, Peptostreptococcus,* or even from the aerobic *E. coli.* Underlying osteomyelitis needs to be excluded, generally with an MRI scan, and the vascular status may need to be determined by use of Doppler ultrasound with wave-form analysis or with transcutaneous oximetry. Milder infections (i.e., limited cellulitis) may be managed with thorough debridement of the infected wound and antimicrobial therapy. First- or second-generation cephalosporins (such as cefazolin or cefuroxime) may be used for presumed monomicrobial infections. For more serious infections broad-spectrum coverage is frequently indicated (i.e., parenteral piperacillin-tazobactam, imipenem, or trovafloxacin). The presence of osteomyelitis may require removal of infected bone (i.e., toe amputation, with or without ray resection). Amputation may sometimes be necessary, and the level is dictated by the extent of bone involvement, the status of the vascular supply, and the extent of soft-tissue involvement. In general, the extent of surgery needs to be balanced by thorough removal of infected tissue on one hand and the preservation of ambulatory capability on the other.

Table 2
Most Common Pathogens Isolated from Deep Tissue
in Moderate to Severe Diabetic Foot Infections[a]

Aerobes
    Gram-negative bacilli
        Proteus mirabilis
        Escherichia coli
        Pseudomonas aeruginosa
        Enterobacter aerogenes
        Others

    Gram-positive cocci
        Enterococcus spp.
        Staphylococcus aureus
        Group B streptococcus
        Others

Anaerobes
    Gram-negative
        Bacteroides fragilis
        Bacteroides spp. (other than fragilis)
        Porphyromonas spp.
        Prevotella spp.
        Fusobacterium spp.
        Others

    Gram-positive cocci
        Peptostreptococcus magnus
        Peptostreptococcus anaerobius
        Other *Peptostreptococcus* spp.

    Gram-positive bacilli
        Clostridium spp.

[a]Data derived from ref. *27*.

3. CONCLUSION

The diabetic patient has a distinct predisposition to many infection processes because of a combination of several factors (1) the presence of a disordered metabolic state, (2) impairment of various facets of the immune function, (3) the presence of neuropathy, and (4) the presence of vascular compromise. With aging, the predilection, severity, and mortality related to infections are greater; thus, the elderly diabetic is at special jeopardy for infections. The clinician needs to maintain acute awareness of these infectious complications and to be able to recognize them early. However, early detection of infection may be difficult in the elderly (*see* Chapter 3). Management of these infectious problems will require aggressi metabolic control of the diabetic state, combined with appropriate antimicrobial therapy and surgical intervention. Good control of the diabetic state may help restore a disordered immune state. Education of the diabetic with regards to proper foot care may help forestall future foot problems.

REFERENCES

1. Davidson, M. B. (1991) An overview of diabetes mellitus, in *The High Risk Foot in Diabetes Mellitus,* (Frykberg, R. G., ed.), Churchill Livingstone, New York, pp. 1–22.
2. Root, H. F. (1934) The association of diabetes and tuberculosis. *N. Engl. J. Med.* **210,** 1–13.
3. Hansen, R. O. (1966) Bacteriuria in diabetic and non-diabetic outpatients. *Acta Med. Scand.* **176,** 721–730.
4. Osi, B. S., Chen, B. T. M., and Yu, M. (1974) Prevalence and site of bacteriuria in diabetes mellitus. *Postgrad. Med. J.* **50,** 497–499.
5. Leslie, C. A., Sapico, F. L., and Bessman, A. N. (1989) Infections in the diabetic host. *Compr. Ther.* **15(7),** 23–32.
6. Sapico, F. L., Leslie, C. A., and Bessman, A. N. (1991) Infections in the diabetic host, in *Difficult Medical Management,* (Taylor, R. B., ed.), W. B. Saunders, Philadelphia, pp. 368–373.
7. Bagdade, J. D., Root, R. K., and Bulger, R. J. (1974) Impaired leucocyte function in patients with diabetes mellitus. *Diabetes* **23,** 9–15.
8. Repine, J. E., Clawson, C. C., and Goetz, F. C. (1980) Bactericidal function of neutrophils from patients with acute bacterial infections and from diabetics. *J. Infect. Dis.* **142,** 869–875.
9. Tan, J. S., Anderson, J. L., Watanakunakorn, C., et al. (1975) Neutrophil dysfunction in diabetes mellitus. *J. Lab. Clin. Med.* **85,** 26–33.
10. Alexewicz, J. M., Kumar, D., Smogorzewski, M., et al. (1995) Polymorphonuclear leukocytes in non-insulin-dependent diabetes mellitus: abnormalities in metabolism and function. *Ann. Intern. Med.* **123,** 919–924.
11. Lawrence, S., Charlesworth, J. A., Pussell, B. A., et al. (1984) Factors influencing reticulophagocytic function in insulin-treated diabetes. *Diabetes* **33,** 813–818.
12. Plouffe, J. F., Silva, J., Fekety, F. R., Jr., et al. (1978) Cell-mediated immunity in diabetes mellitus. *Infect. Immun.* **21,** 425–429.
13. Vergani, D., Johnston, C., B-Abdullah, N., et al. (1983) Low serum C4 concentrations: an inherited predisposition in insulin-dependent diabetics. *Br. Med. J.* **286,** 926–928.
14. Bouter, K. P., Diepersollt, R. J., and Van Romunde, L. K. (1991) Effect of epidemic influenza on ketoacidosis, pneumonia, and death in diabetes mellitus: a hospital register survey of 1976–1979 in the Netherlands. *Diabetes Res. Clin. Pract.* **12,** 61–68.
15. Miller, B. (1992) Preventive therapy for tuberculosis. *Med. Clin. North Am.* **77,** 1263–1275.
16. Leher, R. I., Howard, D. H., Sypherd, P. S., et al. (1980) Mucormycosis. *Ann. Intern. Med.* **93,** 93–108.
17. Doroghazi, R. M., Nadol, J. B., Hyslop, H. E. Jr., et al. (1981) Invasive external otitis. *Am. J. Med.* **71,** 603–614.
18. Sade, J., Lang, R., Goshan, S., et al (1989) Ciprofloxacin treatment of malignant external otitis. *Am. J. Med.* **87(Suppl. 5A),** 385–415.
19. Kodsi, B. E., Wickremesingke, P. C., and Kozinn, P. J. (1976) *Candida* esophagitis. A prospective study of 27 cases. *Gastroenterology* **71,** 715–719.
20. Mentzer, R. M., Jr., Golden, G. T., Chandler, J. G., et al. (1975) A comparative appraisal of emphysematous cholecystitis. *Am. J. Surg.* **129,** 10–15.
21. Michaeli, J., Mogle, P., Perlberg, S., et al. (1984) Emphysematous pyelonephritis. *J. Urol.* **131,** 203–208.
22. Bailey, H. (1961) Cystitis emphysematoma. *Am. J. Roentgenol.* **86,** 850–862.
23. Thorley, J. D., Jones, S. R., and Sanford, J. P. (1974) Perinephric abscess. *Medicine* **53,** 441–451.
24. Whitehouse, F. W. and Root, H. F. (1956) Necrotizing renal papillitis and diabetes mellitus. *JAMA* **162,** 444–447.
25. Wise, G. J., Goldberg, P., and Kozinn, P. J. (1976) Genitourinary candidiasis: diagnosis and treatment. *J. Urol.* **116,** 778–780.
26. Tuazon, C. U., Perez, A., Kishaba, T., et al. (1975) *Staphylococcus aureus* among insulin-injecting diabetic patients. *JAMA* **231,** 1272.

27. Sapico, F. L., Witte, J. L., Canawati, H. N., et al. (1984) The infected foot of the diabetic patients: quantitative microbiology and analysis of clinical features. *Rev. Infect. Dis.* **6(Suppl.),** S171–S176.

23

Vaccinations

David W. Bentley

1. INTRODUCTION

This review focuses primarily on the major vaccines that all persons 65 yr of age and older should receive: tetanus-diphtheria toxoid, influenza virus vaccines and pneumococcal vaccine. See detailed discussions below and Table 1 for a summary. There are, however, other vaccines, e.g., cholera, hepatitis A and B, meningococcal, plague, rabies, typhoid, and yellow fever, that are recommended in circumstances that place an older person into a special high-risk group. For further details, see the recommendations for the use of these vaccines for persons ≥65 yr old by the National Vaccine Advisory Committee (1), The American College of Physicians Task Force/Infectious Disease Society of America (2), and the most recent reports from the Centers for Disease Control and Prevention's Advisory Committee on Immunization Practices (ACIP) on the specific immunobiologics that are published with the Morbidity and Mortality Weekly Report (see their web site:www.cdc.gov/publications). Recommendations regarding immunization of older travelers appear in the Centers for Disease Control and Prevention's annual publication, *Health Information for the International Traveler* (3), or their website (www.cdc.gov/travel).

2. TETANUS–DIPHTHERIA TOXOID

2.1. Clinical Relevance

Tetanus continues to cause serious health problems for older persons. Although the number of reported cases of tetanus in the United States is low (approximately 50–65 cases annually), the estimated completeness of reporting ranges from 40% for mortality to even lower for morbidity (4). Of the approximately 125 cases reported during 1995–1997, 35% occurred in persons ≥60 yr with a case fatality rate as high as 20%. Only 13% of patients reported having a record of the primary series for tetanus toxoid before disease onset. Of the approximately 125 cases, 50% occurred following puncture wounds, but many were related to minor injuries, e.g., lacerations (22%) and abrasions (12%). Three of 93 patients had an acute injury related to surgery performed 4–8 d before the onset of illness. Of the acute wounds, 25% occur at home and 15% occur indoors elsewhere (5). Approximately 40% of persons sustaining an acute injury seek medical care. Of these, only 40% received tetanus toxoid prophylaxis for wound care and <25% with debrided wounds received tetanus immune globulin as recommended

From: *Infectious Disease in the Aging*
Edited by: Thomas T. Yoshikawa and Dean C. Norman
© Humana Press Inc., Totowa, NJ

Table 1
Recommended Immunizing Agents for Persons Aged ≥ 65 Years[a]

Vaccine type	Usual schedule	Indications	Major precautions and contraindications
Tetanus-diphtheria (Toxoids [Td])	Two IM doses 4 wk apart; third dose 6–12 mo after second dose; booster every 10 yr	All elderly persons; tetanus prophylaxis in wound management (*see* Table 2)	History of neurologic reactions or immediate hypersensitivity reactions after a previous dose
Influenza vaccine (inactivated whole-virus and split-virus vaccines)	Annual vaccinations with current vaccine Administered IM Optimal time is October-November but may be given any time during the influenza season	Persons at high risk influenza or its complications[b]; immunocompromised or immunosuppressed persons[d]; all healthy elderly persons	History of anaphylactic hypersensitivity to eggs
Pneumococcal polysaccaride vaccine (23 valent)	One dose, 0.5 mL, IM or SC. Revaccination for those at highest risk of invasive pneumococcal infection 5 yr later or if first dose given before age 65 and ≥5 yr since first dose	Persons at high risk pneumococcal disease and its complications[c]; immunocompromised or immunosuppressed persons[d]; all healthy elderly persons	Previous anaphylactic reaction to the vaccine or any of its components

[a]Data from refs. *9, 15,* and *23.*

[b]Persons at high risk for influenza and its complications: chronic cardiovascular and pulmonary disorders, diabetes, renal dysfunction, hemoglobinopathies and/or persons living in chronic care facilities.

[c]Persons at high risk for pneumococcal disease and its complications: chronic cardiac and pulmonary diseases, anatomical or functional asplenia, chronic liver disease, alcoholism, diabetes mellitus, CSF leaks, and/or living in chronic care facilities.

[d]Persons immunocomprised or immunosuppressed: HIV infection, leukemia, lymphoma, Hodgkin's disease, multiple myeloma, generalized malignancy, chronic renal failure, or nephrotic syndrome; or immunosuppressed as the result of therapy with corticosteroids, alkylating drugs, antimetabolites, or radiation.

Abbreviations: IM = intramuscular; SC = subcutaneous; CSF = cerebrospinal fluid; HIV = human immunodeficiency virus.

(5). Previous reports have noted that 15% of cases of tetanus are associated with chronic wounds, e.g., skin ulcers, abscesses, gangrenous extremities or recent surgery *(4).*

Because there is no natural immunity to the extracellular toxin (tetanospasm) of *Clostridium tetani,* tetanus occurs almost exclusively in persons who are unimmunized, inadequately immunized, or whose history of immunization is unknown. Protection depends on the presence of circulating antibody to the extracellular toxin prior to fixation of the toxin to its ganglioside binding site. Protective serum antitoxin levels are present in 30–45% of community-residing older persons *(6)* and in 30–50% of elderly nursing home residents *(7).* In both settings, the lowest prevalence is in nonveterans. There are several historical clues to the presence of nonprotective titers and the increased risk of disease: (1) never completing the primary immunization series, (2) receiving fewer than two doses of tetanus toxoid or (3) an unknown history *(5)*.

Although a similar low prevalence of diphtheria protective antitoxin antibody levels can be demonstrated in older persons, diphtheria is not as serious a problem for older persons as is tetanus. Thus, this section will not comment further on diphtheria but recommendations for the use of the immunizing agent for older persons, tetanus–diphtheria toxoid, will provide protection against diphtheria as well. The recent outbreaks of diphtheria reported in adults from regions of the former Soviet Union illustrate the disease's epidemic potential in susceptible adults who are inadequately immunized *(8)*.

2.2. Immunizing Agent

The current recommended immunizing agent for older persons is Tetanus–Diphtheria (Td) Toxoid Adsorbed for Adult Use, which is a combined preparation containing 5 Lf units of tetanus toxoid and 2 Lf units of diphtheria toxoid. The dose and administration of Td toxoid should be according to the manufacturer's package insert; adbsorbed preparations should be administered intramuscularly *(9)*. Td toxoid is an effective immunizing agent for older persons. In nursing home residents, protective tetanus antitoxin antibody levels following immunization occur in approximately 40% of nonimmune older persons after the first dose, in 85% following the second dose 4–8 wk later, and in 100% after the third dose 6–12 mo later. The duration of protective levels is somewhat reduced in older persons: approximately 25% of persons have no protective antitoxin antibody in 8 yr, but 90% can be protected after a single booster immunization *(10)*. There are no clinical efficacy studies in older persons. Information on adverse reactions following Td toxoid in older persons is scant. The only contraindications to Td toxoid is a history of neurological reactions (febrile or nonfebrile convulsions, encephalopathy, or focal neurologic signs) or severe hypersensitivity reactions (urticaria or anaphylactic reaction) associated with a previous dose *(9)*.

2.3. Current Recommendations

Vaccination with Td toxoid is recommended for all older persons. The routine immunizing schedule for older persons requires a series of three doses called primary immunization. It is recommended for all older persons who are unimmunized, inadequately immunized, or whose history of immunization is unknown. The booster immunization, also with Td toxoid, is administered every 10 yr after the last dose, provided the primary series has been completed.

The guidelines for tetanus prophylaxis in the management of wounds are the same for all adults and have been further simplified (*see* Table 2) *(9)*. With a clean wound, older persons should receive a single booster at the time of acute treatment. If the immunization history regarding the primary series is doubtful (or, as in most instances, unknown), and the injury is more than a clean wound, older persons should receive Td toxoid and passive immunization with human tetanus immunoglobulin. *In either case, the primary immunization series should then be completed.*

2.4. Implementing Current Recommendations and Improving Utilization

Despite these well-publicized recommendations, tetanus has continued to occur in the United States, primarily in older persons ≥60 yr of age who are highest risk for

Table 2
Summarized Recommendations of Advisory Committee on Immunization Practices (ACIP) for Tetanus Prophylaxis in Routine Wound Management—United States, 1991[a]

History of adsorbed tetanus toxoid (doses)	Clean, minor wounds		All other wounds[b]	
	Td[c]	TIG[d]	Td	TIG
Unknown or <3	Yes	No	Yes	Yes
≥3[e]	No[f]	No	No[g]	No

[a]Data from ref. 9.

[b]Such as, but not limited to, wounds contaminated with dirt, feces, soil, saliva; puncture wounds; avulsions; and wounds resulting from missiles, crushing, burns, and frostbite.

[c]Td = tetanus–diptheria toxoids, which are for adults preferred to tetanus toxoid alone.

[d]TIG = Tetanus immune globulin.

[e]If only three doses of *fluid* toxoid have been received, then a fourth dose of toxoid, preferably an absorbed toxoid, should be administered.

[f]Yes, if more than 10 yr have elapsed since the last dose.

[g]Yes, if more than 5 yr have elapsed since the last dose. More frequent boosters are not needed and can accentuate side effects.

disease and death. This group (especially elderly women) is at highest risk because they lack protective immunity; many have not received the primary series as children (or in the military service for women), and routine periodic (every 10 yr) booster doses of tetanus toxoid are frequently omitted *(6)*. Cost effectiveness studies, however, suggest that efforts to increase tetanus protection in older persons by establishing primary immunization programs is a questionable use of health-care resources *(11)*. More effective strategies to improve Td toxoid vaccine coverage in older persons are needed. Implementation of two following recommendations could help accomplish this.

2.4.1. Identify Persons with High-Risk Conditions

Tetanus immunization programs, for community-residing older persons, would be more cost effective if they were focused on older persons at high risk for tetanus-prone injuries or conditions, especially at the time of the injury. This is probably best done by identifying *all older persons with soft-tissue injuries* as being at high-risk for tetanus. National and regional surveys have documented the problem of inappropriate undertreatment of elderly patients with tetanus-prone wounds who subsequently develop tetanus *(5)*. Because >90% of tetanus morbidity and mortality are associated with soft-tissue injury, the emphasis on appropriate wound management *and* the completion of the primary series is an effective strategy in reducing the number of cases in older persons.

Because more than 65% of elderly preoperative surgical patients may lack protective serum antitoxin levels *(12)*, the Td toxoid history of older persons should be established prior to elective surgery, especially involving the gastrointestinal tract and amputation of gangrenous extremities. Unless a satisfactory vaccination history is documentable, older patients undergoing high-risk tetanus-prone surgery should receive Td toxoid and human tetanus immunoglobulin *and complete the primary series following surgery*. The recently reported cost-effective strategy of a single Td booster at age 65 *(13)* would seem appropriate but only for those who have received the primary series.

Residents of nursing facilities (nursing home) with cutaneous ulcerations or vascular complications should receive the primary series unless there is documentation of the complete primary series *and at least one subsequent booster dose of Td toxoid (including booster doses as wound prophylaxis).* The question of primary immunization programs for all older persons in nursing facilities has been debated, but information to date suggests that the incidence of tetanus in nursing facility residents is remarkably low. Thus, the recommendation that nursing facility medical directors should establish institutionwide policies for tetanus immunization *(14)*, similar to those that promote influenza and pneumococcal immunization, seems premature.

2.4.2. *Improve the Delivery of Vaccines*

The low incidence of tetanus in the United States in infants, children, and young adults is a result of widespread immunization programs supported by pediatricians, mandated for schools, and implemented per military care regulations. Thus, older persons remain largely unprotected because there are no dedicated programs for them. Therefore, all clinicians must emphasize to their high-risk older patients the need for adequate immunization with Td toxoid. For those who have received the primary series, linking a single routine Td toxoid booster with a dose of pneumococcal vaccine at age 60 or 65 is an attractive strategy *(8)*.

3. INFLUENZA VACCINES

3.1. *Clinical Relevance*

Although persons ≥65 yr old comprise approximately 13% of the United States population and have low rates of infection with influenza virus (10% of total influenza infections), they account for nearly 50% of the hospitalizations (20,000 to >300,000 per epidemic) and 90% of the deaths (20,000 to >40,000 per epidemic) attributed to influenza. The highest estimated rates are among persons ≥65 yr old and persons of any age with underlying cardiovascular disease in combination with either diabetes mellitus or chronic pulmonary disease *(15)*.

Prevention of influenza virus infection by immunization is a formidable task in older persons. Influenza A viruses, the primary cause of severe illness, are classified into subtypes on the basis of their hemagglutinin (H) and neuroaminidase (N) antigens. Sufficient antigen variation or drift within the same subtype, e.g., A/Texas/77 (H3N2) versus A/Bangkok/79 (H3N2), may occur over time so that infection or immunization with one strain may not induce immunity to related strains of the same subtype. Major antigenic shifts, which herald pandemic influenza, produce "new" viruses to which the population has no immunity, e.g., the shift in 1957 from H1N1 to H2N2. Influenza B viruses also cause disease in older persons and, although they are much more antigenically stable than influenza A viruses, antigen variation does occur. Consequently, influenza vaccine presently must be administered each year and include the inactivated expected virus strains.

3.2. *Immunizing Agent*

Inactivated influenza vaccines consist of highly purified egg-grown inactivated viruses in either a whole virus or split (subvirion) virus trivalent preparation containing two type A strains and one type B strain. For the 1999–2000 influenza season in the

United States, the standard trivalent inactivated influenza vaccine contained 15 μg each of A/Beijing/262/95-like (H1N1), A/Sydney/5/97-like (H3N2), and B/Beijing/184/93-like hemagglutinin antigens in each 0.5 mL dose of vaccine. A single intramuscular 0.5 mL dose is required each year for older persons (15).

Acute local reactions with mild to moderate soreness around the vaccination site occur in approximately one-third of vaccines and last 1–2 d. Systemic reactions, including fever with or without a flu-like illness, occur in less than 1% of vaccinees, begin 6–12 h postvaccination, and persist for 1–2 d but are not associated with higher rates of systemic symptoms in older persons compared to placebo injections (16).

Precautions to vaccination include immediate hypersensitivity reactions or documented immunoglobulin E (IgE)-mediated hypersensitivity to egg protein; older persons with these findings should consult a physician for appropriate evaluation to help determine if vaccine should be administered. Persons with a previous history of Guillain-Barré syndrome (GBS) have an increased likelihood of coincidentally developing GBS after influenza vaccination, but whether influenza vaccination specifically might increase the risk for recurrence of GBS is not known. However, many experts believe that for most older persons who have a history of GBS and are at high risk for severe complications from influenza, the established benefits of influenza vaccination justify yearly vaccination. There are no studies to suggest an increased risk of reaction in persons with multiple sclerosis or other chronic neurologic demyelinating diseases. Although influenza vaccinations can reduce the clearance of theophylline and warfarin, studies have not demonstrated any adverse clinical consequences attributed to these drugs in vaccinees (15).

The proportion of elderly vaccinees who develop "protective" antibody titers postvaccination, i.e., serum hemagglutination inhibition (HAI) antibody titers of 1:40 or greater, ranges from more than 85% for H3N2 vaccine antigens in healthy community-based persons to 46–100% for H3N2 antigens and 20–69% for B antigens in ambulatory older persons in long-term care facilities. The antibody titers postvaccination for elderly nursing facility patients demonstrate considerable heterogeneity and are significantly lower than healthy young and healthy older persons (17). This suggests that older persons with chronic diseases, medications, or other conditions frequently associated with residence in long-term care facilities may be expected to respond less satisfactorily to inactivated influenza vaccines. T-cell-mediated immune mechanisms, e.g., influenza A-specific cytotoxic T lymphocyte activity, are also important in influenza viral clearance and appear reduced in older adults (18). Recent successful investigational efforts to improve the immunogenic response of older persons to influenza vaccine have included a concurrent four-week series of subcutaneous injections of thymic hormone, thymosin α_1; the use of conjugated diphtheria toxoid-hemagglutinin vaccine; and combined live intranasal and inactivated influenza vaccines. However, the only currently licensed vaccine is the annual inactivated influenza virus formulation (19).

How effective is the vaccine? In a prospective cohort observational study of community-residing older persons during an influenza A epidemic, vaccination was associated with a reduction in the rates of hospitalization for pneumonia and influenza (57%), all acute and chronic respiratory conditions (39%) and congestive heart failure (43%) (20). The first randomized double-blind placebo-controlled trial in a similar population in the Netherlands demonstrated a risk reduction of nearly 60% for clinical influenza with serological confirmation *(21)*. A case-control observational study of influenza outbreaks in nursing facilities indicated that, although the efficacy of influenza vaccine in preventing uncomplicated illness was relatively low (28–37%). The vaccine was substantial in reducing complications, including hospitalization or pneumonia (50–60%) and death (80%) *(22)*.

3.3. Recommendations

Presently, all persons 65 yr of age and older should receive annually the inactivated parenteral influenza vaccine. The elderly subgroups that should be prioritized for organized vaccination programs include: (1) persons with chronic disorders of the cardiovascular or pulmonary systems, (2) residents of nursing facilities and other long-term care facilities, (3) persons who require regular medical follow-ups or hospitalization during the preceding year because of chronic metabolic conditions (including diabetes mellitus), renal dysfunction, hemoglobinopathies, or immunosuppression (including immunosuppression caused by medications) and (4) otherwise healthy older persons. Because most residents in long-term care facilities have reduced antibody responses, it is important that this elderly high-risk group receive influenza vaccine no earlier than mid-October. In addition, all persons who have extensive contact with these higher-risk older persons should also receive influenza vaccination annually. These people include physicians, nurses, and other health-care team personnel, as well as formal and informal providers of care in the home setting *(15)*.

Strategies for implementing current recommendations and improving utilization of influenza vaccine (together with pneumococcal vaccine) will be discussed as in Subheading 4.4.

4. PNEUMOCOCCAL VACCINE

4.1. Clinical Relevance

The overall annual incidence of pneumococcal bacteremia is 50–80 cases per 100,000 in persons 65 yr of age and older; approximately 85% of these cases are associated with pneumonia. Despite appropriate antimicrobial therapy and intensive medical care, the overall case-fatality rate for pneumococcal bacteremia in older patients is 30–40%; nearly 50% of these deaths could potentially be prevented by the use of pneumococcal vaccine *(23)*. Moreover, the continued emergence of drug-resistant *Streptococcus pneumoniae* and its clinical importance further emphasizes the need for preventing pneumococcal infections by vaccination *(24)*.

4.2. Immunizing Agent

The current recommended immunizing agent is pneumococcal vaccine, polyvalent. In July 1983, a 23-valent preparation was licensed in the United States to replace an earlier 14-valent preparation. The vaccine contains purified polysaccharides antigens representing 85–90% of the serotypes (1-5, 6B, 7F, 8, 9N, 9B, 10A, 11A, 12F, 14, 15B, 17F, 18C, 19A, 19F, 20, 22F, 23F, and 33F [Danish nomenclature]) that cause invasive pneumococcal infections in the United States. The vaccine is formulated so that each 0.5 mL dose contains 25 µg per component in a diluent of isotonic saline containing 0.25% phenol (PNEUMOVAX®) or 0.01% thimerosal, a mercury derivative, (PNU-

IMUNE) as preservative. The dose is administered subcutaneously or intramuscularly. Pneumococcal vaccine and influenza vaccine can be given at the same time, if different sites are used, without decreasing the antibody response of either vaccine or substantially increasing the side effects *(23)*.

Vaccine-associated reactions occur within 24 h of injection in approx 30% of vaccinees and consists primarily of mild local side effects, e.g., discomfort, erythema and induration and persists for <48 h. Intradermal administration may cause more severe local reactions and is contraindicated. Fever of 100°F (37.7°C) or greater occurs in 2% of vaccines and generally lasts <24 h. Severe systemic reactions, e.g., fever (≥103°F [39.4°C]), headache, myalgias, and chills, or anaphylactoid reactions were not reported in >7000 vaccinees *(25)*. No neurologic disorders, e.g., GBS, have been associated with administration of the vaccine *(23)*.

The mechanism of protection following vaccination is similar to natural infection and depends on the production of opsonizing antibodies that promote phagocytosis of the homologous types. The level of type-specific antibody, which is protective against each type, has not been determined, and there is considerable variation in individual vaccinee's response. Most adults respond to the vaccine in 2 wk with a maximum response in approx 4–6 wk. Antibody concentrations and responses in older persons, especially those with alcoholic cirrhosis, chronic obstructive pulmonary disease, and insulin-dependent diabetes mellitus, are lower than in healthy young adults. In older immunocompromised patients, e.g., those with anatomic asplenia, leukemia, lymphoma, multiple myeloma, nephrotic syndrome, Hodgkin's disease, or acquired immunodeficiency syndrome, the antibody response is often further diminished or absent. The duration of "protective" serum antibody levels in older persons following vaccination is unknown but does decline after 5–10 yr and declines more rapidly in those immunocompromised/ immunosuppressed *(23)*.

A meta-analysis evaluating the results of nine postlicensure, randomized-controlled studies did not demonstrate pneumococcal vaccine efficacy against nonbacteremic pneumococcal disease persons in high-risk groups, including persons aged ≥65 yr. Problems with evaluating vaccine efficacy in these studies include lack of sensitivity and specificity in diagnosing nonbacteremic pneumococcal pneumonia and other biases *(25)*. The effectiveness of vaccination of persons ≥65 yr old against invasive (bacteremic) pneumococcal infections, as demonstrated in observational nonrandomized case-control studies or serotype prevalence studies based on a national pneumococcal surveillance system, was 80% and 75%, respectively *(23)*.

4.3. Current Recommendations

All persons 65 yr of age and older should receive pneumococcal vaccine. These include both (1) immunocompetent persons 65 yr or older who are otherwise healthy and those who are at increased risk of pneumococcal disease or its complications because of chronic illness, e.g., congestive heart failure, chronic pulmonary disease, diabetes mellitus, cirrhosis, alcoholism, or cerebrospinal fluid leaks; and (2) immunocompromised older persons with conditions noted previously. Persons undergoing elective splenectomy or immunosuppressive treatment, including long-term systemic corticosteroids, should be vaccinated at least 2 wk, or as early as possible, prior to treatment *(23)*.

Revaccination is recommended once for persons ≥65 yr old who are at risk for serious pneumococcal infections and are likely to have a rapid decline in pneumococcal antibody levels. This group includes those older persons noted above who are immunocompromised or immunosuppressed. In addition, all other persons aged ≥65 yr should receive a second dose of pneumococcal vaccine if they received the vaccine ≥5 yr previously and were aged <65 yr at the time of the primary vaccination. Routine revaccination following a second dose is not recommended at this time *(23)*. Although revaccination with pneumococcal vaccine 6 yr after primary vaccination provides a less satisfactory "booster" response in older persons, this is not associated with an increase in adverse side effects *(26)*. Older persons with unknown vaccination status should be administered one dose of vaccine *(23)*.

4.4. Implementing Current Recommendations and Improving Utilization of Influenza and Pneumococcal Vaccines

Despite the well-supported recommendations for influenza and pneumococcal vaccines, the combined cause-of-death category of pneumonia and influenza is the fifth leading cause of death in the United States among persons aged ≥65 yr. Recent self-reported vaccination levels for persons aged ≥65 yr for 1995–1997 indicate that annual influenza vaccination increased from 58–65% and overall pneumococcal vaccination increased from 37–45%. Overall, persons aged 65–74 yr are less likely than persons aged ≥75 yr to report receipt of influenza (63% versus 69%) or pneumococcal (42% versus 51%) vaccinations. Levels for influenza and pneumococcal vaccines administrations are lower among non-Hispanic blacks (50% and 30%, respectively) and Hispanics (58% and 34%, respectively) and for those who had no visit to a physician during a previous year (47% and 29%, respectively) *(27)*. These findings indicate a substantial improvement in coverage levels, but for some groups the levels remain low, especially for pneumococcal vaccine. More effective strategies to improve influenza vaccine and pneumococcal vaccine for all persons aged ≥65 are needed and should include the following.

4.4.1. Identify Persons with High-Risk Conditions

Older persons with underlying chronic diseases, especially cardiac and respiratory conditions, are at highest risk for complications of influenza and pneumonia. These patients, plus older persons with other high-risk medical conditions for which influenza and pneumococcal vaccines are recommended, are easily identified because they require regular medical follow-ups in the community, frequent hospitalizations, or admissions to long-term care facilities. All clinicians should review the older patient's vaccination status at each of these sites to establish and implement effective immunization programs with influenza and pneumococcal vaccines for older persons.

4.4.2. Improve the Delivery of Vaccines

Community-based primary care physician offices are primarily responsible for providing influenza vaccines to most elderly vaccinees, and, in all likelihood, these same offices are the most frequent sites for older persons to receive pneumococcal vaccine. All primary care clinicians should schedule a prevention visit for all patients when they reach age 50 yr to assess vaccination status and provide appropriate vaccines and other preventive measures as recently recommended *(1,2)*. This scheduled visit should then be extended regularly after the age of 50 yr. The finding that more than 75% of pneumo-coccal vaccinations are administered in September through December (the same season as recommended for influenza vaccine) emphasizes the important opportunity for improving vaccination rates during a single office visit during late autumn or early winter.

New strategies to improve the delivery of these vaccines include direct payments to physicians for each vaccine dose administered to older persons with high-risk conditions. Financing through Medicare since 1993 has substantially expanded immunization rates for influenza vaccine especially in physician's offices, and should prove more cost effective than setting up large public clinics in which vaccination rates are variable and low (28). Despite Medicare reimbursement since 1981, the lower utilization rates for pneumococcal vaccine continue, which suggests the need for additional efforts in promoting the use of pneumococcal vaccine. Methods by which office practices have increased vaccination rates include telephone and postcard reminders for patients and computer-generated reminders and peer comparisons for physicians and office staff (29,30).

Although physicians' offices and public clinics will remain the principal setting for immunization against influenza and pneumococcal disease, acute-care hospital-based immunization programs (including emergency rooms and walk-in clinics) can also provide a major opportunity for improving the vaccination status of older persons. Nursing facilities and other residential long-term care facilities should also be included as sites for promoting vaccinations. In nursing facilities that require written informed consent, however, influenza vaccination rates of residents are approximately 60% versus approx 90% for residents in those facilities that do not have this requirement (31). If this barrier persists, and if appropriate means of "informing" residents and their families are not developed, then nursing facilities and other long-term care facilities will provide less than optimal sites for implementing vaccine recommendations for older persons.

4.4.3. Improve the Acceptance of Older Persons

Easy access to vaccines, however, does not guarantee satisfactory vaccination rates. Older persons frequently do not receive influenza and pneumococcal vaccines for several reasons including the perception of not needing vaccination, lack of a physician's recommendation, concern about adverse events following vaccination, and perception of vaccine ineffectiveness (32). The lack of acceptance by older persons of influenza and pneumococcal vaccines is frequently related to the lack of information and proper guidance by their physicians. Furthermore, although physicians know the importance and appropriateness of vaccination for older persons, they greatly under prescribe them for their own patients.

To help allay fears and doubts about the effectiveness and safety of vaccines, older persons need the support of their families and their physicians and other members of the health care team regarding future vaccinations. Older persons (and their families) should receive full and accurate information concerning the efficacy and safety of the vaccination. Explanations must be presented in a clear and meaningful way regarding the relative risks of suffering serious side effects versus the relative risk and dangers to persons their age (and with their health problems) of contracting the disease and its complications. This can best be accomplished with direct discussions with the patient's physician or other members of the health care team. In addition, these discussions can take place in special settings, e.g., nutrition and recreation centers, high-rise apartments, church socials, and the like. Additional studies are needed to help vaccine promoters assess the types of education and motivation needed for targeted persons to become immunized.

The foregoing suggestions for implementing existing recommendations for immunization of persons aged ≥65 yr will require continued efforts to improve utilization of the targeted vaccines for this high-risk group. All physicians, and other members of the health care team, can play a major role now by acting as effective role models in implementing the current recommendations during the care of their older patients. This would be especially effective in promoting hospital-based immunization programs with house staff and in promoting long-term care facility-based programs with nursing personnel.

ACKNOWLEDGMENTS

The author wishes to thank Carolyn Cole and Carol McCleary for their excellent secretarial assistance.

REFERENCES

1. Fedson, D. S., for the National Vaccine Advisory Committee (1994) Adult immunization: summary of the National Vaccine Advisory Committee Report. *JAMA* **272**, 1133–1137.
2. American College of Physicians Task Force on Adult Immunization/Infectious Diseases Society of America (1994) *Guide for Adult Immunization*, 3rd ed., Philadelphia, PA, American College of Physicians.
3. Centers for Disease Control and Prevention (1999) *Health Information for International Travel 1999–2000*, U.S. Pubic Health Service, Dept. of Health and Human Services, Atlanta, GA.
4. Prevots, R., Sutter, R. W., Strebel, P. M., et al. (1992) Tetanus surveillance—United States, 1989–1990. *M.M.W.R.* **41**, 1–9.
5. Bardenheier, B., Prevots, D. R., Khetsuriani, N., et al. (1998) Tetanus surveillance—United States, 1995–1997, in CDC Surveillance Summaries. *M.M.W.R.* **47(No. SS-2)**, 1–13.
6. Gergen, P. J., McGuillan, G. M., Kiely, M., et al. (1995) A population-based serologic survey of immunity to tetanus in the United States. *N. Engl. J. Med.* **332**, 761–766.
7. Weiss, B. P., Strassburg, M. A., and Feeley, J. C. (1983) Tetanus and diphtheria immunity in an elderly population in Los Angeles county. *Am. J. Public Health* **73**, 802–804.
8. LaForce, F. M. (1993) Routine tetanus immunizations for adults: once is enough. *J. Gen. Intern. Med.* **8**, 459–460.
9. Centers for Disease Control and Prevention (1991) Diphtheria, tetanus, and pertussis: recommendations for vaccine use and other preventive measures: recommendations of the Immunization Practices Advisory Committee (ACIP). *M.M.W.R.* **40(No. RR-10)**, 1–28.
10. Solomonova, K. and Vizev, S. (1981) Secondary response to boostering by purified aluminum-hydroxide-adsorbed tetanus anatoxin in aging and in aged adults. *Immunobiology* **158**, 312–319.
11. Hutchison, B. G. and Stoddart, G. L. (1988) Cost-effectiveness of primary tetanus vaccination among elderly Canadians. *Can. Med. Assoc. J.* **139**, 1143–1151.
12. Simonsen, O., Block, A. V., Klaerke, A., et al. (1987) Immunity against tetanus and response to revaccination in surgical patients more than 50 yr of age. *Surg. Gynecol. Obstet.* **164**, 329–334.
13. Balestra, D. J. and Littenberg, B. (1993) Should adult tetanus immunization be given as a single vaccination at age 65? A cost-effectiveness analysis. *J. Gen. Intern. Med.* **8**, 405–412.

14. Richardson, J. P., Knight, A. L., and Stafford, D. T. (1990) Beliefs and policies of Maryland nursing home medical directors regarding tetanus immunization. *J. Am. Geriatr. Soc.* **38,** 1316–1320.
15. Centers for Disease Control and Prevention (1999) Prevention and control of influenza: recommendations of the Advisory Committee on Immunization Practices (ACIP). *M.M.W.R.* **48(No. RR-4),** 1–28.
16. Margolis, K. L., Nichol, K. L., Poland, G. A., et al. (1990) Frequency of adverse reactions to influenza vaccine in the elderly: a randomized, placebo-controlled trial. *JAMA* **264,** 1139–1141.
17. Beyer, W. E. P., Palache, A. M., Baljet, M., et al. (1989) Antibody induction by influenza vaccines in the elderly: a review of the literature. *Vaccine* **7,** 385–394.
18. Powers, D. C. (1993) Influenza A virus-specific cytotoxic T lymphocyte activity declines with advancing age. *J. Am. Geriatr. Soc.* **41,** 1–5.
19. Bentley, D. W. (1996) Immunizations in older adults. *Infect. Dis. Clin. Pract.* **5(8),** 490–497.
20. Nichol, K. L., Margolis, K. L., Wuorenma, J., et al. (1994) The efficacy and cost effectiveness of vaccination against influenza among elderly persons living in the community. *N. Engl. J. Med.* **331,** 778–784.
21. Govaert, T. M. E., Thijs, C. N., Masurel, N., et al. (1994) The efficacy of influenza vaccination in elderly individuals. A randomized double-blind placebo-controlled trial. *JAMA* **272,** 661–665.
22. Patriarca, P. A., Weber, J. A., Parker, R. A., et al. (1985) Efficacy of influenza vaccine in nursing homes: Reduction in illness and complications during an influenza A (H3N2) epidemic. *JAMA* **253,** 1136–1139.
23. Centers for Disease Control and Prevention (1997) Pneumococcal polysaccharide vaccine: recommendations of the Immunization Practices Advisory Committee (ACIP). *M.M.W.R.* **(46(No.RR-8),** 1–24.
24. Nuorti, J. P., Butler, J. C., Crutcher, J. M., et al. (1998) An outbreak of multidrug-resistant pneumococcal pneumonia and bacteremia among unvaccinated nursing home residents. *N. Eng. J. Med.* **338,** 1861–1868.
25. Fine, M. J., Smith, M. A., Carson, C. A., et al. (1994) Efficacy of pneumococcal vaccination in adults: a meta-analysis of randomized controlled trials. *Arch. Intern. Med.* **154,** 2666–2677.
26. Mufson, M. A., Hughey, D. F., Turner, C. E., et al. (1991) Revaccination with pneumococcal vaccine of elderly persons 6 yr after primary vaccination. *Vaccine* **9,** 403–407.
27. Centers for Disease Control and Prevention (1997) Influenza and pneumococcal vaccination coverage levels among persons aged ≥65 yr—United States, *M.M.W.R.* **46,** 797–802.
28. Centers for Disease Control and Prevention (1993) Final results: Medicare influenza vaccine demonstration—selected states, 1988–1992. *M.M.W.R.* **42,** 601–604.
29. Smith, D. M., Zhou, X., Weinberger, M., et al. (1999) Mailed reminders for area-wide influenza immunization: a randomized controlled trial. *J. Am. Geriatr. Soc.* **47,** 1–5.
30. Barton, M. B. and Schoenbaum, S. C. (1990) Improving influenza vaccination performance in an HMO setting: the use of computer-generated reminders and peer comparison feedback. *Am. J. Public Health* **80,** 534–536.
31. Patriarca, P.A., Weber, J.A., Meissner, M.K., et al. (1985) Use of influenza vaccine in nursing homes. *J. Am. Geriatr. Soc.* **33,** 463–466.
32. Vaccination levels among Hispanics and non-Hispanic whites aged ≥65 yr—Los Angeles County, California 1996. (1997) *M.M.W.R.* **46,** 1165–1171.

24

Nutrition and Infection

Kevin P. High

Nutritional factors have been suggested to mediate, at least in part, the immune dysfunction and increased risk of infection common in older adults *(1,2)*. A variety of nutrients directly and indirectly influence immune function and presumably infection risk *(see* Fig. 1 from ref. *[3])*. However, few nutritional interventions have as yet shown clear clinical benefits. This chapter examines the prevalence, clinical manifestations, and diagnosis of malnutrition in elderly adults and summarizes the currently available data regarding the role of nutritional supplements in the prevention or treatment of infectious diseases in the elderly.

1. EPIDEMIOLOGY AND CLINICAL RELEVANCE

Malnutrition is rare in developed countries, but in the United States and other Western cultures the elderly represent a population at special risk (see Table 1) *(4,5)*. Nutrient intake is often reduced in older adults by comorbidities such as dental disorders, stroke, dementia, or cancer. Furthermore, elderly adults often live alone, rarely prepare food for themselves, may substitute cheaper foods in place of more expensive but more nutritious foods, or live in nursing homes or are homebound with minimal sunlight exposure (that may lead to reduced vitamin D synthesis). Finally, some nutrient requirements increase with age; thus, the elderly are at much higher risk than the general population for nutritional deficiencies (*see* Table 2).

1.1. Global Malnutrition

Global malnutrition (decreased intake or increased requirements for protein and calories) is the most common nutritional deficit of elderly subjects. Among older subjects admitted to acute care hospitals or chronic care facilities, up to 65% are undernourished *(6–8)*. This malnutrition is associated with significant adverse clinical outcomes. Volkert and colleagues *(9)* found a close correlation between nutritional status on admission and subsequent risk of hospital death, but the association remained after hospital discharge and the mortality rate remained higher over an 18-mo follow-up. Sullivan and Walls *(10)* also found an increased risk of morbidity and mortality in undernourished elderly admitted to a Veterans Affairs (VA) geriatric rehabilitation unit (GRU), and further demonstrated that much of the risk is due to infection. They evaluated 350 randomly selected patients admitted to the GRU and determined the value of 96 medical, functional, socioeconomic, and nutritional variables for predicting life-threatening complications. Only five variables were predictive of life-threatening complications,

From: *Infectious Disease in the Aging*
Edited by: Thomas T. Yoshikawa and Dean C. Norman
© Humana Press Inc., Totowa, NJ

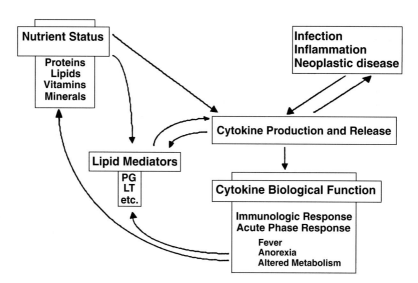

Fig. 1. Interactions of nutritional factors with immune function in elderly adults. Reprinted with permission of ref. *(3)*. PG = postaglandins; LT = leukotrienes

three of which were nutritional (serum albumin, body mass index, and amount of weight loss in the prior year; the other two variables were renal function and activities of daily living). Seventy-one life-threatening events occurred, of which 28 (39%) were clearly infectious (complicated pneumonia or sepsis). These authors further validated their model in a prospective cohort and found the five variable model listed to be 88% sensitive, 61% specific, and 65% accurate for predicting life-threatening events. Thus, it appears that evidence of malnutrition is a strong predictor of morbidity and mortality in older institutionalized adults.

If not present at the time of admission, undernutrition may become evident in elderly patients during hospitalization. Sullivan and colleagues *(11)* prospectively studied a VA population (98% male) of 497 patients who were well nourished at the time of admission to an acute care hospital. Patients were admitted for a variety of ailments with 54% admitted to the medical service and 46% to the surgical service. One hundred-two of the these patients (21%) had an average daily in-hospital nutrient intake of <50% of their calculated caloric needs. As expected, the undernourished group had lower discharge values for serum cholesterol, albumin, and pre-albumin, and lost slightly more weight than the well nourished group. Importantly, this group also experienced higher risk of death in-hospital (relative risk [RR] 8.0, 95% confidence internal [CI] [2.8–22.6]) and at 90 d (RR 2.9 [1.4–6.1]), and were more likely than their well-nourished counterparts to require discharge to a nursing or rehabilitation facility (RR 2.3 [1.1–4.6]). Major contributing factors to the undernutrition of hospitalized elderly included: "nothing by mouth" orders without nutrition via another route and ineffective use of canned supplements and nutritional support services. The major flaw in this observational cohort study is that it does not distinguish whether the undernutrition caused the adverse events or whether sicker patients were more likely to have poor intake and adverse outcomes (i.e., a confounding relationship). If anything, the undernourished group appeared to be healthier at baseline than the well-nourished group (more likely to have been admitted electively and better self-assessment of baseline health).

Table 1
Common Nutritional Deficiencies in the Elderly

Nutrient	Estimated prevalence[a] NH/Hosp (%)	Comm (%)	Physical symptoms and signs and laboratory evidence of deficiency
Protein/calorie	17–65	10–25	Anorexia, depression, muscle wasting, dermatitis, depression, peripheral edema, low serum albumin, lymphopenia
Vitamin A	2–20	2–8	Skin dryness, corneal changes, night blindness
Vitamin B_{12}		7–15	Dementia, depression, neuropathy, megaloblastic anemia
Vitamin D	20–40	2–10	Weakness, osteoporosis/osteomalacia
Vitamin E	5–15		Cerebellar ataxia, decreased relexes, myopathy
Zinc		15–25	Loss of taste, lethargy, poor wound healing

[a]True prevalence is difficult to estimate and dependent on measure employed (i.e., intake, serum levels, tissue levels, change in physiologic measures). See text.
NH = nursing home; Hosp = hospital; Comm = community.

Table 2
Metabolic Changes with Aging and Risk Factors for Malnutrition in the Elderly

Increased protein requirement
  Decreased protein synthesis
  Decreased nitrogen retention

Increased micronutrient requirement
  Synthesis of vitamin D in the skin declines
  Decreased renal hydroxylation of vitamin D to dihyroxyvitamin D
  Atrophic gastritis and decreased stomach acid decreases absorption of
    Vitamin B_{12}, calcium, iron, and folate

Decreased nutrient intake
  Loss of taste and smell
  Food avoidance: milk products, limited menu
  Dental disorders/ ill-fitting dentures
  Comorbidities (e.g., chronic obstructive pulmonary disease, congestive heart
    failure, cancer, depression, dementia)
  Social isolation/living alone; rarely prepare meals
  Economic factors: choosing between medications/food/rent
  Medications: digoxin/other appetite suppressants

Other recent studies suggest that undernutrition is not confined to hospitalized elderly, but occurs in community-dwelling, apparently healthy elderly (reviewed in *[5]*). Wilson and colleagues *(12)* reviewed the records of 1017 outpatients in St. Louis and found evidence of undernutrition in 85 (8%). The elderly (age ≥65 yr) were more likely to be undernourished than younger subjects (11% vs 7%, RR 1.6 [1.5–2.51]). Undernutrition was only recognized 43% of the time in older adults, and only 14% had an intervention to correct the underlying cause. Intentional weight loss and a prescribed diet were the most common causes of undernutrition in younger patients, but rare in the elderly. Depression (30%), poorly controlled diabetes (9%), cancer (9%), oropharyngeal disease (7%), dementia (5%), and drug reactions (3%) were common, potentially treatable causes in elderly adults.

1.2. Micronutrient Deficiency

Micronutrients can be broadly classified into vitamins (e.g., vitamins A, B-complex, C, D, E) and trace elements (e.g., zinc, selenium). Estimating the prevalence of micronutrient deficiencies in the elderly is difficult for several reasons. First, age-specific requirements for dietary intake or physiologic functions have not been firmly established. Second, dietary intake data may not accurately reflect serum levels of micronutrients, and serum levels may not accurately reflect tissue levels. Finally, "adequacy" may depend on the outcome measured.

A good example of these principles is vitamin A. Vitamin A is a fat-soluble vitamin, stored in the liver, and essential for both ocular and immune function. A French nursing facility study *(13)* evaluated four measures of vitamin A deficiency in elderly adults: oral intake, urinary excretion in response to an oral vitamin A load, corneal cytology, and serum levels. These measures assessed vitamin A deficiency to be present in 55%, 21%, 6%, and 2% of nursing facility residents, respectively. The relevant serum level to determine vitamin A deficiency is also unclear. Ocular function may begin to decline when serum vitamin A is <0.7 μmol/L, whereas poor immune function may become apparent at levels <1.05 μmol/L *(14)*. The World Health Organization definition for vitamin A deficiency is determined by ocular complications.

Deficiency of several other vitamins that influence immune function is also prevalent in elderly adults (*see* Table 2). Vitamin D deficiency is particularly common in the elderly due to a combination of social factors. Inadequate dietary intake (due to decreased consumption of milk and other dairy products) may be compounded by minimal sunlight exposure. A 1995 U.S. study *(15)* suggested that 54% of homebound and 38% of nursing facility resident elderly were vitamin D deficient by serum measures (i.e., serum concentration <25 nmol/L). Vitamin D is typically an immunosuppressive vitamin, so there are no supplementation trials with immune response outcomes in the elderly, but some have speculated that vitamin D deficiency might contribute to the increased incidence of autoantibodies in the elderly. Obviously, vitamin D is extremely important for the prevention of osteoporosis and other metabolic disorders in older adults.

Atrophic gastritis, present in up to one third of elderly adults, is associated with vitamin B_{12} deficiency. Low serum vitamin B_{12} is present in 7–15% of older adults and associated with reduced responses to pneumococcal vaccine *(16)*.

Vitamin E deficiency is often defined by oral intake rather than serum or tissue levels, a practice that may significantly underestimate prevalence. In a study of free living, healthy elderly, Chandra *(17)* found 8.3% of elderly adults had serum vitamin E levels below the 95% confidence interval for "normal" adults (12–48 μmol/L). Additional data suggest that using these serum values may still underestimate the prevalence of clinically significant vitamin E deficiency as maximal immune responses in older adults have been correlated with serum levels >48.4 μmol/L *(18)*.

Two trace elements, zinc and selenium, have received significant attention in recent years with regard to immune function and deserve comment. Zinc intake falls throughout life and declines below the U.S. recommended dietary allowance (RDA) of 0.2 mg/kg (12–15 mg/d) in the majority of older adults. One study of 118 healthy elderly in the Detroit area showed a mean zinc intake of 9.06 mg/d *(19)*. Serum zinc levels in that study were comparable in young and older adults, but cellular levels (granulocytes and lymphocytes) were significantly lower in older adults. Selenium, a component of glutathione peroxidase, can have significant effects on immune function and has been touted as a cancer preventive agent in recent studies. Selenium deficiency is common in some parts of the world, particularly Asia and New Zealand, where selenium deficiency in the soil is common. In the U.S., selenium deficiency is rare, and although some studies suggested it may be present in elderly nursing facility residents or hospitalized patients receiving chronic tube feedings, currently available tube feeding formulations almost always contain selenium in sufficient quantities.

2. CLINICAL MANIFESTATIONS

There are several major risk factors for malnutrition in the elderly that may serve as clinical clues to the diagnosis. Poverty, social isolation, dependence or disability, chronic/multiple medications, and dental disorders all increase the risk of malnutrition in elderly adults. Obviously, many comorbidities are also risk factors (e.g., depression, stroke, congestive heart failure) and have specific symptoms and signs associated with the underlying disorder. Clinical clues of global undernutrition in elderly patients include: low body weight, muscle wasting, sparse/thinning hair, flaking dermatitis, cheilosis/angular stomatitis, poor wound healing, and peripheral edema. Specific symptoms, signs, and laboratory abnormalities associated with micronutrient deficiency are shown in Table 1.

3. DIAGNOSTIC TESTS

There are several office assessments of nutritional status that have been validated in elderly adults and thoroughly reviewed elsewhere *(20)*. That extensive reference includes nomograms, chart forms, drug/nutrient interaction checklists, and nutrition-screening protocols ranging from simple waiting room questionnaires to detailed anthropometric measures and laboratory assessments. One helpful screen is to assess weight and height and calculate body mass index (BMI; weight in kg/(height in cm)^2). Barrocas and colleagues *(20)* suggest that older adults who experience ≥5% loss of body weight in 1 mo, a body weight ≥20% below ideal body weight or a BMI >27 or <22 have a more thorough assessment of nutritional status.

4. NUTRITIONAL THERAPY FOR PREVENTION OF INFECTION

4.1. Supplementation to Enhance Immune Responses and Prevent Infection

Despite volumes of very strong evidence that malnutrition is common in the elderly and associated with poor immune function, there are very few studies that have shown nutritional support can improve clinical outcomes in this population. These studies are very difficult to perform, rarely done in hospitalized patients or nursing facility residents, and require large sample sizes to be powered for statistical significance for clinical endpoints, and, thus, usually employ surrogate laboratory markers. A few trials did reach significant clinical endpoints and are noted below in this subheading; the remainder of trials utilized measures of immune function (antibody titers, delayed-type hypersensitivity [DTH] responses, lymphocyte functional assays, and the like) (*see* Table 3) *(17–19, 21–41)*.

Table 3
Summary of Supplementation Trials and Immune Response in Elderly Adults

Ref.	Sample Size	Time (mo)/ Trial type	Nutrient(s)	Major findings/comments
Multivitamin/mineral supplement or commercial formula				
(21)	47	12/R	Multivitamin/mineral supplement	↑ NK cells, slowed decline of CD4$^+$ cells
(22)	30	1/RP	100 mg vit C, 50 mg vit E, 8000 IU vit A	↑ T cells, CD4$^+$ cells, CD4/CD8 ratio, and lymphocyte responses
(17)	96	12/RP	Multivitamin/mineral supplement	↑ IL-2, lymphocyte responses; ↓ number of days with illness
(23)	56	6-12/RP	Multivitamin/mineral supplement	↑ DTH responses at 12 mo
(24)	21	2/Pre-Post	Commercial formula	↑ DTH responses
(25)	58	3/Obs	Macro-, micronutrient supplement	↑ DTH responses
(26)	34	12/Pre-Post	Targeted intervention for deficiency	↑ T cells; Zn^{++} deficient patients appeared to benefit most
Zinc supplementation				
(27)	103	3/RP	15, 100 mg zinc as zinc acetate[a]	No change in DTH or mitogen responses
(28)	63	12/RP[b]	15, 100 mg zinc as zinc acetate[a]	↑ DTH responses, NK cell activity, and lymphocyte proliferation
(29)	118	3/RP[c]	Vit A 800 mg retinyl palmitate and/or Zn^{++} 25 mg sulfate	Retinol: ↓ CD3, CD4; Zn^{++}: ↑ CD4$^+$, cytotoxic T cells (CD3$^+$, CD16$^+$ and CD56$^+$)
(30)	84	1/RP	220 mg bid zinc sulfate	No change in antibody responses to influenza vaccine
(31)	5	1/Pre-Post	55 mg zinc sulfate	↑ DTH responses

(19)	13	6/Pre-Post	Zn++ 30 mg gluconate	↑ IL-1, DTH
(31)	8	4.5/Pre-Post	Zn++ 30 mg (elemental) bid	↑ Lymphocytes, polymorphonuclear neutrophils, DTH responses
(33)	30	1/Obs	220 mg zinc sulfate	↑ T lymphocytes and DTH responses, no change in mitogen responses
Vitamin E supplementation				
(34)	32	1/RP	800mg vitamin E	↑ DTH responses, IL-2 responses, ↓ PGE-2 production
(35)	80	1-4.5/RP	60, 200, 800 IU vitamin E	↑ DTH responses at all three doses, ↑ mitogen responses only in the 800 IU group
(18)	88	8/RP	Vit E 60,200 or 800 mg qd	↑ DTH responses and primary responses to T-dependent antigens; no effect on booster or T-cell-independent responses
Vitamin A/β-Carotene supplementation				
(36)	20	3/RP	15, 30, 45, 60 mg β-Carotene	↑ CD4+ and NK cells, and number of IL-2 receptors
(37)	109	One dose/RP	Vit A 200,000 units	No change in infection rates or antibiotic use
(45)	21	144/RP	β-Carotene 50 mg qod/ASA 325 mg qod/both/neither	↑ NK cell activity w/out altering NK cell percentage, IL-2 or IL-2 receptor
Other/miscellaneous supplementation				
(39)	20	1/RP	500 mg injection of vitamin C	↑ DTH responses
(40)	158	--/Pre-Post	400 mg vitamin C	↑ IgG, IgM, and C-3 (complement) levels
(41)	15	1-2/Obs	50 mg vitamin B_6	↑ CD4+ cells and lymphocyte responses

[a]With additional multinutrient supplement.
[b]Partial crossover design.
[c]Factorial design.

Abbreviations: RP = randomized/placebo controlled; Pre-Post = pre-test, post-test; Obs = observational; ↑ = increase; ↓ = decrease; IL-2 = interleukin-2; PGE-2 = prostaglandin E-2; DTH = delayed-type hypersensitivity; Zn^{++} = zinc; NK = natural killer; qd = once daily; bid = twice daily; qod = every other day; IU = international unit; Ig = immunoglobulin

Multivitamin/mineral supplements have been given in a variety of study designs as outlined in Table 3. All these studies report enhancement of at least some surrogate markers (e.g., DTH responses, cytokine production). The only interventional study to clearly show benefit for preventing clinical events in elderly outpatients was published by Chandra *(17)*. Chandra provided a custom supplement of retinol; β-carotene; thiamine; riboflavin; niacin; pyridoxine; folate; vitamins B_{12}, C, D, E; iron; zinc; copper; selenium; iodine; calcium; and magnesium. All subjects were healthy elderly in the community. The design was 12 mo, double-blind, randomized, and placebo-controlled, and all subjects received supplements regardless of baseline nutritional status. The groups were well matched for nutritional variables and measures of immune response at baseline. Assessment of clinical illness was performed by a single physician blinded with regard to treatment assignment. After 12 mo, there was less overall vitamin deficiency in the supplemented group. Furthermore, CD4+ T-cell percentage, natural killer (NK) cell activity, mitogenic responses, and interleukin-2/interleukin-2 (IL) receptor expression were enhanced in the supplemented group. Most importantly, clinical illness was reduced. Over the 12 mo follow-up, the supplemented group had an average number of "illness days" of 23 vs 48 in the placebo group ($p = 0.002$; *see* Fig. 2), and antibiotic use was lower as well (18 vs 32 d, respectively; $p = 0.004$).

One study in institutionalized elderly utilizing a multivitamin/mineral supplementation strategy also showed decreased infection rates over a 2-yr supplementation trial *(42)*. In that study, nursing facility residents were randomly assigned to receive daily placebo, trace elements (20 mg zinc + 100 μg selenium), vitamins (120 mg vitamin C, 6 mg β-carotene, and 15 mg vitamin E), or both vitamins and trace elements. There were no immunologic studies performed, but the mean number of infections (respiratory and urinary tract infections were counted) was reduced in both groups taking trace elements vs placebo. Interestingly, the trace element group alone had the lowest rate of infection, and the vitamin + trace element group had similar rates of infection as the vitamin alone group. Importantly, this was a very small study (approximately 20 patients/group) with four groups, and it is difficult to draw firm conclusions from a study of this size.

Roebothan and Chandra *(26)* also investigated targeted supplementation in a group of 47 malnourished elderly adults in Newfoundland. In this approach, subjects were provided with supplements limited to those micronutrients in which they were deficient at baseline. If a subject was globally malnourished, they received a commercial high-protein/calorie supplement fortified with a variety of micronutrients. Zinc or zinc plus a global protein/energy deficiency were the most common deficiencies noted. The group was not large enough to determine clinical outcomes, but this targeted approach also improved some immune outcomes, though the evaluation was not as extensive as that employed in the study described earlier *(43)*. Although a targeted approach is more scientifically satisfying, it is probably not practical in the clinical setting, and a blanket recommendation for all elderly to take a single multivitamin/mineral supplement each day seems reasonable.

4.2. Zinc Supplementation Studies

Studies in older adults have given several forms of zinc that range in dose from 15 mg/d of zinc acetate to 220 mg of zinc sulfate twice a day. Often zinc was administered with other single vitamins or a multivitamin supplement (*see* Table 3). Most dem-

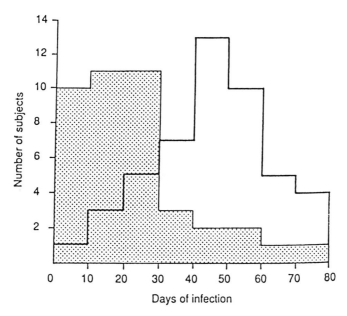

Fig. 2. Days of infection in supplemented (shaded area) and unsupplemented (open area) elderly. Reprinted with permission of ref. *(17)*.

onstrated enhanced DTH responses, and many show enhanced lymphocyte numbers and function of NK cells, but no benefit for boosting humoral immune responses. Only the nursing home study *(42)* described in Subheading 4.1. demonstrated statistical significance for reducing infections.

4.3. Vitamin E Supplementation Studies

Vitamin E, an antioxidant vitamin that has been touted as a preventive measure for many human conditions including heart disease and cancer, has also been extensively studied in the elderly as a booster of immune responses. It is not clear how vitamin E augments immune responses, perhaps via altering cytokine generation from T-cells or macrophages (*see* Fig. 1). Vitamin E supplementation has consistently improved DTH responses in elderly subjects with doses as low as 60 mg/day (*see* Table 3). Additional benefit of augmented responses to primary immunization with T-cell-dependent antigens may also occur at higher doses. Meydani and co-workers *(18)* examined three different daily doses of vitamin E (60, 200, or 800 mg/d) in healthy elderly and determined vitamin E's influence on DTH responses, hepatitis B vaccine (a T-cell-dependent antigen, primary immune response), tetanus/diphtheria vaccine (T-cell-dependent antigens, secondary (booster) immune response), and pneumococcal vaccine (a T-cell-independent antigen). Recipients of any of the three vitamin E doses demonstrated enhanced DTH responses, with the greatest benefit among those receiving 800 mg/d. Primary T-cell antigen responses (hepatitis B vaccine) were augmented in all three groups as well (no dose response). There was no clear benefit of vitamin E administration with regard to vaccine responses to recall antigens (diphtheria and tetanus), nor T-cell-independent antigens (pneumococcal polysaccharides), although subjects provided 200 mg/d did realize a greater increase in tetanus titers than the placebo group.

Based on these and other data, the authors felt there may be a "threshold" effect and that supplementation with 200 mg/d might represent an optimum regimen. However, the study was too small to conclusively decide this issue. The study was also underpowered to achieve significance for clinical endpoints, but in the discussion section, the authors state that self-reported infections were 30% lower in the three vitamin E-treated groups vs the placebo group ($p = 0.10$).

4.4. β-Carotene and Vitamin A

Vitamin A is absolutely essential for proper immune function *(44)*, but long-term supplementation can lead to hepatotoxicity. Thus, there are a few studies with vitamin A, and these have shown mixed results (*see* Table 3). The vitamin A precursor, β-carotene, is not associated with liver toxicity and therefore is often used in supplementation trials. The Physicians' Health Study findings suggest that β-carotene can enhance NK cell activity in elderly men (65–86 yr of age) even over very prolonged follow-up (144 mo) *(45)*. No clinical benefit was noted with β-carotene supplementation in this study with regard to the protocol endpoints of heart disease and cancer, and other studies raise some concern regarding blanket recommendations for β-carotene supplements in all elderly (*see* Subheading 4.5.).

4.5. Cautions Regarding Nutritional Supplementation

The public often regards vitamin therapy with the notions that if "some is good, more is better," and nutritional products are not likely to do harm. Unfortunately, this is not always true, and caution should be exercised in recommending vitamin therapy in the absence of clear data to support its use. An excellent example of risk associated with vitamin intake is β-carotene. As described in Subheading 4.4., β-carotene can enhance NK cell function and consumption of foods high in β-carotene has been associated with decreased risks of cancer. Furthermore, vitamin A, a prominent metabolite of β-carotene, has some demonstrated efficacy in reducing second squamous cell cancers in patients with head and neck cancers. Thus, β-carotene, vitamin A (or both) supplementation trials in smokers at risk for lung cancer were initiated in two prevention studies, one in Europe, the other in the U.S. Both studies were stopped prematurely due to *increased* deaths in the β-carotene/retinol supplemented groups vs placebo control patients *(46,47)*. These studies highlight the dangers that may follow seemingly harmless nutritional interventions without appropriate clinical trial data to support its use.

5. NUTRITIONAL THERAPY DURING ESTABLISHED INFECTION

Nutritional therapy has been employed in a large number of studies for many serious illnesses, but few have specifically focused on elderly subjects with infectious diseases. Several investigators have examined vitamin C (ascorbic acid) for the prevention and treatment of respiratory tract infections. One such study was performed in hospitalized elderly patients with bronchitis or pneumonia *(48)* and compared vitamin C 200 mg/d vs placebo in 57 patients. Supplementation rapidly increased plasma and cellular vitamin C levels, and may have slightly improved respiratory functional status, particularly in those with the most severe illness on admission. However, variable follow-up, small numbers of patients, and unplanned subgroup analyses suggest these data must be interpreted with caution.

Less severe, but very common, infections have also been the subject of nutritional interventional studies. In particular, zinc supplementation has been suggested to be beneficial for wound healing, especially for venous stasis ulcers, a common condition in the elderly. A recent meta-analysis *(49)* suggests that zinc supplementation, if helpful at all, is only likely to be of value in those patients with low serum zinc at the initiation of therapy. The appropriate dose and duration are not known, but in most studies 200–220 mg or zinc sulfate three times a day was given as the therapeutic regimen.

6. NUTRITIONAL THERAPY DURING CONVALESCENCE AFTER INFECTION

Perhaps the most poorly studied aspect of nutritional therapy is its use after a serious illness. Data from surgical patients suggest that the nutritional demands of the elderly remain during the period of convalescence with weight loss continuing for up to 8 wk after hospital discharge. Few studies of sufficient power and appropriate design have been performed in the elderly that examine the influence of nutritional supplements on the risk of infectious diseases following other serious illness. Community-acquired pneumonia (CAP) is a common serious illness in the elderly and a recent study from Spain *(50)* suggests that up to 85% of elderly patients with CAP are malnourished at the time of admission (vs 53% of age/gender-matched controls admitted for other reasons in that study). Woo and co-workers *(51)* studied the effects of nutritional supplementation during convalescence from CAP in a group of elderly patients in Hong Kong. Most of these patients were not institutionalized but lived in the community with spouses or family. Patients were randomly assigned to receive 500 mL daily of a commercially available supplement (Ensure®) or no supplement for 1 mo following discharge. As expected, several nutritional variables showed greater improvement in the supplemented group than in the nonsupplemented group. In addition, supplemented elderly were more likely to be physically active and had a higher functional status and less difficulty sleeping during follow-up visits (up to 3 mo) than nonsupplemented elderly. The study was not powered to detect differences in survival or recurrent infection, and did not perform any measures of immune function.

7. CONCLUSIONS AND RECOMMENDATIONS

Based on the data outlined, it is clear that the elderly are a population at special risk for malnutrition that may lead to increased risk of infection. Global malnutrition is particularly prevalent in hospitalized elderly and may become worse during the hospitalization. Reversible causes of malnutrition such as depression, dental disorders, poorly controlled diabetes, and medication-induced anorexia are common in elderly outpatients and undertreated. Among micronutrients, deficiencies of vitamins A, B_{12}, and E and the trace elements zinc and selenium appear to be most prevalent and of greatest importance for immune function in elderly subjects. The majority of data favor a daily multivitamin/trace-mineral supplement in elderly adults with additional vitamin E if necessary to achieve a daily vitamin E dose of 200 mg/d. Specific replacement therapy should be provided for those individuals with documented deficiencies of other micronutrients (particularly vitamin B_{12}), but specific data regarding protective efficacy for infection is lacking. Commercially available nutritional supplements may be of benefit in hospitalized elderly and during convalescence from serious infectious illnesses such as pneumonia. Future studies should be of sufficient size to achieve statistical significance for clinically meaningful endpoints.

REFERENCES

1. Bell, R. A. and High, K. P. (1997) Alterations of immune defense mechanisms in the elderly: the role of nutrition. *Infect. Med.* **14,** 415–424.
2. Lesourd, B., Mazari, L., and Ferry, M. (1998) The role of nutrition in immunity in the aged. *Nutr. Rev.* **56,** S113–S125.
3. Meydani, S. N. (1990) Dietary modulation of cytokine production and biologic function. *Nutr. Rev.* **48,** 361–369.
4. Singh, M. A. and Rosenberg, I. H. (1999) Nutrition and aging, in *Principles of Geriatric Medicine and Gerontology* (Hazzard,W. R., Blass, J. P., Ettinger, Jr., et al., eds.), McGraw-Hill, New York, pp. 81–96.
5. Morley, J. E., Mooradian, A. D., and Silver, A. J. (1988) Nutrition in the elderly. *Ann. Intern. Med.* **109,** 890–905.
6. Morley, J. E., Silver, A . J., Miller, D. K., et al. (1989) The anorexia of the elderly. *Ann. N. Y. Acad. Sci.* **575,** 50–58.
7. Constans ,T., Bacq, Y., Bréchot, J.-F., et al. (1992) Protein-energy malnutrition in elderly medical patients. *J. Am. Geriatr. Soc.* **40,** 263–268.
8. Rudman, D. and Feller, A. G. (1989) Protein-calorie undernutrition in the nursing home. *J. Am. Geriatr. Soc.* **37,** 173–183.
9. Volkert, D., Kruse, W., Oster, P., et al. (1992) Malnutrition in geriatric patients: diagnostic and prognostic significance of nutritional parameters. *Ann. Nutr. Metab.* **36,** 97–112.
10. Sullivan, D. H. and Walls, R. C. (1995) The risk of life-threatening complications in a select population of geriatric patients: the impact of nutritional status. *J. Am. Coll. Nutr.* **14,** 29–36.
11. Sullivan, D. H., Sun, S., and Walls, R. C. (1999) Protein-energy undernutrition among elderly hospitalized patients. A prospective study. *JAMA* **281,** 2013–2019.
12. Wilson, M. G., Caswani, S., Liu, D., et al. (1998) Prevalence and causes of undernutrition in medical outpatients. *Am. J. Med.* **104,** 56–63.
13. Azais-Braesco, V., Moriniere, C., Guesne, B., et al. (1995) Vitamin A status in the institutionalized elderly. Critical analysis of four evaluation criteria: dietary vitamin A intake, serum retinol, relative dose-response test (RDR) and impression cytology with transfer (ICT). *Int. J. Vit. Nutr. Res.* **65,** 151–161.
14. Semba, R. D., Muhilal, Scott, A. L., et al. (1994) Effect of vitamin A supplementation on immunoglobulin G subclass responses to tetanus toxoid in children. *Clin. Diagn. Lab. Immunol.* **1,** 172–175.
15. Gloth, F. M., Gundberg, C. M., Hollis, B. W., et al. (1995) Vitamin D deficiency in homebound elderly persons. *JAMA* **274,** 1683–1686.
16. Fata, F. T., Herzlich, B. C., Schiffman, G., et al. (1996) Impaired antibody responses to pneumococcal polysaccharide in elderly patients with low serum vitamin B_{12} levels. *Ann. Intern. Med.* **124,** 299–304.
17. Chandra, R. K. (1992) Effect of vitamin and trace-element supplementation on immune responses and infection in elderly subjects. *Lancet* **340,** 1124–1127.
18. Meydani, S. N., Meydani, M., Blumberg, J. B., et al. (1997) Vitamin E supplementation and in vivo immune response in healthy elderly subjects. A randomized controlled trial. *JAMA* **277,** 1380–1386.
19. Prasad, A. S., Fitzgerald, J. T., Hess, J . W., et al. (1993) Zinc deficiency in elderly patients. *Nutrition* **9,** 218–224.
20. Barrocas, A., Belcher, D., Champagne, C., et al. (1995) Nutrition assessment practical approaches. *Clin. Geriatr. Med.* **11,** 675–713.

21. Pike, J. and Chandra, R. K. (1995) Effect of vitamin and trace element supplementation on immune indices in healthy elderly. *Int. J. Vit. Nutr.* **65,** 117–120.
22. Penn, N. D., Purkins, L., Kelleher, J., et al. (1991) The effect of dietary supplementation with Vitamins A, C and E on cell-mediated immune function in elderly long-stay patients: a randomized controlled trial. *Age Aging* **20,** 169–174.
23. Bogden, J. D., Bendich, A., Kemp, F. W., et al. (1994) Daily micronutrient supplements enhance delayed-hypersensitivity skin test responses in older people. *Am. J. Clin. Nutr.* **60,** 437–447.
24. Chandra, R. K., Joshi, P., Au, B., et al. (1982) Nutrition and immunocompetence of the elderly: effect of short-term nutritional supplementation on cell-mediated immunity and lymphocyte subsets. *Nutr. Res.* **2,** 223–232.
25. Chavance, M., Herbeth, B., Lemoine, A., et al. (1993) Does multivitamin supplementation prevent infections in healthy elderly subjects? A controlled trial. *Int. J. Vit. Nutr. Res.* **63,** 11–16.
26. Roebothan, B. V. and Chandra, R. K. (1994) Relationship between nutritional status and immune function of elderly people. *Age Aging* **23,** 49–53.
27. Bogden, D., Oleske, J. M., Lavenhar, M. A., et al. (1988) Zinc and immunocompetence in elderly people: Effects of zinc supplementation for 3 months. *Am. J. Clin. Nutr.* **48,** 655–663.
28. Bogden, J. D., Oleske, J. M., Lavenhar, M. A., et al. (1990) Effects of one year of supplementation with zinc and other micronutrients on cellular immunity in the elderly. *J. Am. Coll. Nutr.* **9,** 214–225.
29. Fortes, C., Forastiere, F., Agabiti, N., et al. (1998) The effect of zinc and vitamin A supplementation on immune response in an older population. *J. Am. Geriatr. Soc.* **46,** 19–26.
30. Remarque, E. J., Witkakmp. L., Masurel, N., et al. (1993) Zinc supplementation does not enhance antibody formation to influenza virus vaccine in the elderly. *Aging Immunol. Infect. Dis.* **4,** 17–23.
31. Wagner, P. A., Jernigan, J. A., Bailey, L. B., et al. (1983) Zinc nutriture and cell-mediated immunity in the aged. *Int. J. Vit. Nutr. Res.* **53,** 94–101.
32. Cossack, Z. T. (1989) T-lymphocyte dysfunction in the elderly associated with zinc deficiency and subnormal nucleoside phosphorylase activity: effect of zinc supplementation. *Eur. J. Cancer Clin. Oncol.* **25,** 973–976.
33. Duchateau, J., Delepesse, G., Vrijens, R., et al. (1981) Beneficial effects of oral zinc supplementation on the immune response of old people. *Am. J. Med.* **70,** 1001–1004.
34. Meydani, S. N., Barklung, M. P., Siu, S., et al. (1990) Vitamin E supplementation enhances cell-mediated immunity in healthy elderly subjects. *Am. J. Clin. Nutr.* **52,** 557–563.
35. Meydani, S. N., Leka, L., and Loszewski, R. (1994) Long term vitamin E supplementation enhances immune response in healthy elderly. *FASEB J.* **8,** A272.
36. Watson, R. R., Probhala, R. H., Plezia, P. M., et al. (1991) Effect of beta-carotene on lymphocyte subpopulations in elderly humans: evidence for a dose-response effect. *Am. J. Clin. Nutr.* **53,** 90–94.
37. Murphy, S., West, K. P. J., Greenough, W. B., et al. (1992) Impact of vitamin A supplementation on the incidence of infection in elderly nursing-home residents: a randomized controlled trial. *Age Aging* **21,** 435–439.
38. Proust, J., Moulias, R., Fumeron, F., et al. (1982) HLA and longevity. *Tissue Antigens* **19,** 168–173.
39. Kennes, B., Dumont, I., Brohee, D., et al. (1983) Effect of vitamin C supplementation on cell-mediated immunity in old people. *Gerontology* **29,** 305–310.
40. Ziemlanski, S., Wartanowicz, M., Panczenko-Kresowska, B., et al. (1986) The effects of ascorbic acid and alpha-tocopherol supplementation on serum proteins and immunoglobulin concentrations in the elderly. *Nutr. Int.* **2,** 1.
41. Meydani, S. N., Hayek, M., and Coleman, L. (1992) Influence of Vitamins E and B$_6$ on immune response. *Ann. N.Y. Acad. Sci.* **669,** 125–139.

42. Girodon, F., Lombard, M., Galan, P., et al. (1997) Effect of micronutrient supplementation on infection in institutionalized elderly subjects: a controlled trial. *Ann. Nutr. Metab.* **41,** 98–107.

43. Posner, B. M., Jette, A. M., and Smith, M. A. (1993) Nutrition and health risks in the elderly: the nutrition screening initiative. *Am. J. Public Health* **83,** 972–978.

44. Semba, R. D. (1998) The role of vitamin A and related retinoids in immune function. *Nutr. Rev.* **56,** S38–S48.

45. Santos, M. S., Meydani, S. N., Leka, L., et al. (1996) Natural killer cell activity in elderly men is enhanced by beta-carotene supplementation. *Am. J. Clin. Nutr.* **64,** 772–777.

46. The Alpha-Tocopherol, Beta-Carotene Cancer Prevention Study Group (1994) The effect of vitamin E and beta carotene on the incidence of lung cancer and other cancers in male smokers. *N. Engl. J. Med.* **330,** 1029–1035.

47. Omenn, G. S., Goodman, G., Thornquist, M., et al. (1996) Effects of combination of beta carotene and vitamin A on lung cancer and cardiovascular disease. *N. Engl. J. Med.* **334,** 1150–1155.

48. Hunt, C., Chakravorty, N. K., Annan, G., et al. (1994) The clinical effects of vitamin C supplementation in elderly hospitalised patients with acute respiratory infections. *Int. J. Vit. Nutr. Res.* **64,** 212–219.

49. Wilkinson, E. A. J. and Hawke, C. I. (1998) Does oral zinc aid the healing of chronic leg ulcers? *Arch. Dermatol.* **134,** 1556–1560.

50. Riquelme, R., Torres, A., El-Ebiary, M., et al. (1997) Community-acquired pneumonia in the elderly. Clinical and nutritional aspects. *Am. J. Respir. Care Med.* **156,** 1908–1914.

51. Woo, J., Ho, S. C., Mak, Y. T., et al. (1994) Nutritional status of elderly patients during recovery from chest infection and the role of nutritional supplementation assessed by a prospective randomized single-blind trial. *Age Aging* **23,** 40–48.

25

Sexually Transmitted Diseases

Helene Calvet

1. CLINICAL RELEVANCE AND EPIDEMIOLOGY

Sexually transmitted diseases (STDs) are not perceived by most health care practitioners as a significant problem for older adults (over age 50) in the United States. In fact, many practitioners do not view older adults as even being sexually active, much less at risk for STDs. Aging, intercurrent illnesses, and psychosocial factors often have significant impact on sexual function or the enjoyment of sex in the elderly. Psychosocial factors, such as attitudes toward sexual behavior, reaction to physiologic changes or illness, performance anxiety, or loss of privacy can contribute to sexual dysfunction in both men and women *(1)*. Aging women may be affected by a number of physiologic changes due to the loss of estrogen, such as shortening of the vaginal vault, thinning of the vaginal mucosa, and reduction or loss in vaginal lubrication *(2)*. These physiologic changes, as well as medical conditions such as arthritis, can lead to dyspareunia, which is reported in up to one third of sexually active women aged 65 and older *(2)*. An even more prevalent problem is erectile dysfunction, which is estimated to affect 10% of all men in the U.S. with higher rates in those over age 40 or with medical conditions such as diabetes mellitus. There are numerous causes of erectile dysfunction, including medical illnesses, medications, normal physiologic changes, and psychosocial factors.

Despite the many barriers preventing sexual activity in the elderly, multiple studies have shown that many older Americans still do engage in sexual activity. The Janus report on sexual behavior found that among Americans 65 and older, 69% of men and 74% of women report some form of sexual activity at least weekly *(3)*. Bretschneider and McCoy *(4)* found in a survey of 100 men and 102 women between the ages of 80 and 102 that 62% of men and 30% of women engaged in sexual intercourse. It is unclear how many of those not engaging in sexual activity are celibate by choice or are affected by health status or partner availability. The availability of medications such as sildenafil may enable men who are celibate due to erectile dysfunction to regain their sexual function.

With the current extent of sexual activity in the older age groups and the possibility of an increase in activity due to medications for erectile dysfunction, safe sexual practices are important for STD and human immunodeficiency virus (HIV) prevention but are practiced by few. Stall and Catania *(5)* found in a survey of over 2000 Americans aged 50 and older living in large metropolitan areas that 11.7% reported at least one risk factor for HIV (multiple sexual partners, high-risk sexual partner, transfusion

From: *Infectious Disease in the Aging*
Edited by: Thomas T. Yoshikawa and Dean C. Norman
© Humana Press Inc., Totowa, NJ

between 1978 and 1984, or injection drug use) *(5)*. Among those stating at least one risk factor for HIV, 73% were sexually active and 83% of these never used condoms. Men in this age group are less likely than their younger counterparts to use condoms because their partners, in general, are past child-bearing age. Older women may not view themselves as being at risk for STDs because they are postmenopausal, and STD risk is often linked to pregnancy risk *(6)*. Also, older sexually active men may have multiple partners available due to the preponderance of widowed females who may be interested in maintaining sexual activity. In fact, by age 85, women outnumber men by almost 3 to 1 *(2)*. In the survey by Stall and Catania, 3.5% of respondents reported having multiple sex partners *(5)*.

The lack of safe sexual practices in older adults and the physiological changes in older women put them at risk for STDs and HIV. Acquired immunodeficiency syndrome (AIDS) in older adults is not insignificant, with the over-50 age group accounting for 10% of the reported cases of AIDS in the U.S. *(7)*. From June 1996–April 1997, there was a 13% increase in the number of AIDS cases reported in those aged 65 and older, almost half of whom were infected by unprotected intercourse *(6)*. Other STDs are also seen in older Americans. In 1997, 4% of the cases of primary and secondary syphilis and 1% of the cases of gonorrhea were reported in persons aged 55 yr and older *(8)*. It is possible that rates are even higher because of underdiagnosis or underreporting.

This chapter focuses on possible differences in the presentations of STDs in the elderly, new advances in the diagnosis of STDs, and epidemiologic trends of STDs in older adults. Also, the latest recommendations for management from the 1998 STD Treatment Guidelines from the Centers for Disease Control and Prevention (CDC) will be highlighted.

2. SYPHILIS

Nationwide statistics for syphilis are most important for early syphilis (primary and secondary) because these represent the recently acquired (incident) cases, and the cases that are most infectious. Primary and secondary syphilis are relatively uncommon in older adults, with only 4% of the cases in the U.S. occurring in persons aged 55 yr and older during 1997 *(8)*. Nationwide efforts for syphilis elimination have led to dramatic declines in syphilis rates in all age groups, but between 1996 and 1997, the rates in persons aged 55 and older decreased only slightly. Regardless of age group, early syphilis is highly infectious, with an estimated 30–60% chance of acquiring infection after a single sexual contact *(9)*. In older women, the risk may be higher due to vaginal thinning in the postmenopausal state leading to more abrasions during sexual intercourse. Syphilis should be considered in the differential of any new genital ulceration, especially if the ulceration is painless, or for unexplained skin rash in a sexually active patient.

The diagnosis of syphilis in the elderly may be challenging for several reasons. First, the prevalence of false-positive nontreponemal serologies, such as the rapid plasma reagin (RPR) or venereal disease research laboratory (VDRL), in the elderly is increased. In all age groups, it is necessary to confirm a positive nontreponemal test result with a treponemal-specific serology, such as the microhemagglutination *Treponema pallidum* (MHA-TP) or fluorescent treponemal antibody absorbed (FTA-ABS), prior to considering treatment (note: the MHA-TP will be replaced shortly by a new, recently FDA-approved test called the *T. pallidum*-particle agglutination, or TP-PA, which is produced by the manufacturer of the MHA-TP). Second, in patients who have untreated syphilis for many years and are presenting with late complications, the RPR and VDRL may be negative, with only a positive treponemal serology as indication of infection. Therefore, the possibility of either false-positive or false-negative screening nontreponemal tests exists in the elderly. Finally, since the elderly have many intercurrent illnesses and are not perceived by medical providers as being sexually active or at risk for syphilis, symptoms or signs of syphilis may be mistaken for other disease states, such as a drug reaction, urinary tract infection, or benign perineal ulceration.

Whereas early syphilis is uncommon in the elderly, latent syphilis is a more frequently encountered problem. A serum RPR is a routine test to perform in the evaluation of dementia, so a common dilemma is how to determine the significance of a positive RPR. If the confirmatory test is positive, then the clinician must decide if the patient requires evaluation for neurosyphilis. According to the 1998 CDC STD Treatment Guidelines *(10)*, cerebrospinal fluid (CSF) evaluation is recommended if the patient has any of the following: (1) neurologic, auditory or ophthalmologic symptoms or signs suggestive of syphilis, such as uveitis, interstitial keratitis, cranial nerve palsies, meningitis, or cerebrovascular accident, which usually occur months to a few years after infection, or tabes dorsalis, general paresis, or psychological or behavioral changes that usually occur many years after infection; (2) suspected treatment failure or relapse of previously known syphilis, demonstrated by a failure to display a fourfold drop in the RPR (or VDRL) titer, or presence of an increase in titer; (3) co-infection with HIV and syphilis of greater than 1 yr duration; or (4) active signs of other forms of tertiary syphilis (aortitis, gummas). Routine lumbar puncture for infection of greater than 1 yr duration or for planned nonpenicillin therapy is not routinely recommended. If the patient undergoes a lumbar puncture, then a second problem that the clinician may encounter is interpreting the CSF analysis. There is no one test that is 100% sensitive for the diagnosis of neurosyphilis. In a patient with positive serum syphilis serology, if the CSF VDRL is positive (without significant contamination of the CSF with blood), most experts would agree that the patient has neurosyphilis. However, in patients with negative CSF VDRL, the clinician should consider treatment if there is any abnormality of the CSF, especially a pleocytosis of >5 white blood cells (WBC)/mm^3, even though this finding is not specific for neurosyphilis. It is important to recognize, however, that the protein level in the CSF may increase with age and other associated conditions, thus the interpretation of the CSF profile with a slightly elevated protein level as the sole abnormal finding may be difficult. Although the FTA-ABS is not a recommended test to perform on CSF because of problems with specificity, a negative CSF FTA-ABS suggests that neurosyphilis is unlikely in these cases *(11)*.

The recommended treatment of syphilis has not changed significantly. Syphilis of less than 1 yr duration (primary, secondary, and early latent) is treated with a single injection of benzathine penicillin, 2.4 million units (MU) intramuscularly (i.m.), and syphilis of more than 1 yr duration (late latent and tertiary) is treated with weekly injections of intramuscularly administered benzathine penicillin, 2.4 MU for 3 wk. The treatment of neurosyphilis is best accomplished with 18–24 MU of intravenous (i.v.) penicillin G for 10–14 d; this recommended dose is slightly higher than that recommended in the 1993 guidelines. An alternative regimen, which can be administered on an outpatient basis, is procaine penicillin 2.4 MU i.m. administered once a day along with probenecid 500 mg orally four times a day, both for 10–14 d *(10)*. Many experts recommend treating patients with neurosyphilis with an additional two injections of 2.4 MU benzathine penicillin weekly immediately following the course of i.v. penicillin in order to achieve the same duration of therapy as for tertiary syphilis.

3. HERPES SIMPLEX VIRUS, TYPE II (HSV-2)

Genital herpes simplex virus (HSV) infection is not a reportable disease but is considered to be extremely common in the U.S. with approximately 45 million adults (approx 22% of the population aged 15–74 yr) estimated to be infected in 1990, based on the serologic results of a random sampling of civilian adults examined as part of the National Health and Nutrition Examination Survey (NHANES III) *(12)*. This represents a 32% increase compared to 1978, when the seroprevalence of HSV-2 was 16% among the adult population during NHANES II *(13)*. The prevalence of HSV-2 infection increased with increasing age, and the odds of having HSV-2 were higher in women (odds ratio [OR] = 1.6), blacks (OR = 5.7), previously married individuals (OR = 2.0 – 2.8), and those with lower family income (OR = 1.2) *(13)*. The highest seroprevalences in NHANES III were seen in black men and women aged 60–74 (61% and 81%, respectively) *(12)*. Therefore, HSV-2 infection is prevalent in older adults and should be considered in the differential diagnosis of a genital or perineal ulceration or rash, especially if it is resistant to usual local care measures.

The majority of people testing positive for antibodies to HSV-2 have subclinical, atypical, or asymptomatic disease, with the minority displaying the classic presentation of vesicular outbreaks. Studies estimate that 70–80% of patients testing positive for HSV-2 antibodies are not aware of the infection, but up to 50% of these individuals will give a history of atypical symptoms that may be due to HSV reactivations *(14)*. Recurrences are very common, averaging four to five per year for HSV-2 in the first few years after acquiring the virus but then tend to become less frequent the longer the time period from initial infection *(15)*. Immune suppression associated with aging or other concomitant morbid conditions in the elderly may lead to an increase in the frequency of recurrences or a recrudescence after many years of no clinically recognizable outbreaks.

The gold standard for diagnosis of HSV infection remains the viral culture; however, the overall sensitivity of culture is estimated to be approximately 50% *(14)*, so a negative culture result does not exclude the diagnosis. The yield from culture is better from early lesions, such as vesicles or fresh ulcers, than from resolving ulcerations, and is more likely to be positive in primary infection than in the recurrent form of the disease. The Tzanck test—staining of cells from the lesion base to look for multinucleated giant cells—may be helpful for diagnosis but is positive only 50% of the time. Currently available serologies are not useful for diagnosis because they do not differentiate between infection with HSV-2 and HSV-1, the latter of which infects the majority of the U.S. adult population. Newer serologies that are type-specific, detecting antibodies to the surface glycoproteins gG1 and gG2, will be useful tools in diagnosing atypical presentations of herpes but are not yet commercially available. Furthermore, polymerase chain reaction (PCR) for HSV DNA is being developed, which, in the future, may supplant virus culture as the test of the choice for the evaluation of genital ulcerations *(14)*.

Table 1
Treatment of Genital HSV-2

Stage of infection	Duration of therapy	Medications		
		Acyclovir	Famciclovir	Valacyclovir
Primary	7–10 d	400 mg po tid	250 mg po tid	1 g po bid
Recurrent	5 d	400 mg po tid or 800 mg po bid	125 mg po bid	500 mg po bid
Suppression	1 yr[a]	400 mg po bid	250 mg po bid	500 mg po qd[b] or 1 g po qd

[a]Therapy longer than 1 yr may be indicated if recurrences continue to occur frequently; however, there is insufficient experience with famciclovir or valacyclovir to recommend therapy with these agents for more than 1 yr

[b]Valacyclovir 500 mg qd dose less effective than other doses of valacyclovir for very frequent recurrences (≥10 per yr) (ref. *10*).

Abbreviations: po, orally; qd, once daily; bid, two times a day; tid, three times a day.

The treatment of herpes simplex infection has been made easier by the availability of famciclovir and valacyclovir, which allow less frequent dosing than acyclovir. However, all three drugs are equally efficacious. (*See* Table 1 for doses and duration of treatment.) If an elderly patient experiences frequent recurrences (>6 per yr), then chronic suppression should be considered. The need for suppressive therapy should be reevaluated after 1–2 yr by a trial off medications. If recurrences are sporadic at that time, then sporadic treatment is in order. If recurrences are frequent again, then another year of suppression is indicated. HIV testing should be considered in the elderly patient experiencing frequent herpetic recurrences who has not recently acquired herpes, as frequent recurrences in long-term disease is unusual.

Counseling of older individuals with HSV genital infection should include information about the natural history, probability of recurrences, benefit of treatment, and chances for transmission. Transmission can occur in the absence of clinical symptoms or signs of an outbreak; in fact, most sexual transmission occurs due to asymptomatic shedding. Therefore, patients with genital herpes should be counseled to use condoms at all times to reduce the risk of transmitting the infection to a partner.

4. CHLAMYDIA

Chlamydia infection was the most common reportable communicable disease in the U.S. in 1998, with almost 540,000 cases reported (*16*). *Chlamydia trachomatis* is an infection predominantly of adolescents, with the highest rate of infection being in the 15–19 and 20–24 yr age groups. The prevalence of infection drops off greatly after age 35, with adults over age 55 accounting for less than 1% of the nationwide cases. The number of *Chlamydia* infections nationwide is increasing, possibly due to improved testing and reporting; concomitant with this rise, the rates of *Chlamydia* isolation in older adults increased from 1996–1997, the greatest increase seen in those aged 65 and older (from 1.9–4.5/100,000 population) (*8*).

The reasons for the predilection of younger age groups to *Chlamydia* are both anatomical and behavioral. *Chlamydia* is an intracellular organism that infects only columnar epithelium, which is often present on the ectocervix of adolescent girls, thus very accessible to infection. In older women, however, the columnar epithelium is located in the endocervix, where it is somewhat protected by cervical mucus. Patterns and rates of partner change also make adolescents and younger women more susceptible to *Chlamydia*. However, older men and women are not immune to the disease. As in men, *Chlamydia* can infect only the urethra in women, causing symptoms of urinary tract infection or urethral syndrome. Chattopadhyay *(17)* found evidence of *Chlamydia* in 4% of 249 culture-negative urine samples with >50 WBC/µL; two of these patients were 65 yr and older *(17)*. *Chlamydia* should be considered as a cause for culture-negative urinary symptoms in the sexually active population.

The diagnosis of *Chlamydia* infections has been revolutionized by the commercial availability of the amplified nucleic acid tests, ligase chain reaction (LCR), PCR, and transcription-mediated amplification (TMA). LCR and TMA have been FDA-approved for testing on urine samples in both men and women, obviating the need for uncomfortable urethral swabs for men or pelvic examinations for women. The sensitivity and specificity of these tests approach 95–98% *(18)*, and are useful for screening males in general and women in nonclinical settings. The LCR from the female cervix is slightly more sensitive than the urine sample, so in situations in which a pelvic examination is to be performed, such as for cervical cancer screening, then a cervical sample for LCR should be sent.

Treatment of *Chlamydia* has also been simplified by single-dose oral therapy with 1 g of azithromycin, which can be administered under observation in the clinic, ensuring compliance. Azithromycin achieves high concentrations in tissues, with therapeutic levels of drug persisting for 1 wk; the single-dose therapy has been found to be as efficacious as the other recommended regimen, i.e., oral doxycycline 100 mg twice a day for 7 d.

5. GONORRHEA

Gonorrhea (GC) can infect not only the urethra and cervix, but the rectum, pharynx, and eye as well, and may disseminate to cause arthritis and/or dermatitis. Reported cases of gonorrhea in adults aged 55 and over account for approximately 1% of the nationwide total. Whereas the national rates of gonorrhea have fallen dramatically since the mid-1970s, there was a stabilization of rates between 1996 and 1997; in fact, rates in adults aged 55 and over actually increased in 1997 (from 9.1–9.5/100,000 population for those 55–64, and from 3.1–4.0/100,000 population for those 65 and older) *(8)*. There is no evidence that the presentation of gonococcal disease in the elderly is any different than in those younger, but like other STDs, the diagnosis may be delayed because it is not considered in the differential diagnosis. It is unclear if the elderly are more susceptible to disseminated GC than others, but there are many case reports of disseminated infection in older individuals in the literature. There is a suggestion that in the case of eye infection, the elderly are more susceptible to corneal involvement *(19)*, but this may due to a delay in diagnosis and treatment.

The diagnostic test for gonococcal urethritis that is most inexpensive and can yield immediate results is the Gram stain, which is highly sensitive in men with symptomatic urethritis. In asymptomatic men and in women, however, the sensitivity of Gram staining is poor, so the diagnostic tests preferred in these groups include culture, DNA hybridization, or the amplified nucleic acid tests (LCR, PCR, or TMA). DNA hybridization and the nucleic acid amplification tests may all be performed on urine samples, have sensitivities equivalent to or exceeding that of culture, and have specificities comparable to culture *(20)*. The treatment of uncomplicated genital gonorrhea infection is easily accomplished with single-dose therapies: ceftriaxone 125 mg i.m., ciprofloxacin 500 mg orally (po), ofloxacin 400 mg po or cefixime 400 mg po *(10)*. Certain areas of the country and the world (the Philippines and Southeast Asia) are experiencing increasing numbers of gonococcal isolates with reduced susceptibility to the fluoroquinolones, so it is important to obtain a travel history from the patient and to be familiar with local resistance patterns if fluoroquinolones are to be used. Concurrent treatment with doxycycline for *Chlamydia* infection is recommended if empiric treatment is being administered.

6. VAGINITIS

Vaginal complaints are a common reason for women of all ages to visit their physician, with an estimated 3.2 million initial visits to physicians offices for this population in 1997 *(8)*. Decreased estrogen production in the postmenopausal woman causes a number of changes in the vagina, which can lead to a variety of symptoms *(21)*. The amount of glycogen in the epithelial cells diminishes, leading to a reduction in the lactobacilli population that help to protect the vagina from other bacteria by their production of lactic acid and hydrogen peroxide. The resulting increase in pH facilitates colonization of the vagina with coliform bacteria, streptococci, and staphylococci. The lack of estrogen also leads to thinning of the vaginal mucosa, loss of rugae, and a progressive loss of elasticity and vascularity. The vaginal vault shortens and narrows, and the vaginal introitus may also become contracted. These changes often lead to dyspareunia, vaginal dryness, itching, burning or pruritis, or vulvar symptoms. Physical signs of vaginal atrophy include pale, smooth shiny mucosa. In the case of atrophic vaginitis, signs of inflammation will also be present, such as erythema, petechiae, friability, bleeding, or discharge *(21)*. It is important for the health care provider to recognize this condition not as an infection or STD but as a syndrome of hormone deficiency, as most women will respond to hormone replacement.

Bacterial vaginosis (BV) and candidiasis are not sexually transmitted infections, but may arise in older women because of the changes in the vaginal microflora that occur in the postmenopausal state. Because these conditions are not STDs, they are not discussed further here, but the reader is referred to the STD Treatment Guidelines for discussion on the diagnosis and treatment *(10)*. Trichomoniasis, caused by *Trichomonas vaginalis*, is an STD, which in women can infect the vagina, cervix, urethra or bladder. Trichomoniasis is not a reportable disease, so accurate data on the incidence of this infection in older women are not available. Common signs due to trichomoniasis include abnormal discharge, which is often discolored and/or frothy, vaginal erythema, and punctate cervical hemorrhages. Symptoms include discharge, itching, or burning of the vagina or vulva, but occasionally women will present with predominantly urethral complaints, such as frequency, urgency, or dysuria. Trichomoniasis, like other STDs, may also be carried asymptomatically for long periods of time, and the host factors that allow the asymtpomatic carriage have not been elucidated.

Trichomoniasis is diagnosed by seeing motile trichomonads on a saline preparation of vaginal secretions. In some cases, the trichomonads may not be readily visualized, so the clinician should suspect the diagnosis if the wet mount has numerous WBCs, the pH is highly elevated, and the "whiff" test (amine odor after addition of 10% potassium hydroxide to vaginal secretions) is mildly positive. A new commercially available culture system, called the InPouch TV test, is available for the diagnosis of trichomoniasis in patients with negative saline preparations. Trichomoniasis is easily treated with a single dose of 2 g oral metronidazole (10), and partner treatment is recommended due to the difficulty in diagnosing the infection in men.

7. HIV/AIDS

In the U.S. people over the age of 50 account for 10% of the reported cases of AIDS *(7)*. The epidemiology of HIV infection in older adults is changing (*see* also Chapter 19) Early in the epidemic, male–male sexual contact and transfusion were the most common risk factors, accounting for 42% and 37% of the cases reported from 1982–88, respectively *(7)*. Although male–male sexual contact remained a significant risk factor in 1989–1991, accounting for 45% of the reported cases, those cases due to transfusion dropped to 20%, and the proportion due to heterosexual contact (11%), intravenous drug use (8%), and undetermined causes (14%) doubled *(7)*. Among the AIDS cases in people aged 50 and older reported to the CDC in 1996, 36% were attributed to male–male sexual contact, 19% to intravenous drug use, 14.5% to heterosexual contact, 2% to transfusion, and 26% to unknown risk factors *(22)*. The proportion of cases due to heterosexual contact was higher than among those aged 13–49 yr (12.7%) *(22)*.

The fact that older patients may not state (or be asked about) risk factors for HIV often leads to a delay in the diagnosis. Gordon and Thompson found that among 24 elderly patients who developed symptoms or signs of HIV infection and sought medical attention, the diagnosis was delayed a median of 3 mo (range 1–10 mo) *(7)*. HIV infection may also go undetected as evaluation for more common conditions causing similar symptoms, such as cancer, infection, or organic brain syndrome are pursued. Patients may also die from other comorbidities instead of their HIV. El-Sadr and Gettler found that among patients over age 60 who were admitted to their hospital from January 1992–February 1993 and died while in the hospital, the HIV seroprevalence was 5%, even though none of the deaths were overtly HIV-related *(23)*. Numerous studies have documented that HIV progresses more quickly in the elderly, and this poor outcome may be related to delay in diagnosis, inability to replace functional T cells that are destroyed, or presence of comorbidities in the elderly *(24–26)*.

Diagnosis and treatment of HIV are beyond the scope of this review. The treatment of HIV in the elderly is more challenging than in the younger population, however, due to drug interactions with other medications the elderly may require and the altered pharmacokinetics of drugs seen with age. Patients should be managed by a clinician who is familiar with the treatment of HIV in order to appropriately monitor for side effects and response to treatment.

REFERENCES

1. Thienhaus, O. J. (1988) Practical overview of sexual function and advancing age. *Geriatrics* **43**, 63–67.
2. Kaiser, F. E. (1996) Sexuality in the elderly. *Urol. Clin. North Am.* **23**, 99–109.

3. Janus, S. S. and Janus, C. L. (eds.) 1993 *The Janus Report on Sexual Behavior.* Wiley, New York, p. 25.

4. Bretschneider, J. G. and McCoy, N. L. (1988) Sexual interest and behavior in healthy 80 to 102 year olds. *Arch. Sex. Behav.* **17,** 109–129.

5. Stall, R. and Catania, J. (1994) AIDS risk behaviors among late middle-aged and elderly Americans. *Arch. Intern. Med.* **154,** 57–63.

6. American Social Health Association (1998) Sex happens after 50 (and so do STDs) *STD News* **5,** 1–2.

7. Gordon, S. M. and Thompson, S. (1995) The changing epidemiology of human immuno-deficiency virus infection in older persons. *J. Am. Geriatr. Soc.* **43,** 7–9.

8. U.S. Department of Health and Human Services, Centers for Disease Control and Prevention (CDC) (1998) *Sexually Transmitted Disease Surveillance* 1997, pp. 1–131.

9. Thin, R. N. (1990) Early syphilis in the adult, in *Sexually Transmitted Diseases*, 2nd ed. (Holmes, K. K., Mardh, P. A., Sparling, P. E., et al., eds.). McGraw-Hill, New York, pp. 221–230.

10. Centers for Disease Control and Prevention (1998) 1998 Guidelines for treatment of sexu-ally transmitted diseases. *M.M.W.R.* **47(RR-1),** 1–116.

11. Hook, E. W. and Marra, C. M. (1992) Acquired syphilis in adults. *N. Engl. J. Med.* **326,** 1060–1069.

12. Johnson, R. E., Lee, F., Hadgu, A., et al. (1994) U.S. genital herpes trends during the first decade of AIDS: prevalences in increased young whites and elevated in blacks. *Sex. Trans. Dis.* **21(suppl),** 109.

13. Johnson, R. E., Nahmias, A. J., Magder, L. S., et al. (1998) Seroepidemiologic survey of the prevalence of herpes simplex virus type 2 infection in the United States. *N. Engl. J. Med.* **321,** 7–12.

14. Schomogyi, M., Wald, A., and Corey, L. (1998) Herpes simplex virus-2 infection: an emerging disease? *Infect. Dis. Clin. North Am.* **12,** 47–61.

15. Corey, L. and Wald, A. (1999) Genital herpes, in *Sexually Transmitted Diseases*, 3rd ed. (Holmes, K. K., Sparling, P. F., Mardh, P. A., et al., eds.) McGraw-Hill, New York, pp. 285–312.

16. U.S. Department of Health and Human Services (1998) Summary—provisional cases of selected notifiable diseases, United States. *M.M.W.R.* **47,** 1078.

17. Chattopadhyay, B. (1992) Carriage of *Chlamydia trachomatis* by elderly people. *Genitourin. Med.* **68,** 194,195.

18. Black, C. M. (1997) Current methods of the laboratory diagnosis of *Chlamydia trachomatis* infections. *Clin. Microbiol. Rev.* **10,** 160–184.

19. Ghosh, H. K. (1987) Gonococcal eye infection in the elderly. *Med. J. Aust.* **146,** 330.

20. Hook, E. W. and Handsfield, H. H. (1999) Gonococcal infections in the adult, in *Sexually Transmitted Diseases*, 3rd ed. ((Holmes, K. K., Sparling, P. F., Mardh, P. A., et al., eds.) McGraw-Hill, New York, pp. 451–472.

21. Pandit, L. and Ouslander, J. G. (1997) Postmenopausal vaginal atrophy and atrophic vagini-tis. *Am. J. Med. Sci.* **314,** 228–231.

22. Centers for Disease Control and Prevention (1998) AIDS among persons aged >50 years—United States, 1991–1996. *M.M.W.R.* **47,** 21–27.

23. El-Sadr, W. and Gettler, J. (1995). Unrecognized human immunodeficiency virus infec-tion in the elderly. *Arch. Intern. Med.* **155,** 184–186.

24. Johnson, M., Haight, B. K., and Benedict, S. (1998) AIDS in older people. *J. Gerontol. Nurs.* **24,** 8–13.

25. Adler, W. H., Baskar, P. V., Chrest, F. J., et al. (1997) HIV infection and aging: mecha-nisms to explain the accelerated rate of progression in older patients. *Mech. Aging Dev.* **96,** 137–155.

26. Skiest, D. J., Rubinstein, E., Carley, N., et al. (1996) The importance of comorbidity in HIV-infected patients over 55: a retrospective case-control study. *Am. J. Med.* **101,** 605-611.

26

Infectious Diseases and Aging

Considerations and Directions for the Future

Thomas T. Yoshikawa and Dean C. Norman

1. THE PROBLEM OF AGING AND INFECTIONS

As has been described in Chapter 1, the aging population will dramatically increase over the next 30 yr. The aging of the current "baby boomers" will nearly double the current number of approximately 33 million Americans aged 65 yr and older to a total of 65 million *(1)*. More and more clinicians will be required to provide health care for older patients as we enter the next millennium. How do we prepare physicians for this challenge? Since our focus is on infections in the older population, how do we develop the best strategy to address the clinical problems described in many of the chapters of this book?

In the tradition of medicine, it seems appropriate to address the broad topic of aging and infections from the perspectives of clinical practice issues, education and training, and research. Recently, these issues have been pursued with many recommendations brought forth for consideration and implementation to a variety of professional and governmental organizations involved with clinical care, training, and funding of research *(2–4)*. These recommendations are summarized in the subsequent sections.

2. CLINICAL CARE ISSUES

The following pathogenetic, diagnostic, therapeutic, and preventive areas of concerns highlight many of the clinical problems requiring further investigation and resolution.

- What is the quantitative impact of age-related immune dysregulation on the predisposition to and recovery from infections? Is the diminution of host resistance associated with aging really a function of aging alone or is it due to overt or undetected age-related diseases? What components of host resistance, i.e., physical barriers (skin, mucosa), phagocytosis (neutrophils, macrophages), humoral immunity (including mucosal immunity), cellular immunity (including natural killer cells), and complement, are impacted the greatest with aging? Are components of host resistance adversely affected with aging during an active infection, i.e., while an infection is active, do the mechanisms of host defense function normally in the elderly compared with younger adults? These and other related questions regarding aging and host resistance are important to answer because future interventional strategies in terms of preventing, mitigating, or eliminating infections may become more focused in areas of immune modulators and boosting of the various components of the host defense system.

From: *Infectious Disease in the Aging*
Edited by: Thomas T. Yoshikawa and Dean C. Norman
© Humana Press Inc., Totowa, NJ

- What is the pathogenetic mechanism for the extremely high prevalence of bacteriuria in elderly women and men? Although the majority of bacteriuria in the elderly are asymptomatic, the incidence and mortality secondary to (symptomatic) urinary tract infection and urosepsis increases substantially with age *(5–7)*. Understanding the pathogenesis of bacteriuria with aging could provide clues to developing effective preventive strategies.
- There is a need to develop a simple, noninvasive, inexpensive, and accurate diagnostic approach to determine the microbial cause of lower respiratory infections, especially pneumonia, in older patients. The vast majority of hospitalizations for community-acquired pneumonia (CAP) (60–85%) occur among patients aged 65 and older *(8,9)*, and mortality related to pneumonia is the highest among the elderly *(10)*. Unfortunately, the microbial etiology of hospitalized community-acquired pneumonia patients is identified in only about 25% of cases, regardless of age *(11)*. Perhaps, with more rapid and precise identification of the cause(s) of pneumonia followed by early specific therapy, the deaths due to pneumonia in older patients can be prevented or substantially reduced.
- Tuberculosis remains a major health problem for older people *(12)*. The current method of detecting early cases of tuberculosis, i.e., tuberculin skin test, is insensitive and lacks specificity in the elderly population *(13)*. A more sensitive and specific, as well as simple, rapid, and expensive method for screening for tuberculous infection and disease will greatly increase the opportunity to eliminate early or inactive disease and reduce the number of active infections.
- We must find newer approaches of intervention(s) that will reduce the mortality and morbidity associated with sepsis and septic shock. Elderly patients experience a disproportionately high incidence of bacteremia and sepsis and their associated complications, especially death *(5,14)*. Because of age-related physiological changes and diseases, preexisting organ dysfunction and limited reserve capacities place the elderly at greater jeopardy to develop multiorgan failure and rapid or eventual demise. Septic shock in the elderly has an associated mortality that can exceed 50% *(15)*.
- There is a need to continue to develop newer antimicrobial agents that have pharmacokinetic and pharmacodynamic characteristics that are especially advantages to the elderly: minimial end-organ toxicities (especially kidneys, liver, brain, bone marrow, ear); microbicidal activity (killing rather than inhibiting organisms); low protein binding (since serum albumin varies considerably in older persons with serious underlying illnesses); relatively long serum half-life that permit once or twice daily dosing; high penetration into a variety of body fluids including cerebrospinal fluid; and availability of both a parenteral and oral preparation with high bioavailability, which allows rapid transition from inpatient therapy to ambulatory management.
- Clarification is needed on the role of prophylactic antibiotics in elderly persons with prosthetic devices such as joint prosthesis, prosthetic cardiac valves, cardiac pacemakers, renal grafts and shunts for hemodialysis, and other foreign implanted material. Although limited, formal recommendations have been made for specific devices under defined clinical conditions (*see* Chapter 17), there is lack of scientific data supporting the administration of prophylatic antibiotics in patients with other implanted foreign devices or material. The cost-benefit and potential adverse effects of antibiotics must be determined.
- Improving the efficacy as well as delivery of current vaccines for the elderly has been discussed in Chapter 23. Nevertheless, it is worthwhile repeating that effective immunizations against infections remain as the most cost-effective approach to reducing the incidence and severity of serious and life-threating infectious diseases. This goal and the first goal mentioned earlier (relationship of aging and host resistance) are inextricably related and will serve as the foundation in the future for much of the newer approaches to the diagnosis, treatment, and prevention of infections in the elderly population.

3. TRAINING AND EDUCATION

Education and training serve as the foundation for implementing changes in the behavior and practice of clinicians. If we are to improve the care of the elderly, particularly in the domain of infections, then efforts must be directed toward pathways and approaches to better inform the practitioner on the current information on aging and infection and the complex issues involved with care of the elderly.

Adult infectious disease fellowship training programs should seriously consider incorporating into their curriculum information that is relevant to the care of the elderly with infection, i.e., biology of aging (especially gerontoimmunology); geriatric pharmacology; and the epidemiology, clinical manifestations, diagnostic approach, treatment, prognosis, and prevention of the most common and important infections afflicting older people. In addition, an understanding of geriatric syndromes (e.g., urinary incontinence, dementia, falls, osteoporosis) and issues of long-term care is essential for the infectious disease specialists who may care for older patients.

Conversely, geriatric fellowship training programs would better serve elderly patients with an intensive curriculum on the broad issues of immune changes with aging, important infections in the elderly, antimicrobial pharmacology, and unique aspects of infectious diseases with aging.

Major professional societies and organizations that sponsor continuing medical education programs for practicing physicians should regularly include in their courses or conferences topics that address the diagnosis, treatment, and prevention of infections in the elderly. Those organizations that also publish a journal should devote a section on geriatric health care issues including infections in the elderly.

4. RESEARCH

To address the clinical issues and problems that need resolution and recommendations (*see* Subheading 2.), there must be support for research. The major support for aging research comes from the National Institute on Aging, the Department of Veterans Affairs, foundations, and industry. However, funding for investigations on issues related to infectious diseases and aging is relatively limited. Support for these types of research should also be sought from other agencies within the National Institutes of Health, i.e., National Institute for Allergy and Infectious Diseases, National Heart, Lung, and Blood Institute, and National Cancer Institute, because of the cross-cutting nature of diseases affecting the elderly and their secondary complication of infection.

Professional societies hosting meetings for presentation of research findings should reserve a section for aging research in their program. Organizations such as the Infectious Diseases Society of America, Interscience Congress on Antimicrobial Agents and Chemotherapy (American Society for Microbiology), and Society for Healthcare Epidemiology of America should consider having a special category of "aging" for abstract presentation. Finally, journals that publish research findings on infectious diseases-related topics should feature a section on investigations in the area of aging (geriatrics and gerontology) and long-term care.

REFERENCES

1. McGinnis, J. M. (1988) The Tithonous syndrome: health and aging in American, in *Health Promotion and Disease Prevention in the Elderly* (Chernoff, R. and Lipschitz, D. A., eds.), Raven Press, New York, pp. 1–15.
2. Yoshikawa, T. T. (1994) Infectious diseases, immunity and aging. Perspectives and prospects, in *Aging, Immunity and Infection* (Powers, D. C., Morely, J. E., and Coe, R. M., eds)., Springer Publishing, New York, pp. 1–11.
3. Yoshikawa, T. T. (1997) Perspective: aging and infectious diseases: past, present and future. *J. Infect. Dis.* **176**, 1053–1057.
4. High, K. and Yoshikawa, T. T. (1999) Introduction: integrating geriatrics into the subspecialty of infectious diseases. *Clin. Infect. Dis.* **28**, 708–709.
5. Gleckman, R. A., Bradley, P. J., Roth, R. M. et al. (1985) Bacteremic urosepsis: a phenomenon unique to elderly women. *J. Urol.* **133**, 174,175.
6. Yoshikawa, T. T., Nicolle, L. E., and Norman, D. C. (1996) Management of complicated urinary tract infection in older patients. *J. Am. Geriatr. Soc.* **44**, 1235–1241.
7. Nicolle, L. E., Duckworth, H., Brunka, J., et al. (1998) Urinary antibody level and survival in bacteriuric institutionalized older subjects. *J. Am. Geriatr. Soc.* **46**, 947–953.
8. Woodhead, M. (1994) Pneumonia in the elderly. *J. Antimicrob. Chemother.* **34(Suppl. A),** 85–92.
9. Fine, M. J., Stone, R. A., Singer, D. E., et al. (1999) Processes and outcomes of care for patients with community-acquired pneumonia. *Arch. Intern. Med.* **159**, 970–980.
10. Riquelme, R., Torres, A., El-Ebiary, M., et al. (1996) Community-acquired pneumonia in the elderly: a multivariate analysis of risk and prognostic factors. *Am. J. Respir. Crit. Care Med.* **154**, 1450–1455.
11. Marrie, T. J. (1999) Clinical strategies for managing pneumonia in the elderly. *Clin. Geriatr.* (Suppl.) August, pp. 6–10.
12. Rajagopalan, S. and Yoshikawa, T. T. (1999) Tuberculosis, in *Principles of Geriatric Medicine and Gerontology*, 4th ed. (Hazzard, W. R., Blass, J. P., Ettinger, W. H., Jr. et al., eds.) McGraw-Hill, New York, pp. 737–744.
13. Battershill, J. H. (1980) Cutaneous testing in the elderly patient with tuberculosis. *Chest* **77**, 188,189.
14. Weinsein, P., Murphy, J. R., Reller, L. B., et al. (1988) The clinical significance of positive blood cultures: a comprehensive analysis of 500 episodes of bacteremia and fungemia in adults. II. Clinical observations, with special reference to factors influencing prognosis. *Rev. Infect. Dis.* **5(1),** 54–70.
15. Weil, M. H., Shubin, H., and Biddle, M. (1964) Shock caused by gram-negative microorganisms. Analysis of 169 cases. *Ann. Intern. Med.* **60(3),** 384–400.

Index